T0203214

BSAVA Manual of Canine and Feline Abdominal Imaging

Editors:

Robert O'Brien
DVM MS Dip.ACVR
Department of Veterinary Clinical Medicine,
University of Illinois at Urbana-Champaign,
1008 West Hazelwood Drive, Urbana,
IL 61802, USA

and

Frances Barr
MA VetMB PhD DVR Dip.ECVDI MRCVS
Department of Clinical Veterinary Science,
University of Bristol, Langford House,
Langford, Bristol BS40 5DU, UK

Published by:

British Small Animal Veterinary Association
Woodrow House, 1 Telford Way, Waterwells
Business Park, Quedgeley, Gloucester GL2 2AB

A Company Limited by Guarantee in England.
Registered Company No. 2837793.
Registered as a Charity.

Illustrations 7.1, 9.5, 9.6, 10.4, 10.31, 12.1 and 13.1 were drawn
by S.J. Elmhurst BA Hons (www.livingart.org.uk) and are printed with
her permission.

A catalogue record for this book is available from the British Library.

ISBN 978 1 905319 10 7

The publishers, editors and contributors cannot take responsibility for information
provided on dosages and methods of application of drugs mentioned or referred to
in this publication. Details of this kind must be verified in each case by individual
users from up to date literature published by the manufacturers or suppliers of those
drugs. Veterinary surgeons are reminded that in each case they must follow all
appropriate national legislation and regulations (for example, in the United Kingdom,
the prescribing cascade) from time to time in force.

17389PUBS22

Printed in the UK by: Severn, Gloucester GL2 5EU – a carbon neutral printer
Printed on ECF paper made from sustainable forests

Other titles in the BSAVA Manuals series:

Contents

Contributors

Laura Armbrust DVM Dip.ACVR
College of Veterinary Medicine, Kansas State University, Manhattan, KS 66506, USA

Elizabeth Baines MA VetMB DVR Dip.ECVDI MRCVS
The Royal Veterinary College, University of London, Hawkshead Lane, North Mymms, Hatfield,
Hertfordshire AL9 7TA, UK

Frances Barr MA VetMB PhD DVR Dip.ECVDI MRCVS
Department of Clinical Veterinary Science, University of Bristol, Langford House, Langford,
Bristol BS40 5DU, UK

Juliette Besso DEDV Dip.ECVDI Eligible ACVR
97 Rue Monge, 75005 Paris, France

Kate Bradley MA VetMB PhD DVR Dip.ECVDI MRCVS
Department of Clinical Veterinary Science, University of Bristol, Langford House, Langford,
Bristol BS40 5DU, UK

Margaret Costello MVB DVR Dip.ECVDI MRCVS
Diagnostic Imaging Service, Culver House, High Street, Arlingham, Gloucestershire GL2 7JN, UK

Lorrie Gaschen PhD Dr.habil DVM DrMedVet Dip.ECVDI
School of Veterinary Medicine, Louisiana State University, Baton Rouge, Louisiana, LO 70803, USA

Gawain Hammond MA VetMB MVM CertVDI Dip.ECVDI MRCVS
Faculty of Veterinary Medicine, University of Glasgow, Glasgow G61 1QH, UK

Nicolette Hayward BVM&S DVR Dip.ECVDI MRCVS
Veterinary Diagnostic Imaging Ltd, Baytree Cottage, Dyrham, Chippenham SN14 8EX, UK

Alasdair Hotston Moore MA VetMB CertSAC CertVR CertSAS MRCVS
Department of Clinical Veterinary Science, University of Bristol, Langford House, Langford,
Bristol BS40 5DU, UK

Francisco Llabrés-Díaz DVM DVR Dip.ECVDI MRCVS
Davies Veterinary Specialists, Manor Farm Business Park, Higham Gobion,
Hertfordshire SG5 3HR, UK

Paul Mahoney BVSc DVR Dip.ECVDI CertVC MRCVS FHEA
The Royal Veterinary College, University of London, Hawkshead Lane, North Mymms, Hatfield,
Hertfordshire AL9 7TA, UK

Wilfried Maï DVM MS PhD Dip.ACVR Dip.ECVDI
School of Veterinary Medicine, University of Pennsylvania, 3900 Delancey Street, Philadelphia,
PA 19104, USA

J. Fraser McConnell BVM&S DVR Dip.ECVDI CertSAM MRCVS
Small Animal Teaching Hospital, University of Liverpool, Leahurst Faculty, Neston,
Wirral CH64 7TE, UK

Martha Moon Larson DVM MS Dip.ACVR
Department of Small Animal Clinical Sciences, VA-MD Regional College of Veterinary Medicine,
Virginia Tech, Blacksburg, VA 24061, USA

Federica Morandi DrMedVet MS Dip.ECVDI Dip.ACVR
Radiology Section, Department of Small Animal Clinical Sciences, University of Tennessee,
Knoxville, TN 37996, USA

Helena Nyman DVM MSc PhD
The University Animal Hospital, Section of Diagnostic Imaging, Box 7040,
750 07 Uppsala, Sweden

Robert O'Brien DVM MS Dip.ACVR
Department of Veterinary Clinical Medicine, University of Illinois at Urbana-Champaign,
1008 West Hazelwood Drive, Urbana, IL 61802, USA

Tobias Schwarz MA DrMedVet DVR Dip.ECVDI Dip.ACVR MRCVS
Department of Veterinary Clinical Studies, Royal (Dick) School of Veterinary Studies,
Easter Bush Veterinary Centre, Easter Bush, Roslin, Midlothian EH25 9RG, UK

Gabriela Seiler DrMedVet Dip.ECVDI Dip.ACVR
School of Veterinary Medicine, University of Pennsylvania, 3900 Delancey Street, Philadelphia,
PA 19104, USA

Foreword

This *BSAVA Manual of Canine and Feline Abdominal Imaging* follows those devoted to the musculoskeletal system and thorax to complete a trio of publications which cover comprehensively all body systems. With its A4 format and quality radiographic illustrations, it is a far cry from the compilation of brief notes and line drawings which comprised the first BSAVA manual of radiography that appeared in the 1970s.

This huge increase in material represents not only advances in knowledge, but also the progress in technology which permits rapid and detailed reproduction of digital images. The introduction of ultrasonography reflects the increasing use of this modality in general practice, but the editors and authors are to be commended for recognising that the skill of radiographic interpretation remains the cornerstone of abdominal imaging for the general practitioner. Nevertheless, the value of integration of imaging modalities is emphasized throughout.

In the 245 pages, the experienced contributors have been given the luxury of covering their allotted topics in considerable detail, with generous use of illustrations. This Manual therefore compares favourably with the recognized reference texts and will be of value to those undertaking specialized training as well as finding an essential place in practice libraries.

Congratulations to the authors, editors and the BSAVA for adding this publication to the expanding list of practice Manuals. It will be much appreciated.

Christine Gibbs BVSc PhD DVR Dip.ECVDI FRCVS
January 2009

Preface

**I'm a great believer in luck, and I find the harder
I work the more I have of it**

Thomas Jefferson

Imaging plays a vital role in the evaluation of a sick patient. First and foremost images are a data set. The information is there. The clever and methodical evaluator can glean a vast amount of information from images. Integration into the work up of the patient requires insight and an abundance of skill and experience. Perseverance and dedication have no equal for the acquisition of a suitable skill set.

In assembling the chapters for the *BSAVA Manual of Canine and Feline Abdominal Imaging* we were fortunate in acquiring the services of many authors. These world experts contributed well written information, wonderful images and a spirit of enthusiasm and competence to this project. Often the contributions were outstanding and truly world-class. We hope that you appreciate their efforts.

We have included many forms of imaging in this text. While the emphasis remains radiography, we included as wide a spectrum as reasonable. Radiography is extremely important and will remain so in the near future. No other modality provides the overview of large portions of the body in such a quick time for most general practices.

Ultrasound imaging has been expanding concomitant with increased prevalence and expertise in general practice. No longer the exclusive realm of academia or referral private practice, ultrasound imaging has now become firmly entrenched in the day-to-day imaging of most practices.

Finally, we hope that this text projects our love of imaging and devotion to the subject material. We hope that you enjoy the text and find it useful. We fully expect that you will accept learning as a life-long mission. This mission helps our patients, their owners and the veterinary profession.

**Bob O'Brien
Frances Barr**

December 2008

Acknowledgements
I wish to acknowledge the unwavering support of my family. To Mo, Niallan, Aidan and Tom. Thanks for the help [ROB].

Approach to abdominal imaging

Frances Barr and Robert O'Brien

Overview of image interpretation

Radiographs should always be examined under optimal viewing conditions; dim surroundings are preferable. Conventional radiographs should be displayed on an X-ray viewer, which provides even illumination over the whole field of view. A small film should be surrounded by black card or the illuminated area restricted by shutters. A 'hot light' can be useful for examination of small, relatively overexposed areas. Digital radiographs should be displayed on a high-resolution screen.

Each radiograph should be examined systematically. Some advocate a zonal system, where each section of the radiograph is examined in turn, before considering the radiographic findings in light of the presenting clinical signs. Others prefer an integrated approach, where knowledge of the presenting signs informs and directs the order in which tissues and organs are inspected. Whichever approach is preferred, it is vital to ensure that all organs and the entire abdominal cavity, including its boundaries, are evaluated. Orthogonal views (lateral and ventrodorsal) are usually required in order to derive the maximum amount of information from an image.

Image interpretation relies on evaluation of the Röntgen signs for each organ. These signs are:

- Number
- Size
- Shape
- Location
- Opacity.

Number

Increase in number

- Another normal structure is mistaken for the organ in question, e.g. the head of the spleen in the dorsocranial abdomen is sometimes taken to be a third kidney.
- A lesion mimics another organ, e.g. a paraprostatic cyst may look like a second bladder, or a mass in the mid-dorsal abdomen may look like a third kidney (Figure 1.1).

Reduction in number

- An organ may be present but not seen. It may be obscured by gas or ingesta, or there may be a

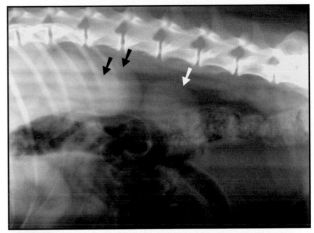

1.1 Lateral radiograph of the mid-dorsal abdomen of a bitch. Note the rounded soft tissue structure (white arrow) lying just caudal to the two superimposed kidneys (black arrows), giving the illusion of three kidneys. This soft tissue structure was confirmed as an ovarian neoplasm.

lack of intra-abdominal fat to delineate the organs. Alternatively, a lack of abdominal detail may indicate fluid within the peritoneal cavity.
- An organ may not be present. It may never have developed (aplasia) or may have been surgically removed.
- An organ may have changed in shape and/or position due to disease in that or an adjacent organ, such that it is no longer recognizable.

Size

It is important to be familiar with normal parameters of size for each organ in the abdomen. These are usually related to the other structures visible on the radiograph, since absolute measurements depend on the size of the animal and the degree of radiographic magnification (for example, small intestinal diameter may be related to vertebral body depth or to rib thickness). It is also important to appreciate the influence of enlargement of an organ on adjacent structures (for example, enlargement of the prostate gland may produce elevation and compression of the rectum). On occasion, an increase in organ size will result in a structure which is not normally visible becoming apparent (for example, abdominal lymph nodes are not usually visible unless enlarged).

Increase in size

- An apparent increase in size due to surrounding fluid or to an adjacent structure with border effacement, e.g. a perirenal pseudocyst gives the illusion of renal enlargement (Figure 1.2).
- A true increase in size due to compensatory hypertrophy or disease.

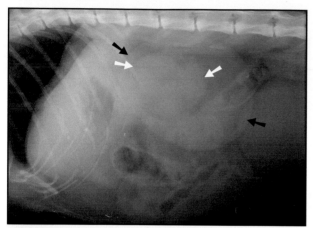

1.2 Lateral abdominal radiograph of an adult cat. The kidneys are superimposed but one (black arrows) appears much larger than the other (white arrows). This is due to a unilateral perirenal pseudocyst.

Decrease in size

- An artefactual decrease in size due to oblique view of the organ with resultant foreshortening. This can be confirmed by examining the orthogonal view.
- A true decrease in size due to hypoplasia or disease.

Shape

- An artefactual change in shape due to oblique view of an organ, leading to geometric distortion. This can be confirmed by examining the orthogonal view.
- A true change in shape due to injury or disease (Figure 1.3).

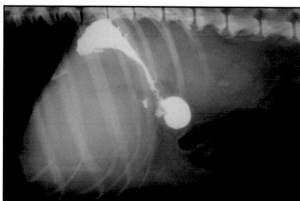

1.3 Lateral abdominal radiograph of an adult dog taken a few minutes after administration of barium. The barium outlines the position of stomach, emphasizing the change in shape of the liver. The normal triangular shape of the liver has been replaced by an irregularly rounded mass. The final diagnosis was a hepatic carcinoma.

Location

- May be due to individual variation and of no clinical consequence, e.g. the colon and bladder are quite variable in position.
- May reflect a pathological process in an adjacent structure, e.g. enlargement of the liver commonly results in caudal displacement of the stomach, or rupture of the abdominal wall may allow displacement of viscera (Figure 1.4).
- The change in position may be, of itself, important, e.g. gastric dilatation and volvulus.

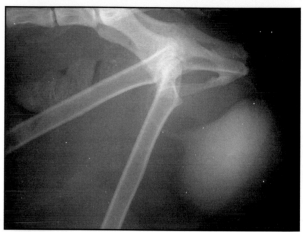

1.4 Lateral radiograph of the caudal abdomen and pelvis of an adult cat after a road traffic accident. Contrast medium has been introduced into the urethra and bladder, confirming that the bladder has become displaced ventrally and caudally through a rupture in the abdominal wall.

Opacity

The opacity of the organ or tissue in question should always be compared with that of adjacent structures to ensure that any change in opacity is real and not an effect of exposure.

Increase in opacity

- Accumulation of ingesta or faecal material. This may be due to recent feeding or a lack of opportunity to defecate. Abnormal accumulation of ingesta/faeces can be due to impaired gastrointestinal function or a physical obstruction.
- Foreign material.
- Urinary tract calculi and choleliths.
- Contrast medium.
- Mineralization of soft tissues, e.g. dystrophic calcification of the gastric wall in chronic renal failure or calcification of the wall of a paraprostatic cyst (Figure 1.5).

Decrease in opacity

- This may be due to fat, which is less radiopaque than other soft tissues.
- A marked decrease in opacity is usually due to gas. It is important to determine whether this is contained with the gastrointestinal tract, is free in the peritoneal cavity, or is within soft tissues (which may indicate a cavitating lesion, tissue necrosis or air embolization).

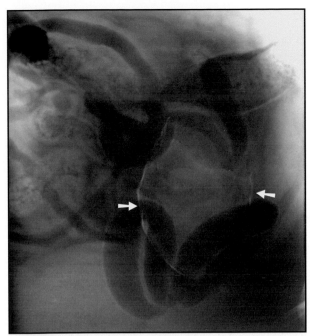

1.5 Lateral abdominal radiograph of the caudal abdomen of a dog. Note the mineralized, thin-walled, oval structure (arrowed), which is highly suggestive of a paraprostatic cyst.

Correlation with clinical signs

Having evaluated the radiograph carefully and systematically, it is then vitally important to consider the radiographic findings in the light of the clinical signs. There may be abnormal findings which are of no clinical significance or of no significance at the current time (e.g. an enlarged prostate gland in an entire male dog with no signs referable to the urinary or lower gastrointestinal tract). There may be abnormal findings which were not expected in the light of the presenting signs but which warrant further investigation (e.g. a small splenic mass in a dog presented for urinary tract signs). Finally, there may be abnormal findings which can be linked wholly or in part to the presenting problems, and either allow a definitive diagnosis to be made or inform further investigations.

The 'surgical' abdomen

There are clinical situations where it is important to make a rapid, yet informed, decision that surgery is required immediately or as soon as the patient can be stabilized, rather than further diagnostic tests. Equally, it is not in the best interests of the patient for exploratory laparotomy to be considered a routine means of investigating unexplained signs. Radiographic features which can indicate the need for urgent surgery include:

- Distension and volvulus of the stomach (see Chapter 9)
- Abnormal small intestinal distension in the presence of normal electrolyte levels (see Chapter 10)
- Free air in the peritoneal cavity (pneumoperitoneum), which cannot be explained by recent laparotomy, abdominocentesis or a

defect in the abdominal wall (Figure 1.6; see Chapter 4)
- Mottled or streaky gas lucencies within abdominal organs indicative of soft tissue emphysema and necrosis
- An overall loss of abdominal detail which may be mottled or granular in appearance, sometimes in association with intestinal ileus or corrugation, is suggestive of an inflammatory or diffuse neoplastic process involving the peritoneal cavity. This should be confirmed by collecting and analysing a sample of abdominal fluid before proceeding to surgery unless the clinical evidence is overwhelming.

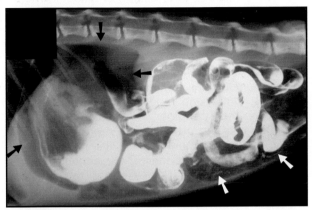

1.6 Lateral abdominal radiograph of a cat taken approximately 30 minutes after administration of contrast medium. Large volumes of air lie free within the peritoneal cavity, especially dorsocranially (black arrows). There has also been leakage of the contrast medium into the peritoneal cavity, especially caudoventrally (white arrows). These findings confirm gastrointestinal perforation; if this condition had been suspected prior to contrast medium administration, the use of barium would have been contraindicated.

Contrast radiography

Careful consideration of the findings on plain radiography in conjunction with the clinical signs may, in some cases, not be sufficient to allow a definitive diagnosis to be made. Contrast techniques may then be one consideration in the further investigation of the case. Contrast procedures allow the further evaluation of:

- Hollow organs such as the gastrointestinal tract, bladder and urethra
- The great vessels (abdominal aorta, caudal vena cava)
- Vascular supply to organs such as the liver and kidneys
- Perfusion and excretion of the kidneys
- Sinus tracts and fistulae.

When planning a contrast procedure it is important to select the appropriate procedure, to be thoroughly familiar with the technique, and to make sure that the appropriate contrast medium and any ancillary equipment is available. (Details of individual procedures are given in the relevant Chapters.)

Overview of additional imaging modalities

The clinician often has additional imaging modalities available and these may be chosen in preference to a contrast study for further investigation of some cases. Diagnostic ultrasonography is now widely available and offers great potential in the evaluation of abdominal disorders. Not only can ultrasonography allow the internal architecture of tissues to be seen, but very small structures (such as the adrenal glands and lymph nodes) can be identified and assessed. Vascular structures can also be evaluated with Doppler techniques allowing the velocity, direction and nature (laminar or turbulent) of blood flow to be determined. Some therefore advocate the routine use of abdominal ultrasonography in preference to abdominal radiography. However, radiography and ultrasonography should be considered as complementary and it is often useful to obtain information from both modalities (Figure 1.7). There are clinical situations where one modality clearly offers more information than the other, so an informed decision should be made to use only one imaging technique, e.g. an ascitic abdomen will yield little information on plain radiography, so abdominal ultrasonography may be preferred. Conversely, free gas in the abdomen post laparotomy may limit the value of ultrasonography in inexperienced hands.

Where available, computed tomography (CT), magnetic resonance imaging (MRI) and scintigraphy may also provide useful diagnostic information (see individual Chapters for further details).

References and further reading

Coulson A and Lewis N (2008) *An Atlas of Interpretative Radiographic Anatomy of the Dog and Cat, 2nd edition.* Blackwell Science, Oxford

Lamb CR, Kleine LJ and McMillan MC (1991) Diagnosis of calcification on abdominal radiographs, *Veterinary Radiology and Ultrasound* **32,** 211–220

Lee R and Leowijuk C (1982) Normal parameters in abdominal radiology of the dog and cat. *Journal of Small Animal Practice* **23,** 251–269

Miles K (1997) Imaging abdominal masses. *Veterinary Clinics of North America: Small Animal Practice* **27,** 1403–1431

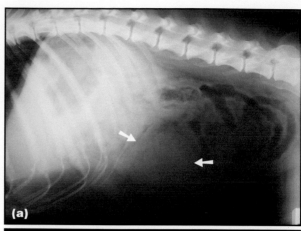

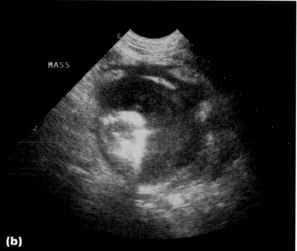

1.7 **(a)** Lateral abdominal radiograph of an adult male dog, presented with collapse and abdominal pain. There is a marked reduction in abdominal detail with corrugation of the small intestinal loops caudally, suggesting peritonitis. In addition, there is the impression of an ill defined mass in the mid-ventral abdomen (arrowed). **(b)** An ultrasound examination of this dog confirmed the presence of a mass. The mass was rounded in cross section and largely hypoechoic with an eccentrically positioned hyperechoic region within. This is typical of a mass of intestinal origin. The final diagnosis was small intestinal carcinoma with perforation and peritonitis.

Abdominal radiography

J. Fraser McConnell

Indications for radiography

The indications for plain abdominal radiography are numerous. However, for some conditions (especially urinary and gastrointestinal disorders) contrast studies may be required to show abnormalities. Radiography is indicated for most conditions where abdominal involvement is suspected, including:

- Abdominal distension
- Organomegaly
- Investigation of palpable masses
- Body wall swellings/hernias
- Weight loss
- Abdominal pain
- Fever of unknown origin
- Investigation of biochemical abnormalities
- Screening for primary or secondary neoplasia
- Scrooning following trauma
- Gastrointestinal signs:
  - Vomiting
  - Diarrhoea
  - Tenesmus
  - Dyschezia
  - Suspected foreign body.
- Urinary signs:
  - Polyuria
  - Dysuria
  - Anuria/stranguria
  - Urinary incontinence
  - Monitoring response to medical treatment for urolithiasis.
- Reproductive tract:
  - Determination of number of fetuses/ pregnancy (in late stages)
  - Vaginal discharge.

Patient preparation

For elective studies the animal should be fasted for 12–24 hours and allowed the opportunity to urinate and defecate prior to radiography. If the size of the gastrointestinal tract and bladder can be reduced in this way there will be less superimposition of the abdominal viscera. The animal's coat should be dry and free of dirt. Wet hair results in a streaky appearance that can be mistaken for small volumes of peritoneal fluid (Figure 2.1) or peritonitis. Flecks of dirt on the coat may be mistaken for soft tissue mineralization and calculi.

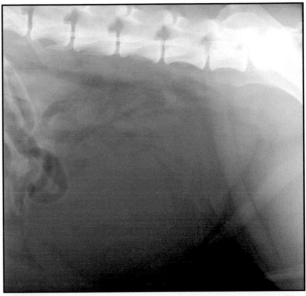

2.1 Lateral radiograph of a dog with a wet coat. The streaky appearance to the caudal abdomen is due to wet hair and can be mistaken for a small volume of abdominal fluid. Note the streaking extends beyond the boundaries of the abdomen.

Radiography

Types of radiography

Conventional film–screen radiography

With conventional (analogue) systems, information is recorded using a continuously variable physical quantity such as time, position or voltage. Conventional film-based radiographs are an example of an analogue system because the degree of film blackening is continuous (without steps).

With conventional film–screen systems, the radiographic image is created by the pattern of photons or light reaching the film. The shade of grey on a particular part of the film is largely determined by the number of photons reaching the film. This relationship between the radiographic exposure (number of photons) and optical density (blackness) of the film is known as the characteristic curve and is sigmoidal (S-shaped) (Figure 2.2). If there are too few (underexposure) or too many (overexposure) photons, the information given by the pattern of photons is lost. Within the useful (straight) part of the characteristic curve there is a continuous (but logarithmic) linear

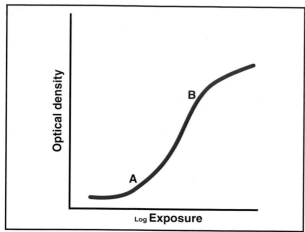

2.2 Characteristic curve for radiographic film. Useful radiographic densities lie between the 'toe' (A) and 'shoulder' (B) regions of the curve. The regions on the curve below A and above B contain no useful information due to underexposure and overexposure, respectively, where no useful information is present on the film. Radiographic exposures should be chosen to use the relatively straight part of the curve (between A and B) where density is proportional to log exposure. The steepness of the slope is known as the film 'gamma', which determines the inherent contrast of the film and also how much latitude there is in choice of exposure.

relationship between the number of photons and the density of the film. When taking conventional radiographs the exposure should be set to use the straight part of the characteristic curve.

Once the film is processed the brightness and contrast of the image are fixed. Although there are potentially hundreds of shades of grey on the film image, the ability of the human eye to differentiate between the shades of grey is limited to around 60. Once the image is formed and the film has been processed there can be no further manipulation of the image. Thus, the radiographic technique must be optimized to give a diagnostic radiograph. One problem with analogue systems is that repeated recording or copying of data often results in deterioration in quality. Therefore, the quality of copy radiographs is usually less than that of the original.

The resolution of the film is dependent upon the crystal size within the emulsion and the intensifying screen. Faster film–screen combinations have larger crystals that require less exposure but have poorer resolution compared with slower (detail) combinations. Detail film–screen combinations should be used for abdominal radiographs in cats and small dogs. For larger dogs rapid film–screen combinations are normally used.

The main disadvantages of conventional film-based systems are:

- Information stored on the film is fixed and cannot be manipulated following the exposure
- There is a limited range of useful exposures that will produce a diagnostic radiograph (narrow dynamic range). If mistakes are made in the choice of exposure or if there are marked differences in the thickness of the tissue being radiographed, then information may be lost

- Expense and problems with processing
- Film is bulky and difficult to archive
- Distribution of images is time-consuming and expensive.

To overcome some of these problems digital radiographic systems were developed.

Digital radiography
The term digital comes from the same source as digit (finger) and a useful analogy is that digital information is similar to counting on fingers. There is a limited number of potential (discontinuous) values that can be measured with a digital system. In digital radiography, the amount of photons/light reaching the detector is converted into a range of discrete values. In contrast, an analogue system can measure an almost infinite (continuous) range of values. With digital radiography, the production of the X-ray beam and interaction of the X-ray photons with the tissues is the same as conventional (analogue) radiography. The difference is in the detection of the X-ray photons and the production of the image.

The digital radiographic image is created from a number of small rectangular picture elements (pixels) arranged in a grid (Figure 2.3). The resolution of the image is determined mainly by the size of the pixels used to make the image. The smaller the pixel the

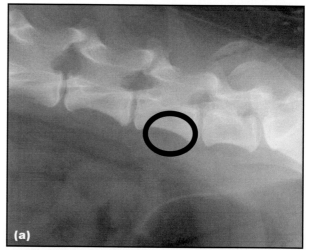
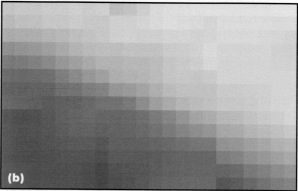

2.3 **(a)** Digital radiographic image of the lumbar vertebrae of a dog. **(b)** At high magnification the pixels (small squares) that form the image can be seen. With some cheap or poor quality digital radiography systems even small degrees of magnification may result in pixellation.

higher the resolution; typical resolution is about 5–10 pixels per mm. For each pixel there is a limited (but large, around 4000) number of potential shades of grey. However, the digital image can be manipulated to use all these potential values, unlike conventional film where the full greyscale is limited by the human eye.

Digital systems convert the pattern of photons reaching the detector into an electrical signal that is digitized. Digital systems are often no better than good quality conventional radiographs and with some systems image quality may be poorer than conventional film-based systems.

With digital radiographic systems there is a direct linear relationship (Figure 2.4) between the exposure and signal, which differs from the sigmoidal relationship seen with film. This means that there are no 'toe' or 'shoulder' regions where information is lost. Once film is black extra photons do not result in new information, whereas in a digital system these extra photons carry useful information. This greater flexibility in exposure factors is one of the major advantages of digital systems. The range of exposures which result in a diagnostic image is known as the dynamic range or latitude. The dynamic range of digital systems is approximately 4–10 times that of conventional film. With digital systems the image can be manipulated after acquisition to alter contrast and brightness. This means it is possible to view areas on the radiograph with marked differences in tissue thickness, or to look at the soft tissues and bones without having to take separate exposures (Figure 2.5).

There are two types of digital radiography, which differ in the way the X-ray photon pattern is converted to an electrical digital signal. These are:

- Computed radiography (CR)
- Direct digital radiography (DR).

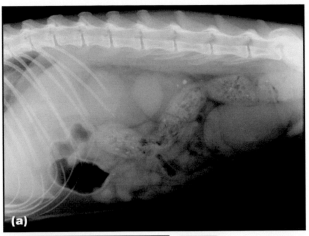

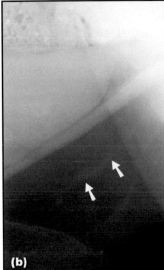

2.5 Computed radiograph of a cat's abdomen. The same image can be manipulated to optimize the assessment of **(a)** bone or **(b)** soft tissues. Digital systems can have better soft tissue contrast than a conventional film-based system. The inguinal lymph nodes and lymphatics (arrowed) can be seen in this cat.

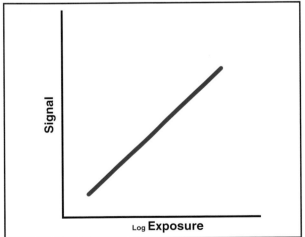

2.4 Response curve of a digital radiographic system. There is a linear relationship between density (signal) and exposure. There are no 'toe' or 'shoulder' regions, which means that useful information is obtained over a much wider range of exposures (wide dynamic range). During post-processing the straight line is usually transformed electronically to produce a sigmoidal curve similar to conventional film but this can be adjusted to produce a range of contrast and brightness. Different post-processing curves are used for different regions to enhance soft tissue or bone.

Computed radiography: CR systems use a cassette that looks similar to a conventional film cassette and which contains a phosphor screen (detector) that can store the latent image for a period of time (Figure 2.6). Within the cassette is an imaging plate made from a photostimulable phosphor (a europium-activated barium fluorohalide compound, $BaFX:Eu^{2+}$). When the X-ray photons hit the imaging plate there is transfer of energy to electrons within the plate. The electrons move to a higher energy state and are trapped within electron traps in a semi-stable state. To read the latent image, the imaging plate is loaded into a cassette reader (this is normally automatic but in some systems is done manually) (Figure 2.7). Within the CR cassette reader a laser moves back and forwards across the detector. The laser gives a small amount of energy to the electrons in the electron traps, allowing them to move back to their resting state and to release energy in the form of light. The light is emitted at a different wavelength from the laser used to read the detector. The light is detected by a photomultiplier tube that converts the light to an electrical signal, which is used to create the image. The intensity of the light emitted from the phosphor is proportional to the number and energy of the X-ray photons hitting the phosphor. After the phosphor has been scanned the latent image is erased by a bright light and the cassette is reloaded.

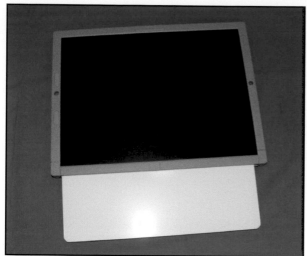

2.6 CR cassette showing the phosphor plate within the cassette. Radiographic technique is the same as for conventional film-based systems. With some CR systems the detector is built into the table, which means some oblique views or horizontal beam studies are not possible.

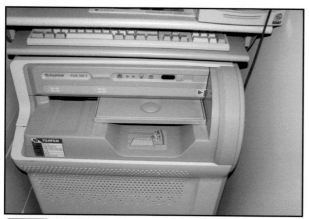

2.7 Cassette reader for a CR system. The cassette is automatically unloaded and the latent image on the phosphor plate is read by a laser. With manual CR systems the image can fade if the phosphor is exposed to bright light.

Direct digital radiography: With DR systems the X-ray photons are converted directly into an electrical charge, usually using a photoconductor or scintillator within a flat panel detector. These systems may give better image quality and image production is faster than a CR system but they are more expensive. There are three main types of DR system:

- Direct conversion of the X-ray photon into an electrical charge using a photoconductor (usually amorphous selenium). The selenium detector has charged flat electrodes on its front and back surfaces. When the X-rays hit the detector a pattern is created on the detector's surface. Electrons are liberated from the negatively charged surface on the front of the detector and are attracted to the positive electrode on the back of the detector. The electrons are detected by a thin film transistor array and are used to create the image

- Indirect conversion using a scintillator that produces light when hit by photons. The light is converted to an electrical signal using a light-sensitive sensor (charged couple device, CCD). This is indirect DR because the X-ray photons result in the production of light which is used to create the digital signal
- Indirect conversion where the scintillator is built into a flat panel detector with photodiodes used to generate the electrical signal. The photodiodes are tiny and thousands are built into the detector. Each photodiode represents 1 pixel on the image.

After the data are acquired they are processed before being displayed by the computer. The type of processing has a great effect on the appearance of the final image and specific algorithms are used for different body areas and systems. These may result in enhancement of edges and reduced noise of the image. In addition to being able to manipulate images after acquisition (e.g. alter window/level, zoom, rotate) there are other potential advantages of digital radiographs, including:

- Wide dynamic range/exposure latitude
- Images are easy to distribute
- No chemicals or film are required
- No darkroom is needed
- Less storage space required for images.

Viewing digital radiographs: Digital radiographs may be printed as hard copies using dry film printers and viewed as conventional radiographs. However, the film and printers are expensive and this negates many of the advantages of a digital system. To gain the greatest advantage from digital radiographs, the images are viewed on computer monitors. The viewing room should be dimly lit to prevent glare from the monitor. The monitor should be calibrated so that the brightness is correct for the ambient light conditions and the monitor luminescence is sufficient (Figure 2.8). Special DICOM compliant monitors are normally used for displaying digital radiographs, and have a resolution of at least two megapixels (MP) and are able to display a wide greyscale range (12 Bit or 4096 shades of grey per pixel) and contrast (e.g. 800:1). These are expensive and contribute to the higher costs of digital radiographic systems. The viewing monitor needs to be capable of displaying the resolution of the imaging system. A standard PC monitor has a resolution of around 1028 x 1280 pixels (1.3 MP) whereas a 35 cm x 43 cm CR plate has a matrix of 1760 x 2140 pixels (3.7 MP) or greater. This means that when the image is viewed full-size on a standard PC monitor there will be some loss of resolution.

As digital images can be enlarged and the size of image displayed may be affected by the size of the monitor, it may initially be harder to recognize differences in the size of organs. Likewise, because the image contrast and brightness can be manipulated and there is a wider greyscale than with conventional film, it may be difficult to determine which opacity is present on the image (e.g. it may be difficult to differentiate gas from fat opacities and mineralization from some soft tissue opacities).

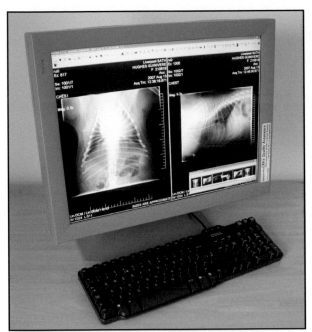

2.8 Diagnostic workstation for viewing digital radiographs. The monitor should be viewed in a room with dimmable lighting to reduce glare on the screen. The monitor should be calibrated for the ambient light conditions. Viewing digital radiographs on a low-resolution computer monitor in poor conditions should be avoided.

Digital radiographs are not free from artefacts and careful technique is required. In addition to the artefacts seen with analogue systems (e.g. movement blur, dirt on the animal's coat, dirty screens, etc.) there are several artefacts specific to digital images. If grids are used with some digital systems there can be artefacts visible on the monitor due to interaction between the grid lines and pixel rows, resulting in a corduroy 'moiré' pattern. In some older systems a dark halo artefact may occur around the edges of metal implants.

Technical considerations

- The abdomen has inherently poor radiographic contrast compared with other parts of the body. The parenchymal organs and fluid have the same radiographic opacity and it is the presence of intra-abdominal fat that allows the serosal surface of the organs to be seen. Radiographic technique should therefore be optimized to maximize radiographic contrast. This is done by using a low kVp (<70) and high mAs technique.
- Due to the inherently poor contrast, the radiographic technique should also be optimized to reduce scatter. Scattered photons reaching the film result in a diffuse increase in density (blackness) of the film, causing reduced contrast. The amount of scatter produced is proportional to the volume of tissue exposed and to the energy of the photons.
  - Scatter can be reduced by reducing the volume of tissue. This can be done by collimating the X-ray beam to avoid thicker portions or compressing the abdomen, but the latter results in distortion of the viscera.
    - Increasing photon energy results in production of less total scatter, but the scattered photons have greater energy so are more likely to exit the patient and reach the film. Paradoxically, the net result of increasing kVp is increased scatter radiation reaching the film and reduced film contrast.
    - A grid reduces the amount of scattered radiation reaching the film. Grids are usually recommended when the depth of tissue is >10 cm but may also be of use in very obese animals at depths <10 cm (e.g. obese cats). The use of a grid requires higher exposure factors and, if patient movement is a problem, then the radiographic technique should be adapted to prevent motion if at all possible. This can be achieved by chemical restraint to reduce movement or not using the grid to allow shorter exposure times.
- Abdominal radiographs should be taken during the end expiratory pause when the diaphragm is cranially positioned, resulting in greater separation of the abdominal organs and when there is less chance of movement blur.
- Exposure times should be short enough to prevent movement blur.

Patient restraint

For the majority of abdominal studies sedation of the patient is preferred, although in sick or compliant animals radiography can be performed without chemical restraint. Gastrointestinal contrast studies should ideally be performed without sedation or general anaesthesia as this may affect gastrointestinal motility. A low dose of acepromazine (ACP) has minimal effect on gastrointestinal motility and in cats a ketamine/diazepam combination or ACP can be used.

Radiographic views

Orthogonal views are required for accurate localization of an object. If only a single radiograph is taken then the actual location of a structure can be difficult to determine (Figure 2.9). There are some differences in appearance between left and right lateral views and between the dorsoventral (DV) and ventrodorsal (VD) views (Figure 2.10). The differences between the left and right lateral views may be marked (Figure 2.11) due to the fact that gas and fluid within the gastrointestinal tract move with patient position. This can in fact be used when investigating gastrointestinal abnormalities. The right lateral view is the view of choice for identification of gastric volvulus, whilst the decubitus lateral view (taken with the animal in left lateral recumbency) is best for showing free abdominal gas (Figures 2.12 and 2.13). It is important that the entire abdomen is included on the radiographs. In large dogs it may be necessary to take two radiographs to image the entire abdomen, one centred on the cranial abdomen and one centred caudally. In cases where pathology may involve structures extending beyond the normal abdominal boundaries (e.g. oesophageal, rectal, genital and urinary tracts) then radiographs to image the pelvic canal/perineum or thorax should be taken.

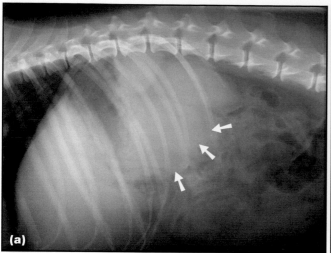

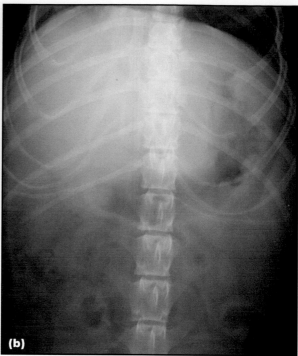

2.9 **(a)** Lateral and **(b)** VD radiographs of a dog with a neoplasm involving the right middle liver lobe. On the lateral view the mass (arrowed) appears to lie caudal to the stomach. The VD view shows that the mass lies lateral to the stomach and displaces the pylorus to the left. If the lateral view alone had been assessed then the mass could have been misinterpreted as being mid-abdominal in location, resulting in an erroneous differential diagnosis list.

View	Observations
Right lateral	Gas within fundus. Greater separation of renal silhouettes. Left kidney relatively more ventral and appears bean-shaped. Right kidney seen more often compared with left lateral view. Greater visibility of the tail of the spleen compared with left lateral view
Left lateral	Gas within pylorus. Duodenum seen more consistently compared with right lateral view. Greater superimposition of the kidneys. Left kidney more ovoid in shape. Left kidney seen more often
Dorsoventral (DV)	Gas within fundus and cardia. Greater superimposition of abdominal viscera
Ventrodorsal (VD)	Gas within body and antrum. Head of spleen and duodenum more consistently seen compared with lateral views. Viscera spread further apart laterally compared with DV view. In narrow deep-chested dogs VD view is often unrewarding compared with lateral views due to crowding of viscera

2.10 Differences between lateral, dorsoventral and ventrodorsal views.

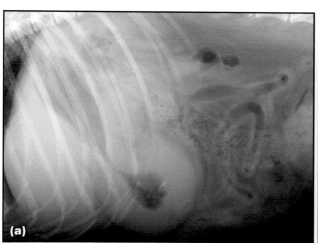

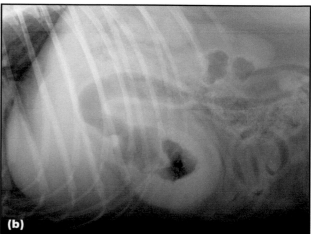

2.11 Lateral radiographs of the abdomen in a dog with a gastric neoplasm. There are marked differences between the **(a)** right and **(b)** left lateral views. The left lateral view shows gas within the pylorus and duodenum. The left lateral view also allows better assessment of the degree of pyloric involvement and duodenal dilatation compared with the right lateral view.

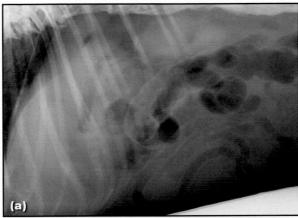

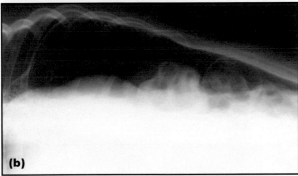

2.12 **(a)** Lateral radiograph of a dog with septic peritonitis and pneumoperitoneum. Free gas is seen caudal to the diaphragm and adjacent to the liver and bowel. **(b)** The decubitus lateral view shows the free gas better than the lateral view. This view is the most sensitive for demonstrating small volumes of free abdominal gas. (Courtesy of Cambridge Veterinary School)

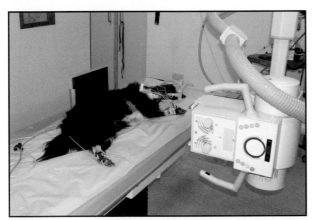

2.13 Positioning for the decubitus lateral view. The animal is placed in left lateral recumbency with the cassette placed adjacent to the thoracolumbar spine. A horizontal beam is used. Care needs to be taken when using a horizontal beam to ensure that personnel are not inadvertently exposed to the X-ray beam. On a radiograph taken with the animal in right lateral recumbency the fundus lies adjacent to the ribcage, making the visualization of gas harder compared with a radiograph taken with the patient in left lateral recumbency.

Assessment of the bladder may be hindered by superimposition of the lumbar spine. Tilting the animal slightly away from VD towards the side where the bladder is lying may reduce superimposition. If diseases affecting the rectum, urethra or contents of the pelvic canal are suspected then radiographs

centred on the pelvis should be taken (Figure 2.14). In male dogs with urethral disease the pelvic limbs should be pulled cranially to reduce superimposition of the urethra by the femurs.

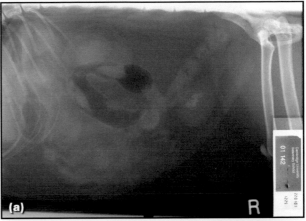

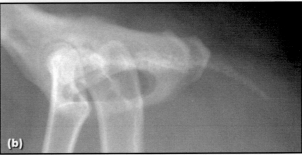

2.14 **(a)** Lateral radiograph of the abdomen in a cat with urolithiasis. Cystic calculi are visible within the bladder. **(b)** A second radiograph centred on the pelvic canal showed a large number of urethral calculi. It is important that the entire area where pathology may occur is included on the radiograph. (Courtesy of Cambridge Veterinary School)

Positioning

Accurate positioning is important to ensure there is not excessive rotation and that the entire abdomen is included on the radiograph (Figures 2.15, 2.16 and 2.17).

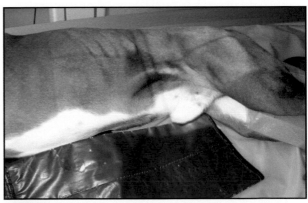

2.15 Positioning for lateral abdominal radiography. The X-ray beam is centred just caudal to the last rib. Dorsally the X-ray beam is collimated to the lumbar spine and ventrally to the body wall. In dogs with a deep chest, such as this Boxer, placing a lead sleeve over the cassette ventral to the body wall helps reduce scatter and may improve contrast. Note the pads between the thighs and caudal retraction of the pelvic limbs.

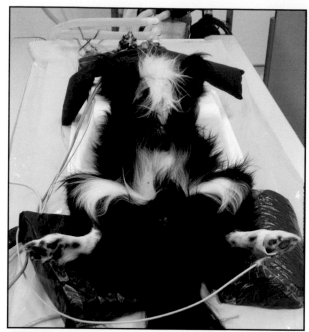

2.16 Positioning for the VD view of the abdomen. Using a trough and padding under the thighs helps prevent axial rotation, particularly in deep-chested dogs. The hindlimbs should be in a neutral frog-legged position.

Lateral view

Centre just caudal to the caudal most part of the last rib (approximately two finger widths further caudally for cats)
Pull pelvic limbs caudally
Pad between femurs and under sternum to reduce axial rotation
Collimate to diaphragm cranially (2–3 ribs cranial to xiphoid) and greater trochanter caudally
Rib heads, transverse processes and hip joints should be superimposed (rotation results in loss of superimposition)

Ventrodorsal view

Centre just caudal to the caudal most part of the last rib (approximately two finger widths further caudally for cats)
Pelvic limbs in neutral frog-legged position
Place thorax within positioning trough/cradle to prevent rotation. Pad under thighs helps to reduce tilting
Collimate to diaphragm cranially (2–3 ribs cranial to xiphoid) and greater trochanter caudally
Lumbar vertebrae and thoracic vertebrae should be in a straight line without lateral curvature. Dorsal spinous processes should be centred over middle of the vertebral bodies and not tilted laterally. Sternebrae should be superimposed over vertebrae

2.17 Accurate positioning for abdominal radiography.

Criteria for correct exposure

A correctly exposed abdominal radiograph should allow clear visualization of the abdominal viscera, intra-abdominal and extra-abdominal fat and the spine. A bright light should not be necessary to evaluate the abdominal viscera in most animals. The lumbar vertebrae should be clearly visible with good contrast between the bone and the adjacent sublumbar muscles and between the sublumbar muscles and the retroperitoneal fat. The ribs overlying the liver and the lumbar vertebrae should be slightly underexposed but should be clearly visible.

An exposure chart should be created for the X-ray machine being used with the film–focal distance, use of grid, film-screen combination and processing kept constant. The most reliable method for choosing a consistently accurate exposure is to use calipers to measure the depth of tissue (Figure 2.18) and to use a variable kVp chart. This is because there is a roughly linear relationship between the depth of tissue and the required exposure. The calipers are placed across the greatest depth of tissue (usually the caudal ribcage) and the depth of tissue is measured. A constant mAs is chosen with a high mA (to maximize contrast) and a short enough exposure time to prevent motion blur. If a fixed mAs is used then for each additional cm of tissue the exposure needs to be increased by 2 kVp (up to 80 kVp) or 3 kVp (80–100 kVp). As a rule of thumb if the mAs is doubled the kVp can be reduced by 10–15% to give an equivalent exposure. Alternately, if the kVp is increased by 10–15% then the mAs can be halved. If there is a large volume of free abdominal fluid or if the animal is very obese, then higher exposure factors (double mAs) may be required.

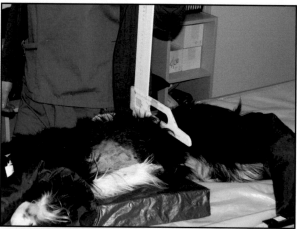

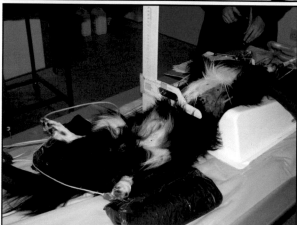

2.18 To ensure a consistently accurate choice of exposure, the depth of tissues can be measured using calipers. For a lateral view the tissue depth is measured just caudal to the ribcage and for a VD view the tissue depth is measured just caudal to the xiphoid. For deep-chested dogs separate radiographs may be required for the cranial and caudal abdomen due to large differences in depth of tissue. It is important that the measurement is made in the same position for each animal to ensure consistency.

If the radiograph is too light or too dark and processing errors, incorrect use of the grid and other non-exposure related faults have been ruled out, then the exposure may be corrected using the guidelines in Figure 2.19.

Radiograph too dark	Radiograph too light
If poor contrast (bones indistinct or absent), reduce kVp by 10–15% If contrast adequate (bones seen clearly), reduce mAs by 30–50%	If the anatomy can be seen, increase mAs by 30–50% If the anatomy cannot be seen, increase kVp by 10–15%

2.19 Changes in exposure to improve image quality.

In deep-chested dogs there is often a large difference in depth of tissue between the cranial and the caudal abdomen, particularly on the VD view. Separate exposures will be needed for the cranial and caudal abdomen using conventional radiography. With digital systems the image can be adjusted to allow assessment of the cranial abdomen and then readjusted to allow assessment of the caudal abdomen.

Due to the wide dynamic range of digital systems, the brightness and contrast of the image are determined by post-processing. Therefore, with digital radiographs the degree of image blackening cannot be used to determine whether the correct exposure has been used. Most digital systems give a value 'exposure level' that is related to patient dose/exposure when the exposure is made. This can be checked against the manufacturer's range of recommended values for the area being radiographed. If the image is underexposed it will often appear grainy and may not show fine detail. Overexposure, unless severe, does not result in a change in the image.

Contrast radiography

The inherent poor contrast within the abdomen and the fact that soft tissue and fluid cannot be differentiated radiographically means that contrast media are required to allow assessment of the luminal surface of the bladder and the gastrointestinal tract, and to allow visualization of the abdominal blood vessels, ureters, kidneys and biliary tract. Contrast studies are most commonly performed to identify anatomy not visible on plain radiographs and to evaluate the integrity of hollow structures or the peritoneal cavity. They may also be used to allow some assessment of organ function (e.g. gastric emptying/transit times).

Contrast media are divided into two main groups:

- Negative contrast media, which are less opaque (darker) on the radiograph than the soft tissues
- Positive contrast media, which are more opaque (lighter) than the soft tissues.

Negative contrast media

Negative contrast media are gaseous and, although they may have a similar or higher atomic number when compared with soft tissues, they appear radiolucent due to their much lower physical density. A variety of gases may be used (air, carbon dioxide,

nitrous oxide). Carbon dioxide and nitrous oxide are theoretically safer than air due to their greater solubility in plasma. There are very rare reports of fatal air embolism following use of air for pneumocystography. Air embolism is most likely if there is increased permeability or ulceration of the mucosal surfaces, so in cases of severe haematuria it may be advisable to avoid the use of air. In cases of suspected air embolism it has been advised that the animal is placed in left lateral recumbency with the caudal part of the body elevated, in order to try and trap air within the right ventricle and prevent arterial embolism or occlusion of the pulmonary artery.

Negative contrast media can only be used for gastric (pneumogastrography), large bowel (pneumocolonography) and bladder (pneumocystography) studies. Negative-contrast studies allow assessment of stomach, colon and bladder position, wall thickness and may show intraluminal objects such as foreign bodies, masses and calculi. Used alone negative contrast media are poor at showing mucosal lesions and perforation of the viscera and do not provide functional information.

Positive contrast media

Positive contrast media all have a higher atomic number than the soft tissues and therefore absorb more photons, resulting in an increased opacity on the radiograph.

Positive contrast media are divided into two groups:

- Barium sulphate
- Iodine based.

Barium sulphate

Barium sulphate has an atomic number of 56 and is:

- Inert
- Relatively palatable
- Prepared as a suspension and has no osmotic potential, and so does not absorb or cause movement of water within the patient
- Good at coating the mucosa.

These properties make barium the contrast medium of choice for most gastrointestinal contrast studies. Barium may be mixed with food for oesophageal studies and pharyngeal studies and when trying to assess gastric emptying, although it is acknowledged to be inaccurate for this purpose. Mixing liquid barium with moderate viscosity 0.5% methylcellulose produces a double-contrast effect, which improves visualization of the small intestine compared with liquid barium alone. As barium is a particulate suspension it should only be given *per os* or *per rectum* and is used for gastrointestinal studies only. Barium is absolutely contraindicated in the urinary, neurological and vascular systems.

Barium sulphate comes in a variety of concentrations, normally classified by weight to volume (w/v) (where a weight of barium is added to water to make a specified volume) or weight to weight (w/w) (where a certain weight of barium is added to water to make a specified weight of suspension). There are a number of formulations available (Figure 2.20).

Barium formulation	Comments
Powder	Mixed with water or food to make a paste or suspension The suspension formed may not be as uniform as pre-diluted suspensions Flocculation of barium more common compared with commercial suspensions
Paste	Used for oesophageal studies to assess the mucosa Better mucosal adherence compared with liquid barium
Liquid suspension	Supplied as pre-made suspension or powder for reconstitution Usually diluted to make 30–60% w/v suspension Preparations designed for human use are often flavoured (e.g. vanilla, cherry), which may be unpalatable for some animals Used on its own for gastrointestinal studies and large bowel studies Mixed with food for oesophageal studies to determine dilatation or strictures Allows assessment of wall thickness and changes to mucosal surfaces Combined with pneumogastrography/ pneumocolonography to produce double-contrast studies, which are the optimal radiographic studies for assessment of mucosal and subtle mural lesions
Barium-impregnated polyethylene spheres (BIPS)	Small (1.5 mm and 5 mm diameter) polyethylene spheres impregnated with barium Two capsule sizes are available (large and small) 10 large and 30 small spheres are administered together 1.5 mm spheres designed to mimic passage of food and allow quantification of gastric emptying and/or (gastro)intestinal transit time 5 mm spheres aim to demonstrate gastrointestinal tract obstruction (given on an empty stomach) Most useful for chronic obstructions but do not give information on cause of obstruction Give no information on wall thickness or mucosal surfaces

2.20 Formulations of barium.

Complications:

- As barium is inert it may persist indefinitely if it leaks into the thoracic or abdominal cavities and can result in a granulomatous reaction. If gastrointestinal or oesophageal perforation is suspected, then a low-osmolar iodinated contrast medium should be used rather than barium.
- In cases where the animal is going to have an endoscopic procedure (oesphagoscopy or gastroscopy) performed soon after the contrast study it is preferable to use water-soluble contrast media.
- If the animal has a swallowing disorder, aspiration of barium may occur. The severity of the sequelae depend on the volume aspirated but the majority of complications arise from aspiration of gastric contents rather than barium.
- Very rarely in dogs and cats, but more commonly in reptiles, barium can form concretions within the bowel that may lead to obstruction.

Iodine-based media

Iodine has an atomic number of 53 and is water-soluble. Iodinated contrast media are based on iodinated benzene rings, either as tri-iodinated monomers or dimers. They are divided into ionic and non-ionic media and are further classified by their osmolality (Figure 2.21). Dimers contain approximately twice as many iodine atoms as monomers but have a similar osmolality. Therefore, at the same iodine concentration dimers have a lower osmolality but a greater viscosity than monomers, so should be warmed to no greater than body temperature to make injection easier. As they are water-soluble, iodine-based contrast media can be given intravenously into body cavities, or instilled into the bladder or gastrointestinal tract. Some water-soluble contrast media designed for gastrointestinal use (e.g. Gastro-grafin) contain preservatives and are contraindicated for all except gastrointestinal use. Iodinated agents are unpalatable and often need to be given by stomach tube when used for gastrointestinal studies.

High-osmolar contrast media: These are cheaper than low-osmolar contrast media and can be used for urinary tract and vascular studies. However, there are some contraindications to their use:

- As they have a high osmotic potential they attract water. If they are used for gastrointestinal studies, the contrast medium is diluted as it passes through the gastrointestinal tract. In neonatal and dehydrated animals this effect can exacerbate the dehydration and low-osmolar agents are preferable
- The high-osmolar agents are more irritant to mucosal surfaces and, particularly in cats with cystitis, they can irritate the bladder mucosa
- If high-osmolar agents are aspirated they can cause pulmonary oedema. Therefore, in cases of oesophageal rupture/broncho-oesophageal fistulae, or if aspiration is likely, a low-osmolar agent should be used.

Low-osmolar contrast media: Ionic and non-ionic low-osmolar contrast media are available, but for abdominal contrast studies the ionicity is unimportant. Use of low-osmolar and non-ionic contrast media results in fewer adverse reactions (cardiovascular effects, allergic reaction and chemical toxicity) compared with the use of high-osmolar, ionic contrast media. Low-osmolar contrast media are preferred to high-osmolar agents for gastrointestinal studies because they are not diluted as they pass though the gastrointestinal tract. In cases of suspected gastro-intestinal or oesophageal perforation, or if endoscopy is going to be performed following radiography, then low-osmolar agents should be used.

Complications: Adverse reactions and complications arising from the use of contrast media are uncommon, but the risks/benefits should be considered before their use and the owners made aware of potential complications. Adverse effects are more common with hyperosmolar media and with ionic media.

Constituent	Properties	Trade name	Indications	
			Vascular and urinary studies	**Gastrointestinal studies**
Iothalamic acid	Monomeric; ionic; high-osmolar	Conray	+	–
Sodium meglumine diatrizoate	Monomeric; ionic; high-osmolar	Urografin	+	–
	Ionic; high-osmolar	Gastrografin	–	+
Sodium meglumine ioxaglate	Dimeric; ionic; low-osmolar	Hexabrix	+	–
Iobitridol	Momomeric; non-ionic; low-osmolar	Xenetix	+	–
Iohexol	Monomeric; non-ionic; low-osmolar	Omnipaque	+	+
Iomeprol	Monomeric; non-ionic; low-osmolar	Iomeron	+	–
Iopamidol	Monomeric; non-ionic; low-osmolar	Gastromiro	–	+
	Monomeric; non-ionic; low-osmolar	Niopam	+	–
	Monomeric; non-ionic; low-osmolar	Scanlux	+	–
Iopromide	Monomeric; non-ionic; low-osmolar	Ultravist	+	–
Iodixanol	Dimeric; non-ionic; iso-osmolar	Visipaque	+	+
Iotrolan	Dimeric; non-ionic; iso-osmolar	Isovist	–	–
Ioversol	Monomeric; non-ionic; low-osmolar	Optiray	+	–

2.21 Iodinated contrast media.

Known or suspected sensitivity to iodine-containing preparations is a contraindication for their use.

Anaphylaxis may occur rarely following intravenous injection of any iodinated contrast medium. Minor side-effects following intravenous injection are not uncommon and include:

- Nausea
- Vomiting
- Hypotension
- Dyspnoea
- Erythema
- Urticaria
- Sensation of heat at the injection site
- Cardiac rate or rhythm disturbances.

Warming contrast media prior to injection and using general anaesthesia reduces the incidence of minor side-effects. Extravasation of high-osmolar agents rarely may lead to soft tissue injury, and a catheter should be used for intravenous administration of such agents. Giving iodinated contrast media results in decreased thyroid uptake of iodine. If the animal is going to receive therapeutic radioiodine (e.g. for hyperthyroidism), then the use of iodinated contrast media should be avoided for 2 months.

Non-ionic, low-osmolar and iso-osmolar agents have fewer adverse effects on the cardiovascular system and are safer in neonates and animals with cardiovascular disease.

Any iodinated contrast medium should be used with care in animals with moderate to severe impairment of renal function as these are primarily excreted via the kidneys. Before giving the contrast medium, renal function should be assessed, the animal rehydrated and any fluid or electrolyte disturbances corrected. Azotaemia is less of a concern than anuria, dehydration or hyperkalaemia. Pre-existing renal disease and dehydration predisposes to contrast medium-induced renal failure, which is thought to be due to renal vasoconstriction or cellular toxicity, and may be irreversible. Contrast medium-induced renal failure may be recognized by increasing serum urea and creatinine levels following injection of the contrast medium. On radiographs there may be persistence of the nephrogram phase, which may become more opaque with time, but absence of this feature does not rule out contrast medium-induced renal failure. The pyelogram phase may be absent and contrast medium may be excreted via the biliary system and be seen in the gallbladder and intestinal tract (Figure 2.22).

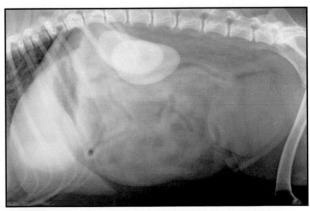

2.22 Lateral radiograph of a dog with contrast medium-induced renal failure. The radiograph was taken 3 days following administration of contrast medium. Note the persistence of opacification of the kidneys and the gallbladder. Absence of these findings does not rule out contrast medium-induced renal failure, which is best diagnosed by biochemical testing and urinalysis. This dog had pre-existing renal disease and cardiac disease, and had been treated with a diuretic for congestive heart failure. Care should be taken when using iodinated contrast media in severely azotaemic animals or hypotensive/dehydrated animals.

Technical considerations

Contrast studies are expensive and need to be performed in a systematic manner to maximize diagnostic yield. The study should be carefully planned, the patient adequately prepared, and the entire procedure completed even if a lesion is seen on early films. This is to ensure that lesions which may be visible only on later films are not missed and to enable artefacts and physiological variation (e.g. peristalsis, air bubbles) to be differentiated from genuine pathology.

In all cases plain radiographs (control films) should be taken prior to a contrast study because:

- The diagnosis may be determined without the need to perform the contrast study
- The contrast media may mask lesions which would be visible on the control films (e.g. some gastric foreign bodies)
- The exposure factors can be checked to ensure that a diagnostic film will be taken following administration of the contrast medium. This is particularly important where dynamic or a rapid series of films are being taken and repeat injections of contrast medium may not be possible (e.g. portovenography, angiography, intravenous urography)
- The preparation of the patient for the study can be assessed: for gastrointestinal studies the stomach can be checked to see it is empty of food, whilst for urinary tract studies the large bowel can be checked to ensure it is empty of faeces which may obscure the ureters or distort the bladder.

Patient preparation

- When performing elective urinary or large bowel contrast studies the animal should ideally have 2–3 enemas the evening ± morning prior to the study. The use of soapy enemas should be avoided as these may produce large numbers of bubbles within the colon. Water a few degrees below body temperature is recommended. The last enema should not be within 2–3 hours of the study.
- For urinary tract studies urinalysis should be performed prior to administration of contrast medium as iodinated contrast media will affect urinalysis.
- Before giving contrast media intravenously, renal function should be assessed, particularly if renal disease is suspected.

Patient restraint

Pneumogastrography and pneumocolonography can be performed without anaesthesia but for all other abdominal contrast studies general anaesthesia (see above) should be used.

Criteria for correct exposure

For negative-contrast studies the exposure factors should be reduced slightly compared with the control film (by approximately 5 kVp) because gas-filled organs attenuate the X-ray beam less than fluid-filled organs. For positive-contrast studies the exposure factors should be increased slightly (by approximately 5–10 kVp) because the positive contrast media attenuates the X-ray beam more than the soft tissues alone.

Integration with other imaging modalities

Radiography should be performed for the majority of abdominal studies because it is cheap, quick, gives a global overview of the entire abdomen and adjacent structures (Figure 2.23) and has a relatively high diagnostic yield. Radiography should generally be performed prior to other imaging modalities because:

- The diagnosis may be determined without the need for more expensive or time-consuming procedures
- Information on the radiograph may allow identification of areas requiring special attention using another modality
- Potential problems with other modalities may be identified; for example, if the stomach and intestinal tract are distended with gas then this may make abdominal ultrasonography difficult
- Certain conditions, such as pneumoperitoneum, ureteric calculi and some foreign bodies, are easier to detect on radiographs compared with ultrasonography.

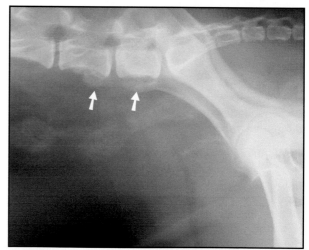

2.23 Lateral radiograph of the caudal abdomen in a dog with prostatic carcinoma and metastases to the lumbar vertebrae (arrowed). Extension of abdominal disease to the spine, body wall, thorax and pelvic canal is often easier to detect radiographically than with ultrasonography. The two modalities give complementary information.

There are limitations with radiography of the abdomen, including:

- The use of ionizing radiation
- The information is largely anatomical (lesions are seen if they cause alterations in the size, shape, position and/or opacity of the abdominal viscera) and often non-specific
- The poor inherent contrast

- A radiograph is a 2D representation of a 3D structure with superimposition of structures, which means that localization of a lesion can be difficult.

Other imaging modalities are used to give functional information or to give additional anatomical information.

- Magnetic resonance imaging (MRI), computed tomography (CT) and ultrasonography can all be used to image the abdomen and offer the advantage of cross-sectional imaging, where images of a slice of tissue are created without

superimposition of structures. They also have greater soft tissue contrast (Figure 2.24) than radiography but still give relatively non-specific anatomical information.

- CT and MRI angiography allow non-invasive assessment of vascular anomalies (e.g. portosystemic shunts) with 3D reconstructions that may help with surgical planning (Figure 2.25).
- In animals with renal disease, especially acute renal failure, the use of iodinated contrast media may exacerbate renal failure or be nephrotoxic. In these cases ultrasonography may be a useful alternative to contrast radiography.
- Nuclear medicine studies (scintigraphy) can be used to provide information about gastric emptying, renal function, liver function or to quantify portosystemic shunting.

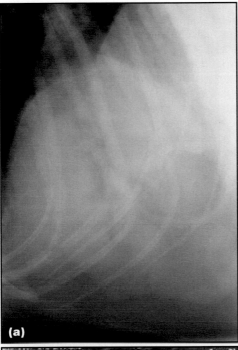

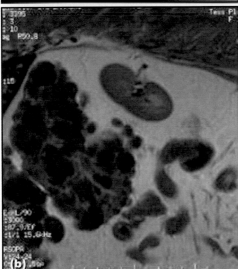

2.24 **(a)** Lateral radiograph and **(b)** sagittal T2-weighted MR image of the cranial abdomen in a dog with cirrhotic liver disease. Although the liver changes (irregular margin and reduced size) are visible radiographically, the MR image gives much better soft tissue contrast. MRI can be used to characterize liver lesions and has greater sensitivity and specificity for many abdominal diseases compared with other modalities. However, it is more expensive and time-consuming, and artefacts may be problematic.

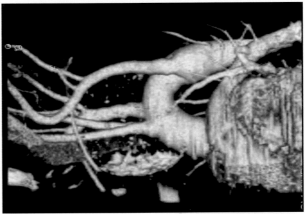

2.25 Sagittal 3D volume rendered CT angiogram of the thoracic vasculature of a dog with a vascular ring anomaly (abnormal left subclavian and carotid arteries are present in this case). 3D volume rendering does not give additional information compared with cross-sectional images but makes it easier to visualize complex vascular malformations.

References and further reading

Armbrust LJ, Biller DS and Hoskinson JJ (2000) Case examples demonstrating the clinical utility of obtaining both right and left lateral abdominal radiographs in small animals. *Journal of the American Animal Hospital Association* **36**, 531–536

Dennis RD and Herrtage ME (1989) Low osmolar contrast media – a review. *Veterinary Radiology and Ultrasound* **30**, 2–12

Jung J, Choi M, Chang J, Won S, Chung W, Choi H, Lee K, Yoon J and Ha H (2003) Effect of methylcellulose on upper gastrointestinal quality in dogs. *Veterinary Radiology and Ultrasound* **44**, 642–645

Kirberger RM (1999) Radiograph quality evaluation for exposure variables – a review. *Veterinary Radiology and Ultrasound* **40**, 220–226

Körner M, Weber CH, Wirth S, Pfeifer KJ, Reiser MF and Treitl M (2007) Advances in digital radiography: physical principles and system overview. *RadioGraphics* **27**, 675–686

Lee R and Leowijuk C (1982) Normal parameters in abdominal radiology of the dog and cat. *Journal of Small Animal Practice* **23**, 251–269

Morcos SK and Thomsen HS (2001) Adverse reactions to iodinated contrast media. *European Radiology* **11**,1267–1275

Robertson ID and Burbidge HM (2000) Pros and cons of barium-impregnated polyethylene spheres in gastrointestinal disease. *Veterinary Clinics of North America: Small Animal Practice* **30**, 449–465

Stacul F (2001) Current iodinated contrast media. *European Radiology* **11**, 690–697

Thomsen HS and Morcos SK (2003) Contrast media and the kidney: European Society of Urogenital Radiology (ESUR) Guidelines. *The British Journal of Radiology* **76**, 513–518

3

Abdominal ultrasonography

Juliette Besso

Basic physics of ultrasound waves

Ultrasound equipment can be considered in two parts: the transducer which sends the ultrasound waves out and receives the returning echoes; and the computer which analyses the data, orders the ultrasound waves emission/reception sequence, allows modifications and displays the information as an image. Ultrasound waves are produced by crystals with piezoelectric properties (Figure 3.1). These crystals vibrate when subjected to an electrical voltage. The vibration amplitude of the crystals, and therefore of the emitted ultrasound waves, is dependent on the natural resonance of the crystals. The crystals are made of natural quartz or a synthetic ceramic, and are located inside the ultrasound transducer.

A pulse of ultrasound waves is emitted about every 1/1000 of a second. Each pulse is a mechanical vibration, characterized by a direction of propagation, a speed, a frequency and a wavelength. Just as light waves follow optical laws, ultrasound waves passing through biological tissues follow similar laws of:

- Reflection
- Refraction
- Absorption.

All biological tissues are characterized by *impedance*, which influences the velocity of sound through the tissue. The junction between two tissues of differing impedance is called the *acoustic interface*. At every interface in the body there is attenuation. Attenuation is the decreased strength (amplitude) of the propagated wave. Attenuation may take the form of reflection, refraction or absorption (Figure 3.2).

At each acoustic interface part of the ultrasound wave is reflected back to the transducer. The piezo-electric crystals within the transducer then assume their 'receiving' function. The returning ultrasound waves (or echoes) received by the crystals produce electrical signals, which are then analysed according to the strength of the echo and the time at which they were received. This information is used to form an image on a screen, where the computer assumes that ultrasound waves travel at a constant speed (1540 m/s) in the soft tissues. Each image results from the gathering of information in multiple directions at all depths, by sweeping through the entire sector and obtaining contiguous information along adjacent lines (*scan lines*). In order to achieve a real-time examination, all this data must be re-acquired in the following split-second repeatedly. The speed of refreshment of the image is called the *frame rate*.

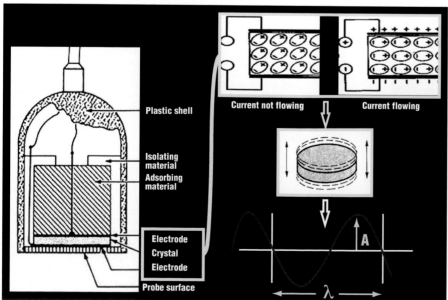

Plastic shell

Isolating material
Adsorbing material

Current not flowing   Current flowing

Electrode
Crystal
Electrode

Probe surface

3.1 The piezoelectric effect: the electrical current induces vibration of the crystals, which in turn generates ultrasound waves. The sinusoidal ultrasound wave has an amplitude (A) and describes a cycle, which is characterized by its wavelength (λ) (distance of a cycle) and its frequency (number of cycles per unit of time).

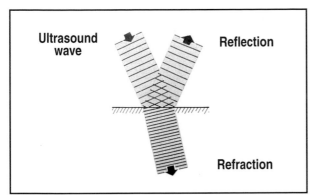

3.2 Ultrasound wave reaching an interface between tissues may become refracted or reflected.

Ultrasound equipment

Transducer types

Transducers vary depending on the number, arrangement and shape of the piezoelectric elements, and mechanical *versus* electronic components. The currently available first-hand and second-hand transducer technology includes: mechanical sector, annular array, linear array, curvilinear (convex) array and phased array transducers (Figure 3.4). Image quality and the type of screen display are highly dependent on the transducers and the associated technology.

For physical reasons, the ultrasound beam is not linear but hourglass-shaped, with an actual thickness in three dimensions. Therefore, each line of information on the screen comes from an hourglass-shaped volume of tissue. The best spatial resolution is achieved where the ultrasound beam is the narrowest: this portion of the ultrasound beam is called the *focal zone* (Figure 3.3). The use of multiple focal zones requires a new ultrasound beam path on the same scan line. Multiple focal zones improve the spatial resolution at the cost of decreased frame rate.

- *Mechanical real-time transducers:* one or several crystals rotate or oscillate over a sector. The screen image is pie-shaped, truncated at the top. One major drawback is the loss of useful information in the near-field due to a near-field artefact, which corresponds to the crowding of scan lines and information in this part of the image. A further drawback is the fixed number (one), size and location of the focal zone. These transducers are fragile and easily broken with rough handling.
- *Annular array transducers:* the crystals comprise concentric rings of various diameters. This allows variation in the number and location of focal zones. The screen image is pie-shaped, truncated at the top and a near-field artefact still exists. These transducers are fragile and easily broken with rough handling.
- *Linear array transducers:* these are electronic array transducers in which small crystals line up to form a linear contact surface. The screen image is rectangular-shaped, with consequently no near-field artefact. The major drawback is the elongated contact surface (i.e. large footprint).
- *Curvilinear array transducers:* identical to linear array transducers but the small crystals are arranged in a curved array. This is a major technological improvement, combining the best of previous technologies. The result is a fanned ultrasound beam with a greater width of exploration, but without a near-field artefact, and a small ergonomic contact surface. Newer technology transducers use phased array techniques to change the size or location of the focal zone.

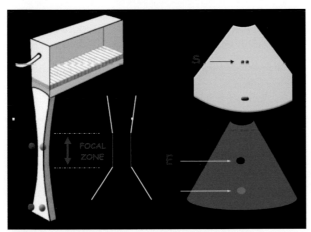

3.3 The narrowest part of the ultrasound beam is known as the focal zone. It affects the sharpness (S) of the object's borders as well as its echogenicity (E).

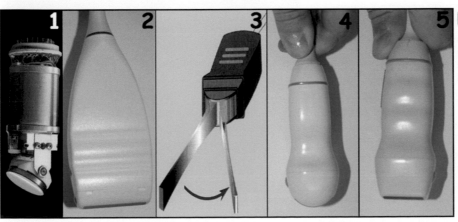

3.4 Types of transducer. (1) Mechanical without shell. (2) Linear array. (3) Diagram of a curvilinear array. (4) Curvilinear array. (5) Phased array.

- *Phased array transducers:* these transducers have a flat row of crystals. However, when groups of crystals are stimulated in an orderly fashion, with variation in the timing and sequence of pulses, ultrasound beams of various angles and shapes can be generated from the same transducer. This is termed 'phasing' or 'electronic steering'. This technology increases field depth, reduces ultrasound beam spread and therefore improves lateral resolution and increases signal-to-noise ratio. This technology is mostly used for cardiac ultrasonography. The contact surface, which is often square and of moderate size, and a near-field artefact remain drawbacks.

Transducers are also characterized by frequency and frequency spectrum. The choice of frequency is a trade-off between depth penetration and spatial resolution. A low-frequency transducer (3–5 MHz) has an excellent penetration but limited resolution. Higher frequency transducers (≥7 MHz) have an improved spatial resolution but poorer penetration. Older technologies had a narrow frequency spectrum: a 7.5 MHz transducer might have a range of 7.45–7.55 MHz. Most mechanical transducers were narrow frequency spectrum transducers, necessitating a change of transducer if a different frequency was required. Current transducers are wide bandwidth frequency transducers; for example, a single transducer may have a frequency ranging from 5 MHz to 9 MHz. This allows the near-field structures to be scanned at the highest resolution and the deeper structures at the best resolution possible consistent with the needed penetration.

Control panel and adjustments

Several controls can be adjusted on the ultrasound machine, which modify images as they are made (pre-processing) and/or after their acquisition (post-processing). It is important to optimize the image settings throughout the scanning process. Depending on the patient, initial settings may be adequate for the entire examination or may need adjusting for the evaluation of a single organ.

- *Depth:* this is the first control to be set. In order to evaluate an organ, it is important to place the organ in the centre of the image and to fill much of the screen. This is particularly important when the focal zone is fixed, as this positions the organ within the inbuilt focal zone, where the resolution is optimal.
- *Focal points:* in most newer machines the position and number of focal zones can be adjusted. A focal point is represented on the screen as an arrowhead or dot on the side of the image. Higher quality machines allow variation in the number of focal points, increasing the area of maximum resolution. For most situations in the abdomen the use of more than two focal zones will decrease the frame rate to an unacceptable level. Exceptions include very superficial organs or more caudal locations less affected by

respiratory motion. The ultrasonographer should always aim for the best definition or spatial resolution by positioning the area of interest within the focal zone.
- *Total gain:* this control amplifies the returning echoes. Increasing the gain makes the screen image whiter at all depths. This increases the signal of both usable information and artefactual noise. Excessive gain produces proportionately more noise than usable information, whilst too little gain can result in useful information being lost (Figure 3.5a). Working in a dark room allows a lower gain setting to be used with proportionately less noise.
- *Time gain compensation (TGC):* this is used to compensate for the variable attenuation of the returning echoes. Ultrasound beam attenuation normally increases with increasing depth but it can also vary because of tissue abnormalities. Gain at different depths can be individually adjusted: generally increased gain in the far-field to decreased gain in the near-field, with a mid-range gain in the middle depth. Newer machines with electronic curvilinear transducers have this compensation as a preset, with TGC controls all aligned at mid-range for a 'fits-all' TGC setting. TGC is very useful with older technology transducers because decreasing the near gain decreases the near-field artefact. Both total gain and TGC should be adjusted to obtain an image of uniform brightness throughout (Figure 3.5b). This is a major step of the ultrasound

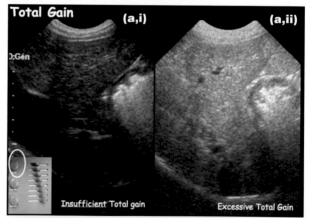

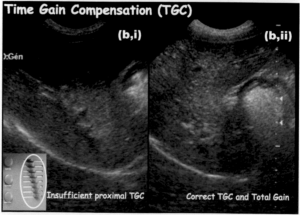

3.5 **(a)** Effects of total gain. (i) Insufficient total gain. (ii) Excessive total gain. **(b)** Effects of time gain compensation (TGC). (i) Insufficient proximal TGC. (ii) Correct TGC and total gain.

examination since an inappropriate setting may hide or falsely create parenchymal anomalies.

- *Frequency:* adjusting the transmitted frequency can improve penetration or resolution as necessary to improve image quality.
- *Sector size:* this allows variation of the angle of the pie-shaped images. Increasing the sector size increases the field-of-view. Decreasing the sector size increases the frame rate and improves resolution. This is most important for echocardiographic applications.
- *Screen brightness and contrast:* these can be adjusted according to personal preference, but are rarely adjusted after machine installation.
- *Power:* the number of ultrasound waves emitted from the transducer. Increasing the power increases the amplitude of transmitted pulses. Poor signal areas (such as deeper structures) may be better evaluated after increasing the power.

Ultrasound image

Echogenicity and principles of interpretation

The *echogenicity*, or grey level, of a tissue is determined by the brightness and concentration of dots on the screen. Each dot on the screen represents a returning echo.

- Most fluids are *anechoic*, appearing black on the screen. They are hypoattenuating: there is little or no attenuation or reflection of the ultrasound beam. They cause distal enhancement artefacts (see below).
- Parenchymal tissues are variably *echogenic*. They reflect a portion of the ultrasound beam.
- Mineralized structures and air are the source of shadowing and reverberation artefacts because they cause complete absorption (bone) or total reflection (air) of the ultrasound beam. This is why ultrasonography does not allow the evaluation of structures containing or covered by gas (for example, normal lungs) or normal bone beyond its surface.

The principal source of tissue echogenicity is collagen. In the normal patient, the abdominal structures can be ranked from least to most echogenic (Figure 3.6). Terms such as *hypoechoic* (less echoic) *iso-echoic* (the same echogenicity) and *hyperechoic* (more echoic) are used to compare organ echogenicity either between two different organs or structures, or to evaluate the echogenicity of one organ compared with normal.

Abnormal areas within the tissue parenchyma are described as lesions. Abnormalities may be detected because of a change in echogenicity. Alternatively, there may be an alteration in the echotexture, resulting in a change in the graininess (fine or coarse) which may be homogenous or heterogenous, or distortion of the normal architecture of the tissue. Changes in echogenicity may occur together with changes in echotexture and architecture, or the two

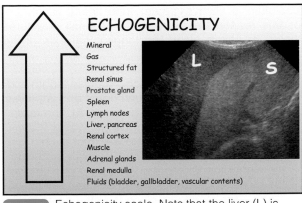

3.6 Echogenicity scale. Note that the liver (L) is hypoechoic to the spleen (S).

may occur independently. When defining a lesion it is important to consider whether it is solitary or one of several lesions, the location, the size in three dimensions, the definition of the margins, the echogenicity and the echotexture. Differentiation can be made, for example, between solid, cystic (thin-walled, round to ovoid, anechoic) and cavitated (with anechoic or very hypoechoic areas, which can be septated, irregularly marginated, ill defined) lesions. Abnormal solid lesions within parenchymal organs may be described as nodules (Figure 3.7). Larger lesions (>3 cm) may be referred to as a mass, but a complete description of the lesion is more important than this arbitrary distinction.

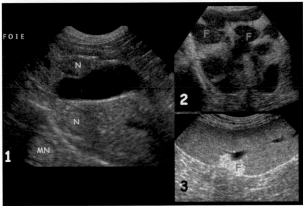

3.7 Nodules and foci. (1) Hepatic nodules (N) are so-called because they distort the architecture of the liver and have a mass effect on the contour of the gallbladder. The echogenicity of the nodules is mixed (both hypoechoic and hyperechoic) in a 'target-like' distribution. The artefactual mirror image (MN) of the real nodule is also visible. (2) Numerous hypoechoic well defined foci (F) in the prostate gland. There is no distortion of the architecture of the prostate gland. This is an unusual site of lymphoma infiltrate. (3) Hyperechoic well defined perivascular focus (F) in the spleen. There is no distortion of the architecture of the spleen. This is a site of benign and frequent myelolipoma.

Image quality

Resolution
Resolution is the ability to distinguish two points as separate, either along the longitudinal (axial) axis or along the lateral axis of the ultrasound beam. Axial

resolution is always greater than lateral resolution; for this reason, measurements of small structures should be taken along the longitudinal axis of the ultrasound beam.

- *Axial resolution* depends on the pulse length and wavelength of the ultrasound beam and improves with increased frequency (Figure 3.8). The pulse length is the number of ultrasound waves within each pulse multiplied by the length of each waveform. The shorter the wavelength (and thus the higher the ultrasound frequency), the shorter the pulse length and the greater the ability to resolve two structures close together as separate echoes. The maximum axial resolution is half the pulse length, i.e values in theory as small as 0.05 mm for a 10 MHz probe.
- *Lateral resolution* depends on the ultrasound beam's width (slice thickness of the structures imaged) and frequency. Since the ultrasound beam is not of even thickness as depth changes, lateral resolution also varies with depth. Lateral resolution is best in the focal zone (where the ultrasound beam is the narrowest, see Figure 3.3). The ultrasound beam is thinner at higher frequency. Both lateral and axial resolution are improved with higher frequency.

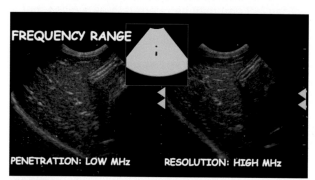

3.8 A curvilinear array transducer used at different frequency ranges, for the same patient, with an identical number and location of focal zones (triangles). The liver parenchyma has a finer texture (more detail is visible) in the resolution mode (right image), particularly in the first 3 cm of depth, but the deeper parts of the liver parenchyma are better seen in the penetration mode (left image).

Penetration

Penetration is often ignored because of the trade-off between penetration and resolution. Sufficient penetration is essential to completely assess deeper structures. Penetration can be increased by using a lower frequency transducer or by using a wide bandwidth frequency transducer with a low-frequency component. This may be termed 'penetration mode' by the manufacturer. Greater penetration can also be achieved by increasing the output power (amount of emitted ultrasound waves) but this also increases needlessly the echoes in the near-field and is limited by safety considerations. Most manufacturers now utilize coded pulse technology to provide increased penetration without concurrent loss of resolution. Differences in technology result in major differences in

penetration between two 7 MHz transducers from different manufacturers or between two different models of 7 MHz transducer from the same manufacturer.

Artefacts

Artefacts are the representation of something that does not exist anatomically. With ultrasonography, artefacts can hamper evaluation and be disturbing, but can also provide useful information about the nature of the structure being examined. In all cases, artefacts must be recognized as such for proper interpretation. Common artefacts include:

- Shadowing
- Refraction
- Reverberation (ring down)
- Distal enhancement
- Mirror image
- Slice thickness
- Side-lobes.

Shadowing

- Shadowing is due to marked ultrasound beam attenuation by mineral, gas and most non-biological material. Very few ultrasound waves pass beyond the level of intense attenuation (the mineral or gas surface), so very few echoes propagate through the interface and therefore return from the deeper tissues.
- Shadowing appears as a linear to cone-shaped hypo- or anechoic area distal to a highly attenuating structure (Figure 3.9). The long axis of the cone is aligned with the long axis of the ultrasound beam. Complete ('clean') shadowing, a uniformly black shadow, occurs when the entire ultrasound beam is absorbed by mineral structures. Incomplete ('dirty') shadowing is seen with a highly attenuating structure. It occurs when complete reflection occurs at a gas surface. It can also occur within an organ when there is significant absorption of the ultrasound beam (e.g. severe hepatic lipidosis).

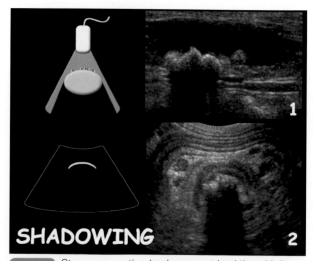

3.9 Strong acoustic shadows cast by (1) multiple calculi lying within the bladder (rectangular image obtained with a linear transducer) and (2) a cloth foreign body within a jejunal intussusception.

- Edge shadowing occurs deep to the margins of a rounded, fluid-filled structure. This is not true acoustic shadowing but arises due to refraction (see below).
- Shadowing hampers evaluation of the structures distal to the origin of the shadow, but it draws attention to the smallest mineralized speck or to an ill defined non-biological structure such as a gastrointestinal foreign body.
- Clean and dirty shadowing cannot be avoided but the ultrasonographer can usually assess deeper structures using an alternate path.

Refraction

- Refraction occurs at the edges of rounded structures such as the gallbladder. This phenomenon is sometimes referred to as 'edge shadowing'. The refracted ultrasound beam is deviated towards the tissue with the slower speed of sound propagation. As the ultrasound beam is bent, there is no sound returning to the transducer from the site immediately deep to the rounded edge, and the lack of information is translated as a black, echo void area on the screen. The rounded shape of the structure is important in the creation of this artefact.
- Refraction appears on the image as a narrow, anechoic line or cone distal to the edges of a rounded structure (Figure 3.10).
- To confirm refraction and thus rule out the presence of mineralization, the transducer can be moved to assess the rounded structure from a different angle; edge shadowing will either move or disappear.

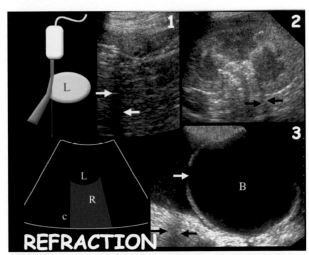

3.10 Refractive (edge) shadowing is visible on the edge of various organs as a narrow black cone (arrowed). C = Cone of reflective shadowing; L = Organ of interest; R = Ultrasound wave passing through the organ. (1) Refraction (arrowed) helps to identify the ovary. (2) The presence of a refraction artefact on the edge of renal pelvis fat (arrowed) may be mistaken for acoustic shadowing (with the corollary erroneous diagnosis of renal calcification). (3) When the bladder (B) is surrounded by abdominal effusion, refraction of the tangential echo (black arrows) results in an artefactual bladder wall interruption (white arrow).

Reverberation

- Reverberation is the result of multiple reflections of an ultrasound beam, bouncing back and forth between two surfaces, or vibrating within a highly reflective surface, usually gas. Some echoes return to the transducer after one, two, three or more bounces; echoes take once, twice, thrice or more times the time to return and the computer takes this into account by placing equidistant echoes along the path (once, twice, thrice as deep) (Figure 3.11). The intensity of this artefact decreases with depth. This artefact is affected by the size and shape of the gas pocket. Small bubbles produce *comet tail* artefacts whereas a more linear gas interface produces repeated hyperechoic lines (*ring down*). Ring down also occurs with any strong linear interface near the transducer face. Ring down causes considerable disruption of the appearance of structures immediately deep to the body wall, and is most noticeable in older, large-breed patients using mechanical and phased linear transducer technologies.

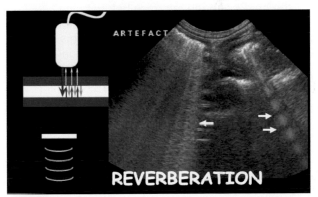

3.11 Multiple streams of reverberation (arrowed) arising from pockets of gas within the jejunum. More specifically, ring down (arrows pointing to the right) reverberations appear as repeated hyperechoic lines.

Distal enhancement

- Distal enhancement is the result of the ultrasound beam passing through a poorly attenuating structure. More sound reaches the tissues beyond this poorly attenuating structure than laterally adjacent areas, which generates more returning echoes.
- It appears as a hyperechoic area distal to a low attenuating structure. The long axis of this hyperechoic area is aligned with the ultrasound beam axis (Figure 3.12). Distal enhancement is commonly seen with normal structures (e.g. gallbladder, urinary bladder), abnormal fluid lesions (e.g. cyst, abscess) and some low attenuating masses (e.g. malignant lymph nodes).
- It cannot be avoided, but distal structures may be assessed more objectively by turning the gain down in the area distal to the fluid accumulation.

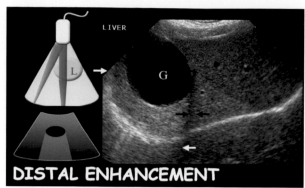

DISTAL ENHANCEMENT

3.12 Distal enhancement is seen deep to the gallbladder (G) as a hyperechoic cone (white arrows). The edge of the gallbladder also creates edge shadowing (black arrows). The part of the ultrasound beam which passes through the gallbladder is less attenuated (and therefore stronger) than the part of the ultrasound beam which passes to one side of the gallbladder.

Mirror image

- Mirror images occur at a highly reflective interface (e.g. the lungs beyond the diaphragm). The ultrasound beam can be reflected between the object and the interface before being reflected back to the transducer (hence taking more time). The computer interprets this delay in returning echoes by representing an identical image of the object symmetrically positioned on the other side of the highly reflective interface (Figure 3.13).
- The mirror image may artefactually position the liver beyond the diaphragm, mimicking a diaphragmatic hernia or lung lobe consolidation.
- Movement of the transducer may significantly alter or eliminate the artefact, allowing confirmation of the true position of the tissues.

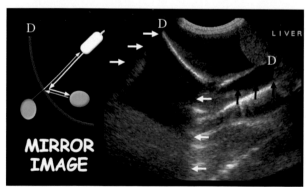

MIRROR IMAGE

3.13 The areas of the image beyond the diaphragm (D) between the white arrows (mirror image 1) and delineated by black arrows (mirror image 2) are artefacts mimicking the presence of pleural effusion. Reverberation artefacts due to air present in the lungs can be seen deep to the black arrows.

Slice thickness

- Slice thickness arises due to the actual thickness of the ultrasound beam. It results in a representation on the screen image of echoes originating from nearby structures in the same 'slice'.

- It may produce echoes in the bladder mimicking intraluminal echoes, which in fact arise either from the bladder wall or from adjacent tissues.
- Displacing the transducer or changing the ultrasound beam angle (for example, turning the transducer 90 degrees) will alter or eliminate the artefact and show the true nature and localization of the nearby tissues.

Side-lobes

- Side-lobes are the artefactual representation of a structure located to one side of the main ultrasound beam. The ultrasound beam is in fact composed of a main beam and smaller, less penetrating accessory beams on both sides, called side-beams or side-lobes. When a highly reflecting structure is located in the path of a side-beam, the returning echoes are strong enough to reach the transducer. The display of this structure 'on the side' is therefore artefactually located in the image plane of the main beam.
- It falsely positions echoes in the bladder, mimicking intraluminal echoes, which in fact are the returning echoes from the nearby colon (Figure 3.14).
- Displacing the transducer or changing the ultrasound beam angle (for example, turning the transducer 90 degrees) will alter or eliminate the artefact and show the true nature and localization of the nearby tissues.

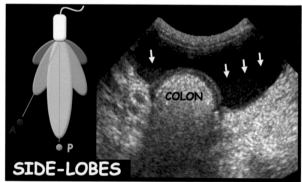

SIDE-LOBES

3.14 The band of echoes lying in the dependant portion of the bladder lumen (arrowed) is artefactual and due to side-lobe artefacts associated with the nearby colon (in this case, in the same image plane). A = Accessory ultrasound beam; P = Primary ultrasound beam.

Doppler ultrasonography

Principles

Doppler ultrasonography is used to detect moving structures (e.g. blood within vessels) and to evaluate flow in terms of direction, speed and volume (Figure 3.15a). The main indications for abdominal Doppler ultrasonography are to: assess the vascularity of organs and masses; detect portosystemic shunts, arteriovenous fistulae and thrombus formations; and search for ectopic ureters.

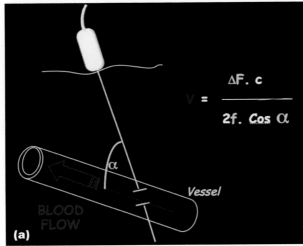

$$V = \frac{\Delta F \cdot c}{2f \cdot \cos \alpha}$$

(a)

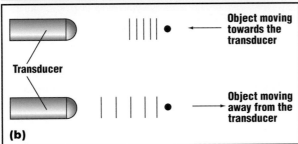

(b)

3.15 **(a)** Equation for evaluating blood flow using Doppler ultrasonography. α = Angle between the ultrasound beam and the blood flow; ΔF = Frequency change (Doppler shift) between incoming and outgoing sound; c = Velocity of sound in the medium; f = Frequency of the initial ultrasound beam; V = Blood velocity. **(b)** If the object (e.g. blood constituents) is moving towards the transducer, the reflected ultrasound waves are compressed and the frequency increases. Conversely, If the object is moving away from the transducer, the reflected ultrasound waves are stretched and the frequency decreases.

Most Doppler ultrasonography techniques work on the same principles. When an ultrasound wave hits a moving target, the frequency of the returning ultrasound beam is different from that of the incident ultrasound beam. This difference is called the frequency shift or Δf (Figure 3.15b) and is in the audible range. Doppler ultrasonography can be displayed as an audible signal through speakers, as a spectral display on the screen (x, y; time, velocity; Figure 3.16) or as a colour display on the 2D screen image (Duplex Doppler; Figure 3.17). The greatest Doppler ultrasonography signal will be collected if the flow is along the ultrasound beam axis. Conversely, the signal will be nil if the ultrasound beam axis and flow are at 90 degrees to one another. Doppler ultrasonography is very sensitive to artefactual motion.

Types of Doppler ultrasonography
There are several types of Doppler ultrasonography:

- Continuous wave (CW)
- Pulsed wave (PW)
- Colour
- Power.

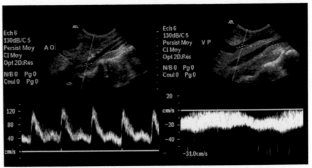

3.16 PW Doppler ultrasonography allows quick differentiation of the pulsed signal of the aorta (bloodstream moving towards the transducer, positive signal) from the wavy continuous signal of the portal vein (bloodstream moving away from the transducer, negative signal) when searching for a portosytemic shunt in the liver hilus. The more parallel is the sample volume to the blood flow, the more accurate is the velocity.

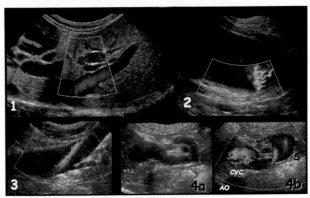

3.17 Colour flow ultrasonography. (1) The lack of colour flow in one tubular structure within the sample volume box is diagnostic for an intrahepatic biliary dilatation. (2) The presence of colour flow in the sample volume box represents a normal vesicoureteral urinary jet in the bladder. (3) The lack of complete colour flow within the sample volume box is diagnostic for a <6-hour-old thrombus in the caudal vena cava. (4) (a) Transverse section of the liver hilus. (b) Colour Doppler ultrasonogram of the same area demonstrating a portocaval shunt (S). Ao = Aorta; CVC = Caudal vena cava.

Continuous wave Doppler ultrasonography
CW Doppler ultrasonography uses two separate crystals; one each for transmission and one for reception. As transmission and reception are separate and therefore continuous, there is no waiting for echoes to return and high velocities can be measured. The information is displayed as a graph of flow velocity over time. The major drawback is the absence of depth information, since the depicted flow may be occurring anywhere along the cursor. CW Doppler ultrasonography is used to assess high-speed flow and is mainly used in echocardiography. All other forms of Doppler ultrasonography are PW and suffer from an upper limit in measuring velocity.

Pulsed wave Doppler ultrasonography
With PW or spectral Doppler ultrasonography the transducer transmits pulses of ultrasound waves, then switches to receive mode between pulses, waiting for echoes to return. It only accepts echoes from a particular depth, defined on the 2D screen

image by a moveable box along a moveable cursor. The frequency shift of this particular sample volume is then calculated and the information is displayed as a graph of mean velocity of the moving targets within the sample against time (see Figure 3.16). PW Doppler ultrasonography therefore has depth discrimination. The direction of flow is indicated by the position of flow compared with the base line of the graph (above the line represents flow towards the transducer). The height of the curve is the peak mean speed of the flow. The area under the curve indicates a laminar flow if clean or a turbulent flow if full. The major drawback of PW Doppler ultrasonography is the limit in measurement of high-velocity flow, although this is rarely an issue for abdominal ultrasonography.

Colour Doppler ultrasonography

The principle is similar to PW Doppler ultrasonography. However, a bigger sample volume appears as a box on the 2D image and the colour display is superimposed on the 2D greyscale image within this box. The box may be adjusted in size and moved to the chosen part of the image. The colour mapping gives both directional and semi-quantitative speed information; for instance, the colour codes can be chosen as red-orange-yellow for increasing speeds of flow going toward the transducer and shades of blue to green for flow going away from the transducer (see Figure 3.17). Colour Doppler ultrasonography is a very good tool for screening larger body regions, regional blood flow within a mass or detecting low flow. Colour Doppler ultrasonography is a very important tool for detecting and characterizing portosystemic shunts.

Power Doppler ultrasonography

Power Doppler ultrasonography works on very different principles to the other types of Doppler ultrasonography. It is a pulsed technology that ignores velocity information, i.e. rather than measuring the frequency shift, it looks at the amplitude of moving blood. The greater the volume of moving blood cells, the brighter the displayed signal. Since there is no measure of the frequency shift, the angle of flow relative to the ultrasound beam axis is no longer an issue. Power Doppler ultrasonography is the most sensitive modality to characterize flow from small vessels or from vessels with a very slow flow (Figure 3.18). Colour mapping may be displayed without directional information, but newer technologies include directional information. Its major drawback is its extreme sensitivity to the smallest motion of the patient or transducer, resulting in flare artefacts.

Contrast ultrasonography

Newer developments in ultrasonography include the access to ultrasonography contrast media. These agents are microscopic encapsulated bubbles that are injected intravenously. The shell is usually an inert phospholipid surrounding the luminal gas. These bubbles are smaller than red blood cells and can travel anywhere that blood travels in the body. The newest commercial contrast agents are very safe and no significant complications have been noted in veterinary imaging.

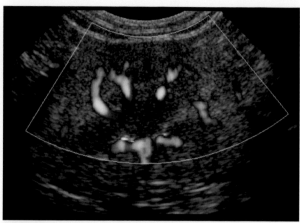

3.18 Power Doppler ultrasonography generally does not give directional information but detects flow from small vessels and vessels with slow flow, such as in this 2.5 kg cat's kidney.

Sophisticated engineering is necessary in the specialized 'contrast software' on the ultrasound machine system to excite the bubbles, allowing the bubbles to be imaged as an indicator of organ perfusion. The three components of contrast ultrasonography are: contrast media; specialized 'contrast software'; and transducers that are contrast medium capable. The advantages of contrast ultrasonography compared with CT and MRI include decreased cost, lack of need for general anaesthesia and lower cost for imaging components.

Contrast ultrasonography is indicated for evaluation of any lesion with a microvascular component, which allows differentiation from normal tissues. These diseases include very common challenging areas in veterinary medicine, and contrast ultrasonography results in improved characterization and detection of liver, splenic and renal nodules, malignant lymph nodes, acute infarction, bowel wall viability and transplant rejection (see Figure 16.9).

Abdominal examination

Indications and contraindications

Ultrasonography is a safe and well tolerated imaging technique. It allows evaluation of the size, shape, contour and internal structure of organs in a non-invasive fashion. In veterinary medicine, abdominal ultrasonography is used to evaluate all abdominal organs, mesentery and omentum, peritoneum and abdominal wall, as well as to determine the origin and extent of abdominal masses. In addition, ultrasonography may be used to guide needles for aspiration or biopsy of fluid or soft tissues within the abdomen.

Ultrasonography has no true contraindications. However, it can be difficult to obtain good quality images in animals with substantial volumes of free air in the peritoneum (e.g. post laparotomy). Barium studies should not be performed before an ultrasound examination because the strong shadowing artefacts generated by barium hamper evaluation.

Patient preparation

Prerequisites

It has been recommended that a patient undergoing an abdominal examination be fasted for several hours prior to the examination in order to limit the presence of food material and gas in the gastrointestinal tract. Reverberation and shadowing artefacts caused by gas and food narrow the acoustic window. However, it is often possible to avoid the artefacts, either by approaching the organ from a different angle or by pressing gently with the transducer to displace bowel segments.

The other concern may be the degree of bladder distension. Bladder wall thickness and luminal lesions are better appreciated when the bladder is full. However, the bladder is not always full and the ultrasonographer will have to evaluate the wall thickness in the light of the degree of distension and be aware of the risk of missing a small focal wall thickening if the bladder is not distended. Another option is to place a urinary catheter and slowly inject warm saline into the bladder; injecting slowly limits the injection of gas bubbles. In addition, intravenous use of furosemide (2 mg/kg) has been suggested to increase bladder filling; this also allows evaluation of ureteral jets of urine into the bladder when looking for ectopic ureters.

Sedation

A very important, but often overlooked, aspect of patient preparation is that of reassurance. A quiet and calm environment, taking time to obtain the patient's confidence, placing the patient in a comfortable position for the examination and using soundless clippers will reduce patient stress. Stress causes panting and aerophagia, and often a moving patient with a tense abdomen. Limiting stress eases the examination process and greatly improves its quality. It also allows most examinations to be done without sedation. However, a few unapproachable patients may require sedation. It is important to be aware of the vasodilatory effect of certain drugs to avoid misinterpretation.

Clipping

Hair, even when wet, traps microbubbles of air, which decrease image quality. Clipping is usually necessary therefore, and must be close to the skin to achieve the best imaging quality. Clipping should extend from the costal arch to the pubis; clipping over the caudal aspect of the ribcage on the right-hand side might be necessary for deep-chested patients for better evaluation of the liver, right kidney and hepatic hilus. Coupling gel should be applied to the skin to ensure good contact between the transducer and the patient. Provided it does not destroy the plastic surface of the transducer, isopropyl alcohol may be applied before the gel in order to remove any remaining hair, dirt and grease. Isopropyl alcohol is also the coupling agent of choice for interventional needle procedures.

Patient positioning

The examination may be performed with the patient in dorsal or lateral recumbency or even standing. Dorsal recumbency allows the organs to lie symmetrically and because it is the closest to the available descriptive and cross-sectional anatomy texts, dorsal recumbency seems the least misleading. In dorsal recumbency, placing the hindlegs in a frog-legged position has many advantages: it is less painful for older patients' hips and it relaxes the rectus abdomini and other abdominal wall muscles, facilitating the examination. Lateral recumbency is a good alternative, particularly for very deep-chested or dyspnoeic patients. Shifting the patient from dorsal to lateral recumbency might improve or complete the evaluation; for example, by redistributing gas or in determining the mobility of the contents of the bladder or gallbladder.

Procedures

In order to become familiar with the technique and normal appearance of the abdominal organs, it is necessary to be as complete and systematic as possible during the ultrasound examination. The proposed sequence given here may vary as long as each organ is evaluated one by one, and always in the same order. Most protocols begin cranially and circle the abdomen, but any protocol is acceptable if it allows a systematic and complete evaluation of the entire abdomen.

Abdominal evaluation may be performed according to the following sequence:

* Liver (includes gallbladder, biliary tract and portal vein/hilar vessels)
* Right kidney
* Right adrenal gland
* Hepatic lymph nodes
* Right pancreatic lobe
* Duodenum
* (Right ovary/uterine horn)
* Spleen
* Left kidney
* Left adrenal gland
* Left pancreatic lobe
* (Left ovary/uterine horn)
* Bladder
* Urethra (as much as can be seen into the pelvic canal)
* (Prostate gland)
* Iliac and hypogastric lymph nodes
* Aorta/caudal vena cava from the iliac bifurcation to the liver
* If a prostatic or uterine abnormality is detected, the examination should be completed by assessment of the ventral surface of the lumbar vertebrae and the intervertebral disc spaces
* Assessment of the gastrointestinal tract includes the stomach (including, if possible, the cardia but certainly the pyloric antrum and pyloric sphincter), pyloroduodenal angle, pancreatic body (unless enormous amounts of gastric gas are present), jejunum, ileum, the ileocaecocolic junction (mainly in cats), colon, colic lymph nodes and jejunomesenteric lymph nodes
* Mesenteric and omental fat
* Abdominal wall and serosal surfaces.

Additional sites

Abdominal ultrasonography may reveal lesions that results in ultrasonographic evaluation of other body parts in order to complete the diagnosis.

Thorax: When evaluating the abdomen, the normal appearance of the diaphragm is a hyperechoic line with uniform and extensive reverberation artefacts, due to the normal inflated lungs, beyond the thin diaphragmatic muscle layer. Abnormal findings may be discovered in the thorax using the liver as an acoustic window (Figure 3.19). These include pleural effusion, abdominal organs such as the liver, spleen or gastrointestinal tract, focal or lobar pulmonary consolidation or a diaphragmatic or caudal mediastinal mass. In each case, the clue to the diagnosis is being able to see something at a location where usually nothing can be seen because of reverberation artefacts.

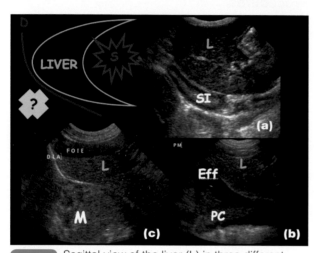

3.19 Sagittal view of the liver (L) in three different patients, which led to the identification of thoracic lesions beyond the diaphragm (D).
(a) Identification of small intestine (SI) cranial to the diaphragm allowed diagnosis of a diaphragmatic hernia.
(b) Pleural effusion (Eff) and pulmonary consolidation (PC) are visible. The mass was confirmed as a pulmonary carcinoma (diagnosis achieved via aspiration from a thoracic window). **(c)** Thoracic mass (M). Analysis of the movement of the mass compared with the surrounding lungs is essential to differentiate a pulmonary from extrapulmonary mass. S = Stomach.

Alternatively, some findings in the abdomen require thoracic evaluation either to achieve a diagnosis or to complete a diagnosis. For example, when hepatic venous congestion is found, evaluation of the heart and pericardium is indicated. If the abdominal evaluation is suggestive of lymphoma or another abdominal neoplasm, it is important to check the thorax for mediastinal masses (including cardiac masses), enlarged thoracic lymph nodes, superficial pulmonary metastases or pleural effusion. Sternal lymph nodes are a common site of metastasis from a cranial abdominal neoplasm or peritoneal lesion.

Oesophagus: In patients presented with 'vomiting', with a normal abdominal ultrasound examination, it can be useful to look for oesophageal or perioesophageal lesions in the neck. Cervical ultrasonography is fairly straightforward, and allows morphological assessment of the oesophageal wall and lumen but will not provide an accurate functional evaluation. It is a simple way of assessing soft tissues around the oesophagus, looking for fistulous tracts, abscesses and foreign bodies. Thoracic oesophageal lesions usually require plain radiography for evaluation, with contrast radiography in some cases.

Other:

- In cases of hypercalcaemia, evaluation of the parathyroid and anal glands is often indicated.
- When a urethral obstruction is suspected, the penile and part of the membranous urethra may be directly assessed. The urethral distension makes it easier to follow and abnormal contents, such as shadowing calculi, may be identified. Care should be taken to access the penile urethra from the side, in order to differentiate shadows from a potential calculus and from the os penis. The site(s) of intraluminal obstruction can be specified. However, ultrasonography is not a sensitive technique to rule out a urethral stricture.
- Identification of a mass in the pelvic area, mainly around the iliac vessels, may lead to evaluation of its extension into the inguinal ring or femoral fossa. Doppler ultrasonography is a simple and painless tool for assessment of vascular repercussions and/or invasion. The assessment of the caudal extent of a pelvic mass may benefit from a perineal ultrasonographic approach but will sometimes need the adjunct of computed tomography.
- The patient population referred for a congenital portosystemic shunt examination is often also at risk for hydrocephalus. Transfontanellar screening to assess ventricular size is quickly and safely performed without the need for anaesthesia.

References and further reading

Kremkau FW (1998) *Diagnostic Ultrasound: principles and instruments, 5th edn.* WB Saunders, Philadelphia
Nyland T and Mattoon J (2002) *Small Animal Diagnostic Ultrasound, 2nd edn.* WB Saunders, Philadelphia

4

The peritoneal cavity

Elizabeth A. Baines

Normal peritoneum

The peritoneum is a serous membrane, predominantly composed of connective tissue, which lines the peritoneal space and is contained largely within the abdominal cavity. In the normal animal the peritoneal cavity is an almost non-existent space, containing only a small volume of lubricating fluid.

The peritoneum is divided into:

- Parietal peritoneum, which covers the inner surfaces of the walls of the abdominal, pelvic and scrotal cavities
- Visceral peritoneum, which covers the surface of the organs, wholly or in part
- Connecting peritoneum, which consists of double sheets of peritoneum extending between organs or connecting them to the parietal peritoneum. These peritoneal folds are known as mesenteries, omenta or ligaments.

The common dorsal mesentery is the peritoneal fold which leaves the dorsal abdominal wall and reflects around most of the freely moveable organs of the abdominal cavity. It provides a route for the coeliac, cranial and caudal mesenteric arteries, sympathetic and parasympathetic nerves, lymphatics and branches of the portal vein to pass to and from the intestine and other organs. It comprises the mesogastrium, mesoduodenum, mesojejunoileum, mesocolon and mesorectum.

The greater omentum, derived from the dorsal mesogastrium, is a fat-streaked, lacy, double reflection of the peritoneum, which covers most of the abdominal contents ventrally and laterally. The two layers of the omentum enclose the lesser peritoneal cavity, or omental bursa, which can be entered via the epiploic foramen.

Organs that lie against the walls of the abdominal or pelvic cavity and are covered in peritoneum on only one surface are described as being retroperitoneal (see Chapter 5). Organs that project freely into the cavities and have an almost complete covering of peritoneum are termed intraperitoneal.

The pelvic cavity contains the pelvic portion of the peritoneal cavity. In the male this is a single rectovesical pouch but in the female this pouch is divided in the dorsal plane by the uterus and broad ligaments, resulting in a dorsal rectogenital pouch and a ventral vesicogenital pouch. In both sexes there is a small pubovesical pouch ventral to the bladder neck. Vaginal processes exist as extra-abdominal extensions of the peritoneal cavity.

Imaging of the peritoneal cavity may be performed with plain radiographs of the abdomen (lateral and ventrodorsal (VD) views) and with ultrasonography, using a variety of acoustic windows. Contrast radiography is less commonly used since the advent of diagnostic ultrasonography.

Dogs

In the normal dog, the parietal peritoneum is not visible. The most commonly visualized parts of the peritoneum are the mesentery and greater omentum by virtue of the fat within these structures. Upon ultrasound examination, the mesentery and omentum of a dog in good body condition appear hyperechoic to the other organs and fairly heterogenous (Figure 4.1). On plain radiographs of the abdomen, in an adult dog of normal body condition, fat acts as a contrasting substance to highlight the serosal surfaces of the soft tissue structures within the abdomen (Figure 4.2).

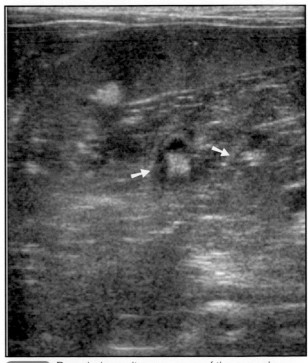

4.1 Dorsal plane ultrasonogram of the normal mesentery in a 9-year-old West Highland White Terrier. Intestinal loops (arrowed) are present surrounded by the fine hyperechoic streaks and amorphous tissue of the mesentery. The spleen is visible in the near-field.

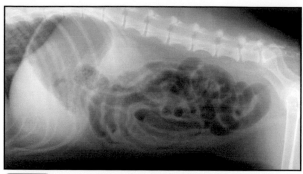

4.2 Lateral abdominal radiograph of a skeletally mature medium-breed dog, showing the normal distribution of fat within the abdomen.

Cats

The adult cat often has moderate to large fat deposits in the peritoneum, particularly within the falciform ligament, and also in the retroperitoneal space (Figure 4.3). The mesentery itself does not accumulate as much fat as in dogs. The small intestines in obese cats may appear compressed centrally on lateral views and to the right of centre on VD views by the more peripheral intraperitoneal fat deposits (Figure 4.4). Upon ultrasound examination, the mesentery and omentum of a cat in good body condition appear hyperechoic to the other organs within the abdomen and fairly heterogenous. There may only be 3–4 mm of mesentery between each small intestinal loop.

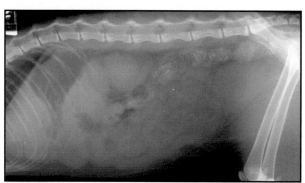

4.3 Lateral abdominal radiograph of a skeletally mature cat. Small fat deposits are present in the falciform and retroperitoneal regions.

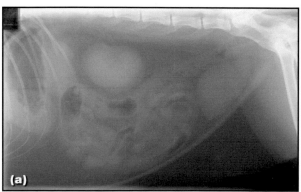

4.4 **(a)** Lateral abdominal radiograph of an obese skeletally mature cat. Large fat deposits are present in the falciform, umbilical, retroperitoneal and inguinal regions, resulting in central displacement of the abdominal organs. (continues) ▶

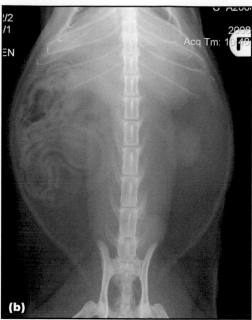

4.4 (continued) **(b)** VD abdominal radiograph of an obese cat. Substantial fat deposits highlight the kidney on the left, and result in displacement of small intestines to the right. (Courtesy of F Barr)

Neonates and juvenile animals

Neonates and juvenile animals up to about 6 months old have minimal intraperitoneal fat deposits. Fat which is present is termed 'brown fat' and has a higher water content than adult fat, so serosal detail is poor within the abdomen (Figure 4.5). This appearance may be confused with free fluid in the peritoneal cavity and so the radiographs must be assessed carefully. Observation of fascial planes in the retroperitoneal space and pelvic canal and assessment of the body contour are required to try to differentiate these conditions (Figure 4.6).

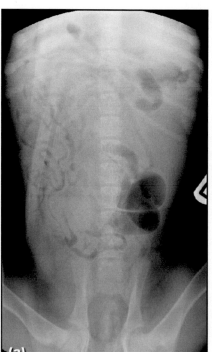

4.5

(a) VD abdominal radiograph of a 4-month-old Hungarian Vizsla. The serosal surfaces of the intestines are poorly visualized due to the lack of intra-abdominal fat. (continues) ▶

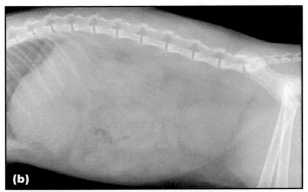

4.5 (continued) **(b)** Lateral abdominal radiograph of a 5-month-old cat. There are only small intra-abdominal fat deposits and serosal detail is poor.

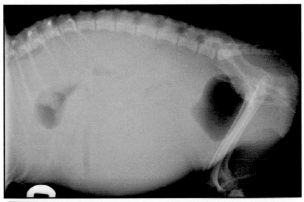

4.6 Lateral abdominal radiograph of a 17-week-old Cavalier King Charles Spaniel with suspected urinary tract rupture. The pendulous body contour with complete effacement of all serosal detail is highly suggestive of free fluid, but the absence of intra-abdominal fat deposits may make interpretation uncertain.

Ultrasonography of neonates is easy compared with adults. The lack of mature fat and immaturity of the body wall minimize many acoustic artefacts associated with attenuation and ring down. In addition, neonatal cats and dogs have proportionately larger parenchymal organs (liver and spleen) than adults and regularly identifiable lymph nodes, especially jejunal lymph nodes.

Body condition

In obese animals, fat deposits accumulate within the falciform ligament and the greater omentum. If fat deposits are huge, the increased radiographic scatter may result in an overall 'flatter' radiographic image (Figure 4.7). Upon ultrasound examination, the increased fat reduces the clarity of the image and can reduce the accuracy of any measurements. A large falciform fat pad will cause quite marked attenuation of the ultrasound beam during ultrasonography of the liver and may result in an inaccurate assessment of the echogenicity of that organ.

In emaciated animals, the absence of fat results in reduced contrast between the different viscera within the abdomen on radiographs, which reduces the ability to discern separate structures. Upon ultrasound examination, the absence of fat reduces many artefacts due to scatter and so clearer images of

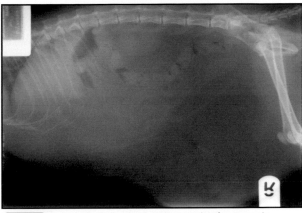

4.7 Lateral abdominal radiograph of a grossly obese skeletally mature cat. Radiographic scatter is increased, resulting in reduced anatomical detail and tissue contrast.

structures such as the small intestine can be made. However, visualization of the adrenal glands, jejunal lymph nodes and the pancreas may be impeded by the absence of highlighting fat.

On radiographs, emaciation may be confused with free fluid in the peritoneal cavity and so the radiographs must be assessed carefully. Emaciated animals often have a reduced dorsoventral (DV) abdominal height, giving them a 'tucked up' appearance, whereas animals with free peritoneal fluid often have a distended abdominal contour. However, if any abdominal organs are enlarged or distended, it becomes very difficult to differentiate between emaciation and free fluid (Figure 4.8) and further imaging modalities, such as ultrasonography, may be required.

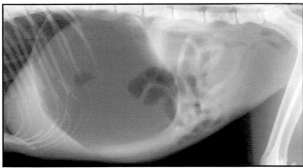

4.8 Lateral abdominal radiograph of an emaciated skeletally mature cat with a distended stomach, resulting in distension of the abdomen. Differentiation between emaciation and free peritoneal fluid is very difficult in this case.

Peritoneal diseases

Clinical signs related to diseases of the peritoneum may include pyrexia, dyspnoea, inappetence, vomiting, constipation, dysuria and abdominal pain, depending on the degree of abdominal distension and the effect of peritoneal enlargement on the other abdominal viscera. Other clinical signs relate to associated disease processes in individual abdominal organs. It is less common for the peritoneum to be the sole organ involved.

Pneumoperitoneum

Pneumoperitoneum is defined as free gas within the peritoneal cavity. The most common cause is iatrogenic, usually secondary to laparotomy, when it can persist for up to a month. Larger volumes of air require more time to resolve.

Pathological pneumoperitoneum occurs after penetrating trauma or rupture of a hollow viscus. Recognition of pneumoperitoneum is most important in cases when there is no history of penetrating abdominal trauma or previous laparotomy. In these instances the presence of pneumoperitoneum usually indicates rupture of the gastrointestinal tract, which is a surgical emergency. Exceptionally large volumes of air may accumulate with gastric rupture. Pneumo-peritoneum can result from gastric volvulus when there is concurrent gastric wall necrosis and is an important negative prognostic sign. Pneumoperito-neum occurs much more rarely following pneumo-cystography and, in this case, can be a sign of severe cystitis as well as bladder rupture.

- The serosal surfaces of abdominal organs are highlighted with gas lucencies, often triangular in shape. Larger volumes of air collect under the ribs, highlighting the lobes of the liver, crura of the diaphragm and cranial poles of the kidneys (Figure 4.9a).
- Free fluid admixed with free air results in some loss of serosal detail, with the homogenous appearance to the abdomen disturbed by small gas bubbles suspended within the fluid.
- Small volumes of free gas can be hard to detect and positional radiography may be required if free gas is suspected.
- Very large volumes of free gas can also be difficult to detect as a large gas bubble covers the whole abdomen. With moderate to large volumes of free air the VD view (Figure 4.9b) usually allows visualization of the peritoneal and pleural borders of the diaphragm. The ability to measure diaphragm thickness accurately is the best sign of pneumoperitoneum.
- A decubitus left lateral view (Figure 4.9c) using a horizontal beam is useful when conventional views are insufficient.

Ultrasonography is often very difficult in cases of pneumoperitoneum. Patients examined ultrasono-graphically prior to radiography will have incomplete examinations due to poor image quality, particularly when scanning from a non-dependent position. However, the source of the rupture may be determined ultrasonographically by imaging from the dependent aspect of the patient.

- Gas, with associated reverberation artefacts, may be identified peripherally, unrelated to the gastrointestinal tract.

Loss of peritoneal detail

Various conditions can affect the peritoneal cavity and result in reduction or loss of peritoneal detail. There is overlap between the imaging findings of the different

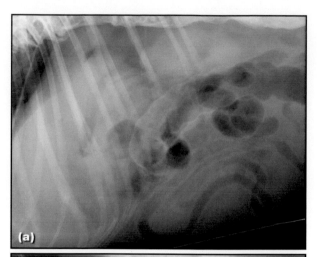

(a)

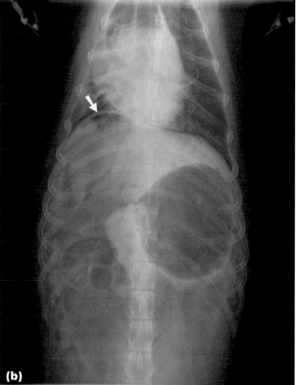

(b)

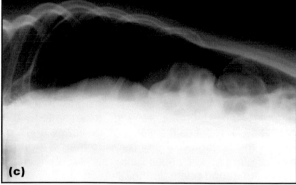

(c)

4.9 **(a)** Lateral abdominal radiograph of a 5-year-old crossbreed dog with gastric perforation secondary to ulceration. Gas lucency can be seen highlighting the crura of the diaphragm and the lobes of the liver dorsally. **(b)** VD view demonstrating gas (arrowed) behind the ventral portion of the diaphragm. (Courtesy of R O'Brien). **(c)** Decubitus lateral view showing the accumulation of free gas against the uppermost lateral body wall.

conditions and so definitive diagnosis is often difficult from radiography alone. However, ultrasonography and guided sampling techniques will provide much more information and often allow a definitive diagnosis to be made.

The major causes of loss of peritoneal detail are:

- Neonate (brown fat)
- Emaciation (lack of fat)
- Free fluid
- Peritonitis (including steatitis)
- Carcinomatosis
- A large mass.

Fluid

Free abdominal fluid may be exudate, transudate (ascites), blood, chyle, urine or bile.

- Radiographs reveal a loss of serosal detail throughout the abdomen, regardless of the cause or nature of the fluid. If the volume of free fluid is small, serosal detail may be reduced and hazy (Figure 4.10), whereas a larger volume of free fluid results in an overall homogenous increase in soft tissue opacity throughout the peritoneal cavity (Figure 4.11), highlighted only by any gas within the gastrointestinal tract or free within the peritoneum.
- Discernible structures, such as gas-filled intestinal loops, may appear to be further apart from each other than normal. This is due to the fluid between and around them pushing them apart.
- If the volume of free fluid is large, the abdomen appears distended.
- Repeat radiography following abdominocentesis may improve image quality, but serosal detail is likely to remain poor.
- Positional radiography to displace the fluid away from organs of interest has been largely superseded by ultrasonography.

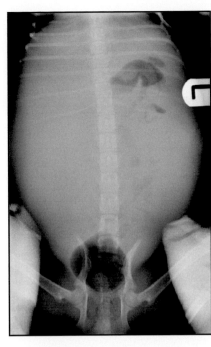

4.11 VD abdominal radiograph of a 17-week-old Cavalier King Charles Spaniel with uroabdomen. There is complete effacement of all serosal detail with distension of the body contours.

- Effusions are usually anechoic and the presence of free fluid within the peritoneal cavity allows assessment of the margins of abdominal structures as the fluid dissects between different organs.
- Ultrasonography is much more sensitive than radiography in detecting small volumes of free fluid. Small volumes are most easily detected in the region of the apex of the bladder and between the liver lobes (Figure 4.12)
- Abdominal organs appear more echogenic than normal when surrounded by anechoic fluid, due to reduced attenuation of the ultrasound beam as it passes through the fluid. They are more clearly visualized with their serosal surfaces highlighted by the fluid.
- A transudate or modified transudate appears anechoic with no suspended material. Haemorrhage or an exudate tends to be more

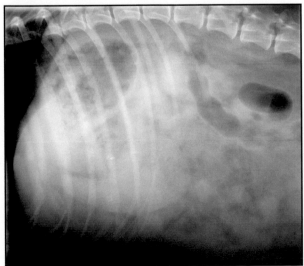

4.10 Lateral abdominal radiograph of a 10-year-old crossbreed bitch with modified transudate secondary to lymphangiectasia. A small to moderate volume of free abdominal fluid is present.

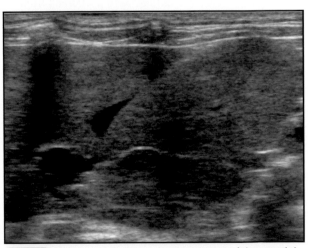

4.12 Parasagittal plane ultrasonogram of the cranial abdomen of a 9-year-old male neutered British Shorthaired cat with alimentary lymphosarcoma. A small anechoic triangular shape can be seen separating the liver lobes, indicating a small volume of free fluid.

echogenic, with swirling echogenicities within due to cellular content, fibrin and/or debris.
- The omentum and mesentery are readily apparent as echogenic tissues surrounding the intestines, floating within the fluid (Figure 4.13).

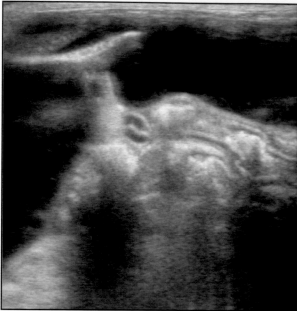

4.13 Dorsal plane ultrasonogram of the mid-abdomen of a 17-week-old male Cavalier King Charles Spaniel with uroabdomen. Loops of small intestine and mesentery can be seen surrounded by anechoic fluid.

Peritonitis

Inflammation of the peritoneum and mesentery results in oedema and hyperaemia of the membrane. This in turn results in an increased hazy or granular soft tissue opacity in the peritoneal cavity, reducing serosal detail. It may be generalized or localized depending on the cause. The reduction in serosal detail is usually exacerbated by some associated abdominal fluid due to exudation (Figure 4.14).

- Abdominal distension is uncommon.
- It can be difficult to differentiate peritonitis from small volumes of abdominal fluid from other causes.

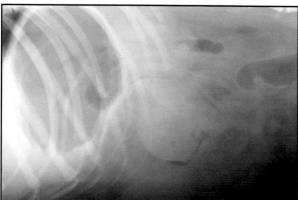

4.14 Lateral abdominal radiograph of a large-breed dog with focal peritonitis. There is a hazy loss of detail with irregular contours in the mid-ventral abdomen with displacement of the small intestines caudally and the spleen ventrally.

- Ultrasonography will demonstrate some free fluid and this fluid will usually contain echoes. There may be hyperechoic fibrin tags and the serosal surfaces of organs may appear irregular.
- The mesentery may appear hyperechoic and more homogenous than normal (Figure 4.15).
- Irrespective of the underlying cause of the peritonitis, gastrointestinal changes may be noted. Corrugation of intestinal loops (Figure 4.16) is indicative of intestinal irritation, whilst static, distended loops indicate ileus.
- Sampling of the fluid, if present, will permit determination of its nature.
- Feline infectious peritonitis (FIP) may cause either an effusive 'wet form' of disease with fibrinous serosal inflammation and pleural and/or peritoneal fluid, or a less effusive 'dry form' of disease characterized by the presence of multiple visceral pyogranulomas. The effusive form appears similar to classic peritonitis, whereas the less effusive form appears similar to carcinomatosis.

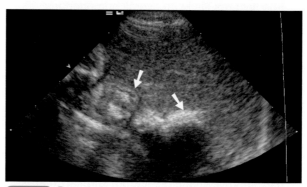

4.15 Dorsal plane ultrasonogram of an 8-year-old female neutered Domestic Shorthaired cat with pyoabdomen. Intestinal loops (arrowed) are poorly visualized within a mass of echogenic fluid.

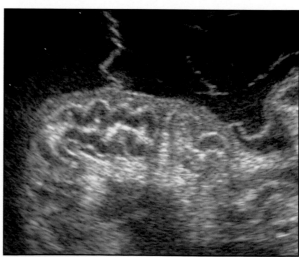

4.16 Dorsal plane ultrasonogram of a 5-month-old Beagle with bile peritonitis after a road traffic accident 2 weeks previously. The small intestinal loops have a corrugated appearance and are surrounded by homogenous, hyperechoic mesentery. There is a moderate volume of free peritoneal fluid. (Courtesy of F Barr)

Steatitis

Steatitis (inflammation of fat tissue) in the cat, secondary to vitamin E deficiency, high fish diet or chronic pancreatitis, results in increased opacity within any fat deposits. On an abdominal radiograph this will be seen as an appearance similar to focal peritonitis, affecting the falciform fat, the perirenal fat and also any large extra-abdominal fat deposits, such as the inguinal area. An appearance of focal peritonitis extending outside the abdomen should alert the radiologist to the possibility of steatitis. Ultrasonographically this fat may be very attenuating, causing shadow artefacts.

Carcinomatosis

Metastatic seeding of neoplasms through the peritoneum results in hazy loss of detail and free fluid. It can be difficult, if not impossible, to differentiate carcinomatosis (Figure 4.17) from peritonitis, especially FIP in cats, and a small volume of fluid on radiography and ultrasonography.

- On ultrasonography the fluid may contain multifocal echoes, and outline roughened serosal surfaces and thickening of the mesentery (Figure 4.18).
- Ultrasonography may identify small hypoechoic foci throughout the mesentery, which may be more supportive of a diagnosis of carcinomatosis, but tissue sampling is required to determine the cause definitively.

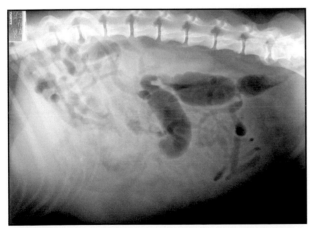

4.17 Lateral abdominal radiograph of a 9-year-old male Golden Retriever with carcinomatosis. Compare this image with that in Figure 4.10. Both radiographs show mottled loss of serosal detail. (Courtesy of C Lamb)

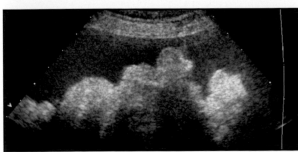

4.18 Dorsal plane ultrasonogram of the abdomen of the dog in Figure 4.17, showing echogenic fluid and hyperechoic irregularly rounded thickened mesentery. (Courtesy of C Lamb)

- Haemangiosarcoma nodules may have a more specific appearance and often mimic the primary mass with a complex echoic pattern.

Other peritoneal lesions

Abdominal mass

A mass within the abdominal cavity is due to enlargement of one or more of the intra-abdominal structures. This enlargement may be physiological (such as pregnancy) or pathological. Causes of pathological enlargement in any organ include cyst, haematoma, abscess, neoplasia and granuloma (the 'CHANG' differential diagnoses list). Additional differential diagnoses in certain organs include torsion, hyperplasia and obstruction.

- If sufficiently large, a mass may be detected on plain radiography. Displacement of other viscera, such as the small intestines, can be useful in assessing the origin of a mass (Figure 4.19) (see Chapter 8).
- An abdominal mass may result in a localized reduction in serosal detail.
- Ultrasonography is especially useful to verify the identity of the enlarged organ and to characterize the echotexture of the mass. This can be variable, depending on the nature of the mass. Fine-needle aspiration under ultrasound guidance will yield more information (Figure 4.20).

Neoplastic mass: Neoplastic masses can arise within the peritoneum and mesentery, but are uncommon. Lipomas are the most common neoplasms of peritoneal or mesenteric origin. Other types of neoplasm originating from the peritoneum include haemangiosarcoma and other sarcomas.

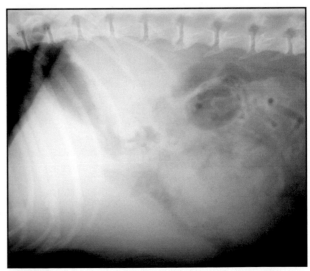

4.19 Lateral abdominal radiograph of a medium-breed dog with splenic haemangiosarcoma. There is a soft tissue opacity mass in the cranioventral abdomen with caudodorsal displacement of the stomach and intestines. The liver is enlarged and irregular and there is hazy loss of serosal detail, indicating free fluid.

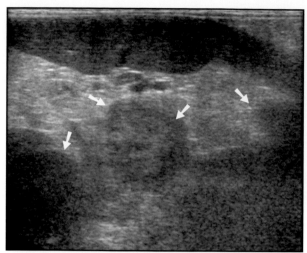

4.20 Dorsal plane ultrasonogram of the abdomen of a 4-year-old male neutered Domestic Shorthaired cat with a palpable abdominal mass. Ultrasonography revealed a large hypoechoic mass (arrowed) in the cranial abdomen, extending throughout the mesentery and involving the common bile duct and pancreas. Ultrasound-guided fine-needle aspiration biopsy revealed carcinoma.

Lipoma: A mesenteric or omental lipoma appears as a relatively radiolucent mass within the abdomen (Figure 4.21). It may be a homogenous fat opacity or be more heterogenous. It can be difficult to differentiate this appearance from that of a peritoneal abscess. Ossifying lipomas ('Bates body') have histological foci of cartilage and bone within the adipose tissue. Radiographically they appear as round, mineral opaque lesions, separate from other structures and surrounded by peritoneal fat. They are usually an incidental finding, and more common in cats than dogs.

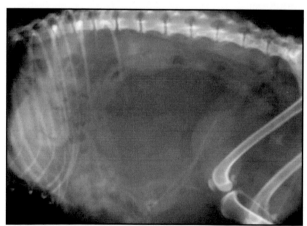

4.21 Lateral abdominal radiograph of an adult dog with a lipoma in the broad ligament. A large relatively radiolucent mass is present in the centre of the abdomen, causing cranioventral displacement of the small intestines and dorsal displacement of the kidneys and descending colon. (Courtesy of F Barr)

Ultrasonography identifies the mass as having a homogenous echogenicity similar to that of visceral fat and allows fine-needle aspiration, which should be diagnostic. Computed tomography (CT) is the most useful way to detect and image fully intra-abdominal lipomas (Figure 4.22). Mineralized lipomas have a distinctive shadow artefact.

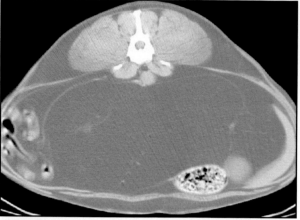

4.22 CT slice at the level of the fourth lumbar vertebra of a 10-year-old male Labrador with multiple lipomas. A large hypoattenuating, fairly well defined mass can be seen causing dramatic peripheral displacement of the small intestines to the right and the descending colon ventrally. The cranial pole of the bladder can be seen just lateral to the descending colon. The spleen is lateral to the colon. (Fat-optimized window: width 500 HU, level –200 HU)

Non-neoplastic mass:

Haematoma: These can occur after blunt abdominal trauma, may be associated with bleeding neoplasms, may develop secondary to cystocentesis or may be idiopathic. On abdominal radiography, a haematoma (if of sufficient size) will appear as a soft tissue opacity mass, which may displace other viscera. Ultrasonography reveals a non-specific hypoechoic or mixed echoic mass. Echogenicity changes with time as the haematoma matures. The nature of the mass is difficult to confirm, even with the absence of a Doppler ultrasonography signal, indicating its non-vascular nature. Sequential ultrasonographic examination may allow differentiation of haematomas (Figure 4.23) from other types of peritoneal mass.

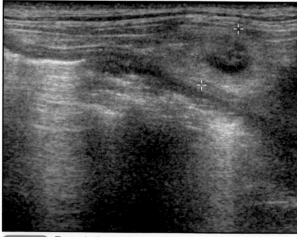

4.23 Dorsal plane ultrasonogram of the mesentery in the left dorsal abdomen of a 7-year-old Lhasa apso, 2 weeks after splenectomy. There is an oval area of hyperechoic mesentery with a hypoechoic centre (between cursors). This was thought to be a mesenteric haematoma and had resolved on re-examination 3 weeks later.

Abscess: Mesenteric or omental abscesses may occur secondary to gastrointestinal perforation, penetrating wounds, parenchymal organ abscessation and surgical swab retention (Figure 4.24).

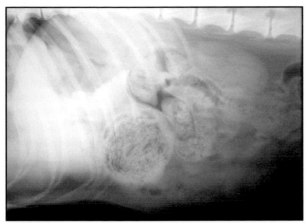

4.24 Lateral abdominal radiograph of a skeletally mature large-breed dog with a retained surgical swab. A large stripy mottled mixed soft tissue and gas opacity is present in the cranioventral abdomen. (Reproduced from Merlo and Lamb (2000) with permission from *Veterinary Radiology and Ultrasound*)

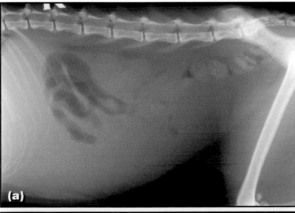

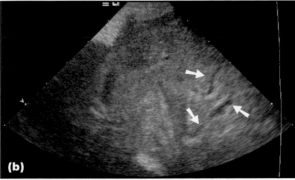

4.25 An 8-year-old female neutered Domestic Shorthaired cat with pyoabdomen. **(a)** Lateral abdominal radiograph. Serosal detail is lost throughout the abdomen and the gas-filled intestines appear more dorsal in the abdomen than normal, suggesting the presence of a homogenous soft tissue opacity mass rather than just fluid. **(b)** Dorsal plane ultrasonogram revealed an echogenic mass of tissue within the abdomen. Poorly defined small intestine loops (arrowed) can be seen within the tissue. Laparotomy and histopathology confirmed the presence of grossly inflamed peritoneum with a moderate volume of thick pus.

- Radiographically the abscess may be visible as a soft tissue opacity causing some displacement of adjacent structures. The mass may appear homogenous (Figure 4.25a) or have a mottled, mixed soft tissue and gas opacity.
- On ultrasonography, abscesses appear as poorly marginated, hypoechoic masses, containing variable amounts of echogenic fluid (Figure 4.25b). They may have thick, irregular walls and have a complex internal compartment.

Intra-abdominal mineralization

Intra-abdominal mineralization may result from tissue death, metabolic disorders, neoplasia and inflammation. Mineralized foci within the peritoneum include mineralized mesenteric lymph nodes (Figure 4.26), usually secondary to infection and focal mineralizations within the omentum or mesentery itself, secondary to cyst, neoplasia, chronic infection or necrosis. Mesenteric cysts appear as small foci with eggshell mineralized rims; they are of no clinical significance (Figure 4.27).

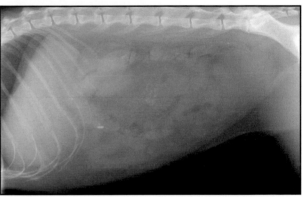

4.26 Lateral abdominal radiograph of an 8-year-old female neutered Domestic Shorthaired cat with mineralized mesenteric lymph nodes, visible as speckled, granular mineralized foci in the mid-abdomen, with peripheral displacement of the intestines.

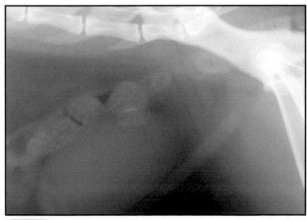

4.27 Lateral radiograph of the caudal abdomen of a skeletally mature cat with a small smooth mineralized focus superimposed on the dorsal aspect of the bladder. This was determined to be nodular fat necrosis of no clinical significance. (Courtesy of C Lamb)

Foreign bodies

Foreign bodies may be found within the peritoneal cavity either due to penetration of the body wall or penetration of a viscus with subsequent migration into the peritoneal cavity. A radiopaque foreign body (Figure 4.28) will be visible on plain radiographs, whilst radiolucent material may be detected ultrasonographically. There may be associated focal peritonitis. Retained surgical swabs often have a characteristic geometrical mixed soft tissue and gas pattern (see Figure 4.24). Ultrasonographically they cause shadow artefacts and may have a hypoechoic rim caused by fibrin deposition, depending on duration *in situ*. A ruptured gallbladder with biliary mucocele may result in a ball of gelatinized bile becoming a free peritoneal foreign body.

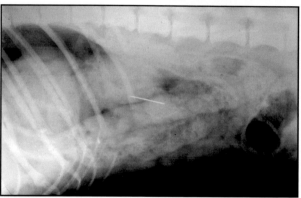

4.28 Lateral abdominal radiograph of an adult dog taken after a laparotomy. A fine linear metallic opacity is present in the mid-abdomen. Small intestinal loops are present ventral to this opacity. There is a moderate to large volume of free gas within the abdomen and the serosal surface of the colon can be clearly seen. (Courtesy of F Barr)

Hernias and ruptures

A defect in the boundaries of the peritoneal cavity may be congenital (resulting in a hernia) or traumatic (rupture). Common sites include:

- Umbilical hernia
- Inguinal hernia
- Perineal hernia
- Rupture of the prepubic tendon
- Paracostal rupture
- Diaphragmatic rupture
- Peritoneo-pericardial diaphragmatic hernia
- Hiatal or paraoesophageal hernia.

Even when a hernia or rupture results in a visible swelling, radiography may be a useful means of determining which organs have become displaced through the defect. Identification of tubular, gas lucencies indicates displacement of intestinal segments through the defect. Displacement of solid or fluid-filled organs and/or fat may be more difficult to identify radiographically, but contrast radiography or ultrasonography may be helpful in this respect.

Contrast radiography

Both positive- and negative-contrast studies have been performed to highlight structures and identify masses within the peritoneal cavity. These techniques have been largely superseded by abdominal ultrasonography.

Pneumoperitoneography

Air, carbon dioxide and nitrous oxide, in combination with a variety of different radiographic positions, have all been used in this technique. The animal is anaesthetized and placed in dorsal recumbency. A catheter connected to a three-way tap is introduced in an aseptic fashion into the peritoneal cavity through, or just to the right of, the umbilicus. Negative pressure should be applied to the catheter to ensure that the liver and spleen have not been penetrated. The selected gas is introduced slowly until the abdominal cavity is moderately distended. No resistance should be felt to injection if the needle is correctly positioned. Pneumoperitoneography should not be used if there is the possibility of peritonitis, nor if diaphragmatic rupture is suspected, as it may cause a pneumothorax. It is also contraindicated if there are severe cardiac or respiratory problems, as the increased intra-abdominal pressure may compromise cardiac or respiratory function.

The radiographs taken will depend on the region of interest within the peritoneal cavity, but the general principle is to use a horizontal beam and position the animal such that the area of interest is dorsal. For example, a decubitus lateral view can be used to highlight the kidneys or an upright VD view to examine the diaphragm.

Pneumoperitoneography is a potentially dangerous technique as fatal air emboli have occurred. Positive-contrast peritoneography is a safer technique, but ultrasonography is definitely the preferred procedure. However, the detection of naturally occurring pneumoperitoneum remains an important part of abdominal radiological interpretation.

Positive-contrast peritoneography

This technique is performed in a similar fashion to pneumoperitoneography, substituting a non-ionic water-soluble iodine-containing contrast medium for the gas. This procedure is rarely used, except in the diagnosis of diaphragmatic rupture or hernia. Contrast medium is introduced at a dose rate of 1.5 ml/kg bodyweight, and the patient is then gently rolled to distribute the contrast medium. Any positive contrast medium on the pleural aspect of the diaphragm supports the diagnosis of hernia. False-negative diagnoses are common with organ entrapment in the hernial rent.

Overview of additional imaging modalities

Increasingly, magnetic resonance imaging (MRI) and CT are available for diagnostic purposes in veterinary medicine. The cross-sectional nature of these imaging modalities enables greater characterization of the peritoneal disease processes. The peritoneal cavity is easily examined with CT (Figure 4.29) and modern MRI equipment, avoiding excessive artefacts due to respiratory movement. Both these modalities improve the accuracy of imaging diagnosis, enabling better decisions for appropriate treatment to be made. The normal CT and MRI abdominal anatomy of both cats and dogs has been published.

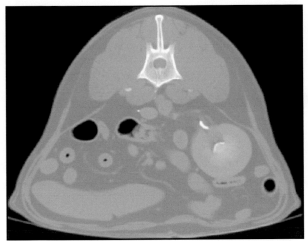

4.29 Post-contrast CT slice at the level of the second lumbar vertebra of an 8-year-old male Weimaraner showing contrast medium in the left renal pelvis and proximal ureter. Intestinal loops can be seen throughout the abdomen surrounded by a small amount of hypoattenuating fat. (Window: width 2000 HU, level –200 HU)

- CT has been very useful in identifying and characterizing masses, particularly intrapelvic and spinal masses, which are inaccessible via transabdominal ultrasonography.
- In the case of intra-abdominal or intrapelvic lipomas, the use of a fat-optimized window allows full assessment of the lipomatous tissue (see Figure 4.22).
- CT is extremely useful to guide surgical intervention or radiotherapy.
- CT is the superior modality for detection of pneumoperitoneum, as even tiny bubbles of air are easily detectable. CT provides an overview of the abdomen not achievable with ultrasonography.
- Intravenous contrast medium may be administered, unless there is a clinical contraindication. Pre- and post-contrast techniques allow assessment of the margins and vascularity of the lesion and examination of the association between the mass and the vessels in the abdomen, allowing differentiation between those masses which are truly invasive and those which are just space-occupying. This is particularly true for masses in the adrenal glands (Figure 4.30) and caudal vena cava (see Chapter 15).
- MRI relies on novel tissue contrast characteristics to produce the image and offers superior soft tissue resolution to that of CT.
- MRI allows imaging in any plane, without repositioning the subject, providing better 3D assessment of the lesion and allowing more complete planning for surgery or radiotherapy.

References and further reading

Assheuer J and Sager M (1997) *MRI and CT atlas of the dog, 1st edn.* Blackwell Science, Vienna

Besso JG, Wrigley RH, Gliatto JM *et al.* (2000) Ultrasonographic appearance and clinical findings in 14 dogs with gallbladder mucocele.

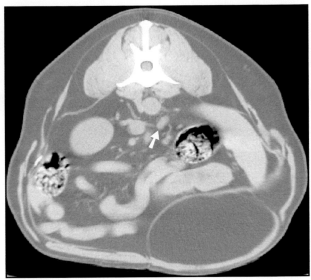

4.30 CT slice at the level of the first lumbar vertebra of a 10-year-old male Labrador with a body wall mass. A large hypoattenuating mass can be seen on the left ventral aspect of the abdomen, between the rectus abdominis and transversus abdominis muscles. The CT study provided information that the mass was external to the peritoneal cavity, facilitating surgical planning. The left adrenal gland (arrowed) can be seen ventrolateral to the aorta. (Fat-optimized window: width 500 HU, level –200 HU)

Veterinary Radiology and Ultrasound **41**, 261–271

Burke RA and Feeney DA (2003) The abdomen. In: *Small Animal Radiology and Ultrasonography.* ed. RA Burke and DA Feeney, pp. 281–286. WB Saunders, Philadelphia

Evans HE (1993) The abdomen. In: *Miller's Anatomy of the Dog, 3rd edition*, ed. HF Evans, pp. 425–435. WB Saunders, Philadelphia

Farrow CS (1994) The abdomen. In: *Radiology of the Cat.* ed. CS Farrow, pp. 145–150. Mosby-Year Book, St Louis

Herrtage ME and Dennis R (1995) Contrast media and techniques. In: *BSAVA Manual of Small Animal Diagnostic Imaging*, ed. R Lee, pp. 147–156. BSAVA Publications, Cheltenham

Kealy JK and McAllister H (2000) The abdomen. In: *Diagnostic Radiology and Ultrasonography of the Dog and Cat, 3rd edn*, ed. JK Kealy and H McAllister, pp. 19–29. WB Saunders, Philadelphia

Kirby BM (2003) Peritoneum and peritoneal cavity. In: *Textbook of Small Animal Surgery, 3rd edn*, ed. D Slatter, pp. 414–418. WB Saunders, Philadelphia

Mahaffey MB and Barber DL (2002) The peritoneal space. In: *Textbook of Veterinary Radiology, 4th edn*, ed. DE Thrall, pp. 516–525. WB Saunders, Philadelphia

Mattoon JS and Nyland TG (2001) Abdominal fluid, lymph nodes, masses, peritoneal cavity and great vessel thrombosis. In: *Small Animal Diagnostic Ultrasound, 2nd edn*, ed. TG Nyland and JS Mattoon, pp. 82–91. WB Saunders, Philadelphia

Merlo M and Lamb CR (2000) Radiographic and ultrasonographic features of retained surgical sponge in eight dogs. *Veterinary Radiology and Ultrasound* **41(3)**, 279–283

Samii VF, Biller DS and Koblik PD (1998) Normal cross-sectional anatomy of the feline thorax and abdomen: comparison of computed tomography and cadaver anatomy. *Veterinary Radiology and Ultrasound* **39**, 504–511

Samii VF, Biller DS and Koblik PD (1999) Magnetic resonance imaging of the normal feline abdomen: an anatomic reference. *Veterinary Radiology and Ultrasound* **40**, 486–490

Smallwood JE and George TF (1993) Anatomic atlas for computed tomography in the mesaticephalic dog: thorax and cranial abdomen. *Veterinary Radiology and Ultrasound* **34**, 65–84

Smallwood JE and George TF (1993) Anatomic atlas for computed tomography in the mesaticephalic dog: caudal abdomen and pelvis. *Veterinary Radiology and Ultrasound* **34**, 143–167

Tanabe S, Yamada K, Kobayashi Y, *et al.* (2005) Extra-abdominal chondrolipoma in a dog. *Veterinary Radiology and Ultrasound* **46**, 306–308

Yasuda D, Fujita M, Yasuda S, *et al.* (2004) Usefulness of MRI compared with CT for diagnosis of mesenteric lymphoma in a dog. *Journal of Veterinary Medical Science* **66** 1447–1451

5

The retroperitoneum

Francisco Llabrés-Díaz

Normal retroperitoneum

The retroperitoneum is an extraperitoneal space situated ventral to the vertebrae and paraspinal muscles; it extends along the length of the entire abdomen from the diaphragm to the anus. The lateral boundaries are the abdominal and pelvic walls. The ventral boundary is the dorsal parietal peritoneum. Therefore, conditions affecting the peritoneum may spare the retroperitoneum.

Organs that project freely into the abdominal, pelvic or scrotal cavities with an almost complete covering of peritoneum are considered to be intraperitoneal. However, those organs situated close to the walls of the abdominal or pelvic cavities and covered on one surface only by peritoneum are considered to be retroperitoneal. Some of these organs are too small to be seen, whilst others are commonly seen on radiographs because they are surrounded by fat (Figure 5.1). The retroperitoneal organs include:

- Kidneys
- Ureters
- Adrenal glands
- Aorta
- Caudal vena cava
- Coeliac and cranial mesenteric arteries, renal and deep circumflex vessels
- Lymph nodes:
  - The lumbar lymphocentre: lumbar aortic and renal lymph nodes
  - The iliosacral lymphocentre: medial iliac, hypogastric and sacral lymph nodes.

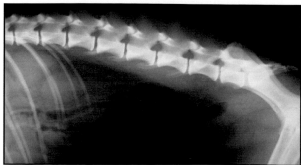

5.1 Lateral abdominal radiograph showing the normal retroperitoneum of a 6-year-old male neutered Whippet. The presence of fat allows identification of some of the retroperitoneal structures, especially the left kidney.

- Cisterna chyli and lymphatic ducts
- Neural structures (including sympathetic nerves and ganglia)
- Loose connective tissue.

Connection with other spaces in the body

The loose connective tissue mesh that fills the retroperitoneum does not provide a complete barrier to disease and therefore rapid spread of pathology can occur. In addition, the retroperitoneum communicates cranially with the mediastinum (Figure 5.2) and

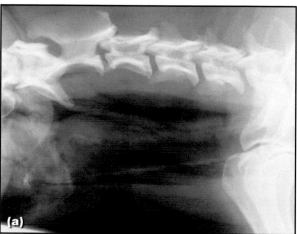

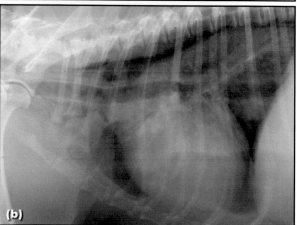

5.2 Radiographs of an 11-year-old male neutered English Springer Spaniel that had suffered iatrogenic damage to the upper respiratory tract. **(a)** Lateral radiograph of the cervical area. Air can be seen tracking along the fascial planes. **(b)** Lateral thoracic radiograph. The clear boundaries of the mediastinal structures indicate the presence of pneumomediastinum. (continues) ▶

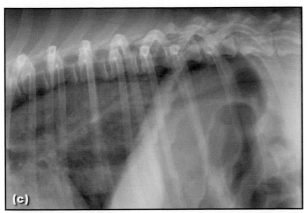

5.2 (continued) Radiographs of an 11-year-old male neutered English Springer Spaniel that had suffered iatrogenic damage to the upper respiratory tract. **(c)** Close-up of a lateral radiograph of the thoracolumbar region. The aorta is clearly seen owing to the presence of air that is extending from the caudal mediastinum into the retroperitoneum.

caudally with the pelvic canal, reaching the anus. This connection is of great importance from a clinical perspective and the presence of radiographic signs of retroperitoneal disease should prompt the investigation of these neighbouring spaces to confirm or rule out the presence of pathology and to investigate the origin of the disease process.

Ultrasonography

The relative indications and advantages of ultrasonography are covered in Chapter 3. Particular considerations related to the retroperitoneum are:

- Ultrasonography is particularly helpful in cases where radiographs have identified an increase in retroperitoneal radiopacity, as it allows determination of the internal architecture (fluid *versus* tissue) and vascularity of the lesion
- Ultrasonography is important for selecting areas to aspirate or biopsy and is extremely useful for obtaining ultrasound-guided samples
- It can be difficult to determine accurately the true extent of diffuse pathology and very large masses with ultrasonography, in comparison with radiographs or advanced imaging techniques. A multi-technique approach is better in this scenario.

Technique

Several ultrasonographic windows to the retroperitoneum are available. Selection is mostly based on the ultrasonographer's personal preference. The author favours a lateral approach to this area with the animal in lateral recumbency. The ventral aspect of the vertebral bodies is easily identified by the presence of acoustic shadowing and indicates the dorsal boundary of the retroperitoneum. A combination of longitudinal and transverse planes with respect to the long axis of the body will enable examination of the entire retroperitoneum. Following the aorta and caudal vena cava in a caudocranial direction is useful.

The normal ultrasonographic appearance of the retroperitoneal organs is covered in the relevant Chapters. The general appearance of the retroperitoneal space, however, is a loose array of echogenicities (Figure 5.3), similar to that of the omentum within the peritoneal cavity. Fluid is not usually apparent in the normal retroperitoneum.

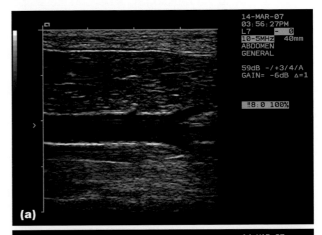

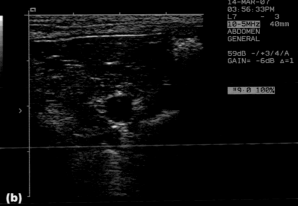

5.3 **(a)** Ultrasonogram of the normal retroperitoneum of a 13-year-old neutered Yorkshire Terrier bitch obtained in a longitudinal plane, parallel to the long axis of the body. Cranial is to the left. The aorta can be seen in the mid-field, surrounded by the normal retroperitoneum. **(b)** Transverse image of the same area. Dorsal is to the left of the image. The shadowing caused by the descending colon is visible to the right of the image.

Overview of additional imaging modalities

Extraordinary anatomical detail, free of superimposed neighbouring structures, can be obtained with computed tomography (CT) and magnetic resonance imaging (MRI). This makes them very useful in cases of diffuse retroperitoneal pathology, especially when surgery is contemplated.

Financial constraints, the limited availability of CT and MRI in some areas and the difficulty in accurately interpreting the resulting images constitute the main drawbacks. CT is quicker than MRI and is generally less affected by movement artefacts. A complete MRI examination of patients with diffuse pathology extending into other anatomical areas, such as the mediastinum, can be very lengthy and frustrating. CT is the advanced imaging technique of choice in these cases.

Technique

A detailed discussion of MRI and CT techniques, including the different sequences (MRI) or windows (CT) available to the radiologist, is beyond the scope of this Chapter, thus only the general concepts are mentioned here.

Magnetic resonance imaging

- As a rule of thumb, STIR images, T2-weighted images and equivalent pre- and post-contrast (using intravenously injected paramagnetic contrast medium) enhanced T1-weighted images should be obtained when investigating diffuse retroperitoneal pathology. These facilitate the detection of pathological and/or contrast enhancing areas, respectively, which appear hyperintense compared with the surroundings.
- Pathology and normal accumulations of fluid appear hyperintense to the surroundings on STIR and T2-weighted images. Fat is also of high signal intensity on T2-weighted images but not on STIR, which is why STIR images are helpful.
- Fat is of high signal intensity on T1-weighted images, whereas fluid is of low signal intensity. Contrast enhanced areas are brighter than on pre-contrast T1-weighted images.
- The array of sequences available to the radiologist and the true multiplanar capabilities of MRI can make this a superior technique to CT, especially if severe soft tissue or vertebral canal disease is present.

Computed tomography

Images from bone and soft tissue windows should be obtained before and after injection of contrast medium (intravenous, iodinated, water-soluble), plus post-processing reconstruction planes, software permitting.

Retroperitoneal diseases

Fluid

Fluid accumulation within the retroperitoneum results in a loss of contrast on plain radiographs, because the soft tissue structures within the retroperitoneum are no longer highlighted by the surrounding fat. A small volume of fluid results in streaking or mottling of the retroperitoneal area. Larger volumes of fluid obscure all retroperitoneal detail (Figure 5.4) and can result in expansion of the retroperitoneal space with ventral deviation of the colon and small intestines.

Blood is radiographically indistinguishable from urine or other fluids, but this differentiation may prove critical for the patient. For example, a traumatic haematoma usually resolves over time, and indeed there is the risk of further haemorrhage if a haematoma is disturbed during exploratory surgery. However, the presence of urine warrants intervention to prevent tissue necrosis and systemic illness.

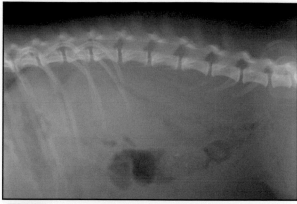

5.4 Lateral abdominal radiograph of a 4-year-old neutered Jack Russell Terrier bitch following a recent road traffic accident. There is retroperitoneal enlargement and loss of detail due to fluid accumulation. Fractures of several vertebral transverse processes are evident and marked swelling of this area also contributes to the retroperitoneal enlargement.

Both radiography and ultrasonography are helpful in determining whether retroperitoneal disease is present. However, ultrasonography is more sensitive than radiography in the detection of a small amount of fluid (Figure 5.5).

- A moderate amount of fluid causes a striated or marble-like appearance due to a combination of areas of fluid and relatively hyperechoic fatty tissue. A little free fluid may accumulate adjacent to the organ of origin; for example, perirenal free fluid is a common sequel to acute renal failure.
- A large accumulation of fluid will be easily detectable on ultrasonography as an anechoic area with variable small internal echogenicities (Figure 5.6), resulting from the cellularity and other characteristics of the fluid.
- Carcinomatosis involving the retroperitoneum is often associated with the presence of fluid, resulting in a striated or marble-like pattern (see above) (Figure 5.7). There may also be an

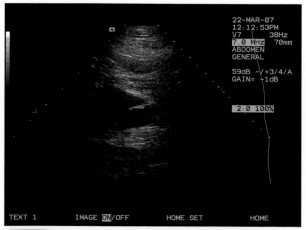

5.5 Ultrasonogram of the retroperitoneum of a 5-year-old male neutered English Springer Spaniel presented with pyrexia and abdominal pain. A small anechoic pocket of fluid was detected caudal to the renal area. A migrating foreign body was suspected but was not found.

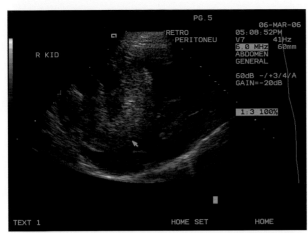

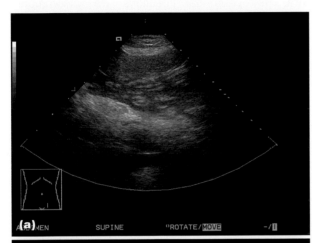

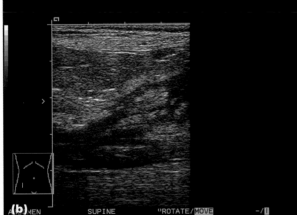

5.6 Ultrasonogram of the cranial retroperitoneum of the dog shown in Figure 5.4. There is fluid accumulation around the right kidney. Cranial is to the left.

5.7 Ultrasonograms of the central retroperitoneum of a 9-year-old male neutered Shih Tzu cross obtained with **(a)** a 7 MHz curvilinear transducer and **(b)** a 10 MHz linear transducer. Cranial is to the left. This pattern is consistent with fluid accumulation and carcinomatosis but is not specific for this condition. The final diagnosis was disseminated caudal retroperitoneal mast cell tumour.

increase in echogenicity of the soft tissues, but a certain level of experience is needed before subtle retroperitoneal changes in echogenicity can be detected confidently.

Ultrasound-guided aspiration will allow determination of the type of fluid present, and thus the best course of action.

Fluid of renal or ureteric origin

- Acute renal failure:
  - This is a non-specific finding with many causes, including obstructive uropathy, toxicity, infection or neoplasia
  - The volume of fluid is usually small and it accumulates in contact with the cranial or caudal capsule of the affected kidney(s)
  - This finding may be unilateral or bilateral, depending on the insult. Systemic injuries, such as intoxication or haematogenous infection, are usually bilateral
  - Ureteral obstruction or pyelonephritis may be unilateral. In cases of unilateral fluid there may be no concurrent signs of renal failure noted on serology or urinalysis.
- Retroperitoneal fluid can also be seen in association with a traumatic episode and secondary leakage of urine:
  - If the fluid becomes encapsulated, the lesion is defined as a urinoma
  - Uroabdomen is diagnosed when the creatinine and potassium levels in the free fluid are higher than those in serum
  - Extravasation of sterile urine can be asymptomatic for 1–2 days. Clinical signs will develop sooner if the extravasated urine is infected
  - A urogenital contrast study (Figure 5.8) may be needed to determine the origin of the leakage into the retroperitoneum before surgery is performed
  - The presence of other lesions secondary to the traumatic episode (e.g. bladder or abdominal wall rupture, pneumothorax, rib fractures or fractures elsewhere, lung contusion, diaphragmatic hernia) should be investigated.
- Ultrasonography should be used to confirm that a retroperitoneal accumulation of fluid exists, assess concurrent lesions and to obtain an ultrasound-guided sample to characterize the nature of the fluid.

Haemorrhage
Possible causes of haemorrhage include:

- Trauma
- Rupture of highly vascularized masses
- Vascular rupture:
  - Neoplastic infiltration
  - Penetrating injuries
  - Vascular anomalies.
- Coagulopathies:
  - Disseminated intravascular coagulation (DIC)
  - Rodenticide toxicity
  - Immune-mediated thrombocytopenia.

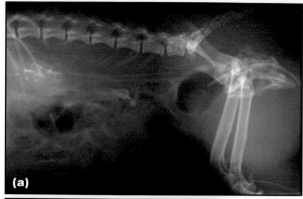

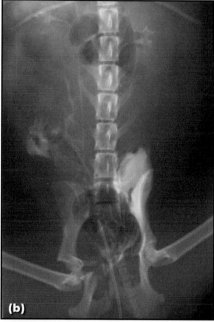

5.8 **(a)** Lateral and **(b)** VD radiographs of the dog in Figure 5.4 after bladder catheterization, air insufflation and intravenous urography. The presence of positive contrast medium outside the bladder neck, extending cranially and surrounding intestinal loops in places confirms the suspicion of uroretroperitoneum and uroperitoneum.

In cases of trauma, it is important to determine whether other areas of the body are affected and, if possible, to ascertain the origin of the bleeding. The spleen, liver and kidneys (in that order) are the most common abdominal sources of haemorrhage; ultrasonography is useful in determining the origin of the haemorrhage. Adrenal gland phaeochromocytomas are the particular neoplasm associated with retroperitoneal haemorrhage. The haemorrhage may originate from rupture of the neoplasm or invasion or thrombosis of neighbouring vessels. Haemoperitoneum may coexist with haemorrhage in the retroperitoneum. Ultrasonography is particularly helpful in this scenario and findings may include:

- Abnormal adrenal gland(s)
- Retroperitoneal fluid
- Detection of metastases.

The presence of hypertension should raise the suspicion of a phaeochromocytoma.

Cullen's sign (periumbilical discoloration or ecchymosis), together with haemoglobinuria, has been reported in a dog with a large retroperitoneal haemorrhage. Retroperitoneal or peritoneal haemorrhage should be ruled out when this infrequent sign is detected. Focal renal subcapsular haematomas may be seen following blunt trauma and this area needs to be specifically assessed using ultrasonography. Advanced imaging may provide more detailed information about damage to skeletal structures or may verify the presence of a mass lesion.

Foreign bodies

Migrating foreign bodies are probably the most common cause of chronic and recurrent cases of retroperitonitis. Other causes include penetrating injuries, extension of local infections, such as severe pyelonephritis, and iatrogenic damage to the urethra. Retroperitoneal infections are uncommonly associated with reactions to ligatures used in neutering surgeries.

Appropriate therapy and prognosis are determined by the underlying cause and whether the process is chronic or acute. Chronic cases are likely to be associated with fever, pain, fluctuating flank abscesses and discharging sinuses. Back pain and neurological deficits are also possible. In these cases, local drainage and systemic antibiotic therapy are likely to resolve the problem only partially, and recurrence is very likely.

Migrating foreign bodies may originate from the oral cavity or sites more caudal in the respiratory or gastrointestinal systems.

- Migrating plant awns may gain access to the cranial retroperitoneum through the oesophageal wall at the sharp point of the oesophageal flexure just cranial to the cardia.
- Alternatively, access to the retroperitoneum is gained by migrating through the dorsal attachments of the diaphragm from the caudodorsal thoracic cavity after inhalation and migration out of the lung. The presence of a cough and transient radiographic changes in the lungs before the development of changes in the lumbar spine supports this hypothesis in some patients.

Radiographic findings

- Normal radiographs do not rule out retroperitoneal extension of the infection during the acute phase of the disease.
- Some or all of the following radiographic patterns can be identified in these cases:
  - Diffuse increase in opacity with a large volume of free fluid or a mass
  - Focal soft tissue opacities, possibly with internal gas opacities, if there is abscessation or an open discharging sinus (Figure 5.9)

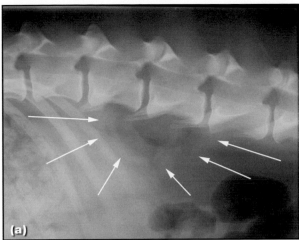

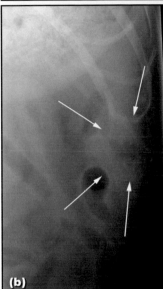

5.9

Close-up of **(a)** a lateral and **(b)** a VD abdominal radiograph of a 4-year-old male neutered German Shepherd Dog with a 2-year history of intermittently discharging, fluctuating lesions of the left flank. The radiographs demonstrate the presence of gas (arrowed) accumulating deep within the flank lesion. A migrating foreign body was suspected. Surgery was declined.

- Although radiographically visible enlargement of the sublumbar muscles has been described, this is considered difficult to identify
- In chronic cases, an irregular periosteal reaction can be seen on the ventral aspect of neighbouring vertebral bodies (spondylitis). The area from T13 to L4 is commonly affected (Figure 5.10). Care must be taken not to confuse spondylitis

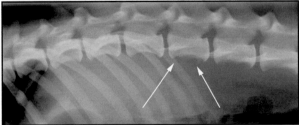

5.10 Close-up of a lateral abdominal radiograph of a 2-year-old male English Cocker Spaniel showing a subtle periosteal reaction arising from the ventral aspect of the second lumbar vertebra. A retroperitoneal abscess was confirmed and surgically debrided following advanced imaging but no foreign body was found.

with the normal roughening of the ventral aspects of the bodies of the third and fourth lumbar vertebrae associated with the diaphragmatic attachments
- If migration started within the thorax at the level of the peripheral attachments of the diaphragm to the pleura, a periosteal reaction might be seen along the ribs, as well as pleural effusion, pleural thickening and/or focal abscesses. These are infrequent findings.
- Associated discospondylitis may be harder to detect on plain radiographs during the early stages of the disease. Advanced imaging can be more helpful in this situation, as well as for detecting involvement of the epidural space (spinal epidural empyema).
- In extensive cases, and when CT or MRI are not available, sinography (fistulography) can be helpful. This technique is useful if foreign material is demonstrated within the sinus and/or there is an unexpected extension of the sinus tract or communication with another organ cavity (fistula). In such cases, the surgical approach and the extension of the surgical field will be significantly influenced by the results of the contrast study. However, false-negative results are possible if the foreign body remains undetected or the entire length of the sinus is not demonstrated. False-positive results are also possible if filling defects interpreted as foreign bodies actually represent tissue fragments, blood clots or focal accumulation of exudate. Therefore, this technique can be misleading in the management of a case and the use of advanced imaging is recommended where available.
- If ultrasonography and sinography are to be used in the same patient, plain radiography and ultrasonography should precede sinography to avoid creating artefacts.

Ultrasonographic findings

- Ultrasonography is useful in determining whether the retroperitoneal radiographic changes are associated with fluid accumulation, abscessation and/or a parenchymal lesion.
- However, the full extent of the pathology is difficult to determine in severely affected patients, especially if the sublumbar and epaxial musculature is affected, as this area is not routinely investigated when performing a retroperitoneal ultrasound examination. The presence of a focal swelling or a discharging sinus should prompt a more extensive ultrasonographic investigation.
- Ultrasonography has been advocated as a useful tool for the detection of shadowing created by foreign bodies. However, shadowing is not a constant feature, especially with decomposed or very small foreign bodies.
- Grass seeds have a characteristic double or triple spindle shape on ultrasonography and fluid may accumulate around them.

- Possible explanations for the lack of
  identification of a foreign body by
  ultrasonography include:
    - Highly cellular fluid around the foreign body
    - Complex cellular or gas echoes within an
      abscess
    - Dense fibrous tissue surrounding the foreign
      body
    - Gas trapped within the sinus tract or
      surrounding the foreign body.
- In some cases, the draining tract can be
  followed ultrasonographically to the foreign body.
  Ultrasonography can also be used to guide the
  retrieval of superficial foreign bodies from within
  the discharging sinus using forceps or to guide
  the surgeon to the foreign body, either by
  positioning a needle close to the foreign body or
  through intraoperative ultrasonography.

Advanced imaging findings

In cases of retroperitonitis, surgical exploration with
extensive flushing and debridement of abnormal tissue is recommended, followed by antibiotic therapy
determined by the results of appropriate culture and
sensitivity tests. Advanced imaging plays a fundamental role in determining the extent of the process,
especially as both sides of the retroperitoneum may
be affected without necessarily showing discharging
sinuses on both flanks.

The speed of CT makes it an appealing technique.
Reconstructions can be obtained in any plane when
using modern systems and software, and this is also
useful. Bone detail is exquisite.

However, overall MRI is a superior technique in
this situation because of the true multiplanar characteristics of this modality and the array of sequences
available. The ability to evaluate the extent of the
abscessation, accompanying soft tissue changes and
involvement of the vertebral column and epidural
space makes this technique attractive (Figure 5.11).

The advantages of some of the sequences
available are discussed above. In general, STIR
images are useful with low-field MRI systems and
are extremely helpful in this clinical scenario (Figure
5.12). Pre- and post-contrast T1-weighted images
offer similar information as well as better anatomical
detail.

With either CT or MRI the following should be
looked for:

- Evidence of retroperitoneal fluid accumulation
- Involvement of neighbouring structures, mainly
  the paralumbar muscles, vertebrae, the
  intervertebral discs and the epidural space, as
  well as the presence of a discharging sinus.
  However, a good alignment of the slices with the
  sinus tract is difficult to achieve and this may be
  responsible for the lack of identification of the
  whole length of the tract on CT or MRI images.

Overall, it is very difficult to demonstrate the
presence of foreign bodies, especially if they are
small.

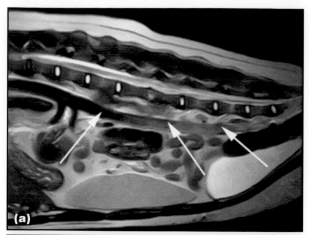

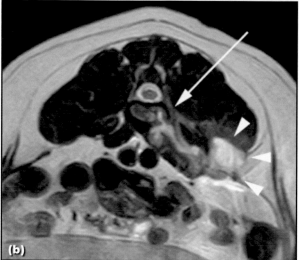

5.11 **(a)** Sagittal lumbar/abdominal and
(b) transverse T2-weighted MR images of a
2-year-old Labrador Retriever bitch presented for back
pain of 6 weeks' duration. The images show not only the
presence of retroperitoneal changes compatible with
abscessation (arrowed in a) but also the active involvement
of the L3–L4 intervertebral disc space (arrowed in b) in the
inflammatory process, extending from a large abscess
within the paraspinal muscles (arrowheads). Part of a
grass seed was retrieved at surgery.

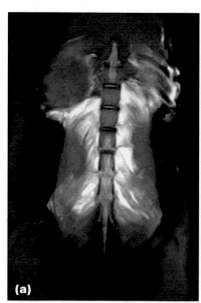

5.12

(a) STIR image in
the dorsal plane at
the level of the
paravertebral
muscles of the dog
in Figure 5.5. This
image shows
extensive
hyperintense
regions within the
muscle, which were
used to direct the
surgeon during the
cleaning and
debriding
procedure.
(continues) ▶

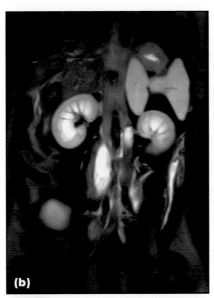

5.12 (continued) **(b)** STIR image in the dorsal plane at the level of the retroperitoneum of the dog in Figure 5.5. This image shows extensive hyperintense regions within the muscle, which were used to direct the surgeon during the cleaning and debriding procedure.

Air

Air in the retroperitoneum is most commonly an extension of pneumomediastinum or a result of trauma. A small amount of gas within an abscess or due to focal infection by gas-producing organisms should be differentiated from extensive pneumoretroperitoneum. Depending on the underlying cause, concurrent pneumoperitoneum may be present. Retroperitoneal air can eventually reach the peritoneal cavity.

Plain radiography is particularly useful in patients with pneumoretroperitoneum.

• A decrease in retroperitoneal opacity, together with the clear depiction of retroperitoneal structures, is seen in cases of diffuse pneumoretroperitoneum (Figure 5.13).
• Focal lesions containing gas (for example some abscesses) will also appear radiolucent, but they may not be easy to detect unless they are large and contain fair amounts of gas (see Figure 5.9).

CT may be used to confirm the presence of a small amount of air; it also allows assessment of the mediastinum and other areas connected with it. Ultrasonography and MRI are not considered primary choices in this situation, except in the investigation of focal lesions containing air.

Masses

Mass lesions are common in the retroperitoneal space. Many are primary or metastatic neoplasms from organs in the retroperitoneal space (e.g. kidney, adrenal gland). Other masses may not have an obvious organ of origin. This is especially true of sarcomas. Haemangiosarcoma is common in the caudal retroperitoneal space without an obvious organ of origin, and may be difficult to identify or characterize owing to surrounding haemorrhage.

Non-neoplastic masses are also possible. The presence of air within the mass should raise the suspicion of an abscess. The presence of mineralization warrants further investigation and a mineralized granuloma or neoplasm should be considered. Mineralized adrenal glands of normal size and shape in cats are usually of no clinical significance. Adrenal gland mineralization is uncommon in dogs as an incidental finding and warrants further studies. Mineralization of an adrenal gland that is abnormal in size or shape in either species requires investigation.

A retroperitoneal mass will displace neighbouring peritoneal structures ventrally and/or to one side. An ovarian mass is peritoneal in origin and, therefore, the neighbouring duodenum or colon will be displaced medially or laterally, but not ventrally. Ventral tipping of the caudal pole of the ipsilateral kidney would be expected.

Periosteal reaction along the mid-ventral margins of the caudal lumbar vertebrae, although not pathognomonic, should raise the suspicion that a caudal abdominal or intrapelvic neoplasm is present with concurrent retroperitoneal extension (Figure 5.14). This periosteal reaction should be distinguished from spondylosis deformans, which affects the vertebral endplates. Spondylitis secondary to foreign body migration will usually affect more cranial lumbar vertebrae (see above).

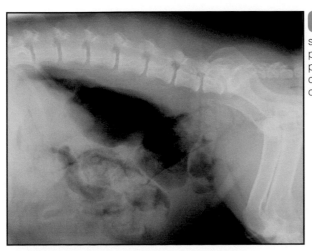

5.13 Lateral abdominal radiograph of an 8-year-old male neutered Scottish Terrier. An irregularly shaped, dorsally located radiolucency indicates pneumoretroperitoneum. This arose when trying to perform a pneumocystogram for the investigation of chronic haematuria. The final diagnosis was transitional cell carcinoma of the prostate gland and bladder neck.

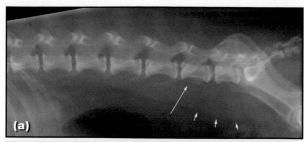

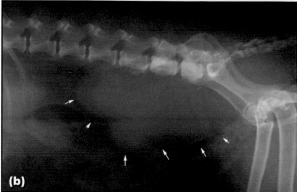

5.14   Close-ups of lateral abdominal radiographs of a 9-year-old male neutered crossbreed dog with adenocarcinoma of the anal glands. An 8-month interval occurred between **(a)** the first and **(b)** the second radiograph. (a) Early enlargement of the medial iliac lymph nodes (short arrows) and periosteal reaction of the sixth lumbar vertebra (long arrow) are evident. (b) Dramatic progression is seen with massive enlargement of the lymph nodes (arrowed).

Although use of radiography and ultrasonography can be sufficient to fully investigate some retroperitoneal masses, those patients with very large masses, or where the lesions, regardless of their size, are very close to critical structures such as the aorta, the caudal vena cava or the neighbouring vertebrae and vertebral canal, will benefit from more advanced imaging.

References and further reading

Armbrust LJ, Biller DS, Radlinsky MG *et al.* (2003) Ultrasonographic diagnosis of foreign bodies associated with chronic draining tracts and abscesses in dogs. *Veterinary Radiology and Ultrasound* **44**, 66–70

Brennan KE and Ihrke PJ (1983) Grass awn migration in dogs and cats: a retrospective study of 182 cases. *Journal of the American Veterinary Medical Association* **182**, 1201–1204

Della Santa D, Rossi F, Carlucci F, Vignoli M and Kircher P (2008) Ultrasound guided retrieval of plant awns. *Veterinary Radiology and Ultrasound* **49**, 484–486

Frendin J, Funkquist B, Hansson K, Lonnemark M and Carlsten J (1999) Diagnostic imaging of foreign body reactions in dogs with diffuse back pain. *Journal of Small Animal Practice* **40**, 278–285

Frendin J, Greko C, Hellmen E, Iwarsson M, Gunarsson A and Chryssantou E (1994) Thoracic and abdominal wall swellings in dogs caused by foreign bodies. *Journal of Small Animal Practice* **35**, 499–508

Gnudi G, Volta A, Bonazzi M, Gazzola M and Bertoni G (2005) Ultrasonographic features of grass awn migration in the dog. *Veterinary Radiology and Ultrasound* **46**, 423–426

Heusquin J, Burton CA and Llabres-Diaz FJ (2007) Outcome of sublumbar abscesses following surgical management guided by diagnostic imaging: study of 14 dogs. *Proceedings of the BSAVA Congress 2007*, p. 528

Holloway A and O' Brien R (in press) Perirenal effusion in dogs and cats with acute renal failure. *Veterinary Radiology and Ultrasound*

Johnston DE and Christie BA (1990a) The retroperitoneum in dogs: anatomy and clinical significance. *Compendium on Continuing Education for the Practicing Veterinarian* **12**, 1027–1033

Johnston DE and Christie BA (1990b) The retroperitoneum in dogs: retroperitoneal infections. *Compendium on Continuing Education for the Practicing Veterinarian* **12**, 1035–1045

Lamb CR, White RN and McEvoy FJ (1994) Sinography in the investigation of draining tracts in small animals: retrospective review of 25 cases. *Veterinary Surgery* **23**, 129–134

Liptak JM, Dernell WS, Ehrhart EJ *et al.* (2004) Retroperitoneal sarcomas in dogs: 14 cases (1992–2002). *Journal of the American Veterinary Medical Association* **224**, 1471–1477

McEvoy FJ, Lamb CR and White RN (1993) An application of sinography in small animal practice. *Veterinary Record* **132**, 183–185

Penninck D and Mitchell SL (2003) Ultrasonographic detection of ingested and perforating wooden foreign bodies in four dogs. *Journal of the American Veterinary Medical Association* **223**, 206–209

Roush JK, Bjorling DE and Lord P (1990) Diseases of the retroperitoneal space in the dog and cat. *Journal of the American Animal Hospital Association* **26**, 47–54

Saunders WB and Tobias KM (2003) Pneumoperitoneum in dogs and cats: 39 cases (1983–2002). *Journal of the American Veterinary Medical Association* **223**, 462–468

Schermerhorn T, McNamara PS, Dykes NL and Toll J (1998) Cullen's sign and haemoglobinuria as presenting signs of retroperitoneal haemorrhage in a dog. *Journal of Small Animal Practice* **39**, 490–494

6

Abdominal vessels

Francisco Llabrés-Díaz

Normal abdominal vasculature

The aorta, caudal vena cava and portal vein are the main abdominal blood vessels. A detailed description of all abdominal vessels is not included here, but the most important are listed below (with larger vessels in **bold type**).

- Branching from the aorta (from caudal to cranial):
  - Median sacral artery
  - Internal iliac arteries
  - **External iliac arteries**
  - Circumflex iliac arteries
  - Caudal mesenteric artery
  - Lumbar arteries
  - Testicular or ovarian arteries
  - **Renal arteries**
  - Phrenicoabdominal arteries
  - **Cranial mesenteric artery**
  - **Coeliac artery**.
- Draining into the caudal vena cava (from caudal to cranial):
  - **Common iliac veins**
  - Lumbar veins
  - Deep circumflex iliac veins
  - Right testicular or right ovarian vein (the left drains into the left renal vein)
  - **Renal veins**
  - Phrenicoabdominal veins
  - **Hepatic veins**
  - Phrenic veins.
- Draining into the portal vein:
  - **Splenic vein** (left-sided)
  - **Cranial** and **caudal mesenteric veins** (central)
  - **Gastroduodenal vein** (right-sided). The pancreaticoduodenal vein, running within the right limb of the pancreas, enters the gastroduodenal vein. The right branches of the gastroepiploic and gastric veins anastamose to create a right loop, which enters the gastroduodenal vein or, in some cases, drains directly into the caudal vena cava. The left branches of the gastroepiploic and gastric veins anastamose to create a left loop, which enters the splenic vein.

The azygous vein crosses the dorsal diaphragm, ventral and to the right of the aorta, joining the cranial vena cava. The normal azygous vein is not visible ultrasonographically in dogs and cats. Figure 6.1 shows the relationship of the major blood vessels in the cranial abdomen of a dog.

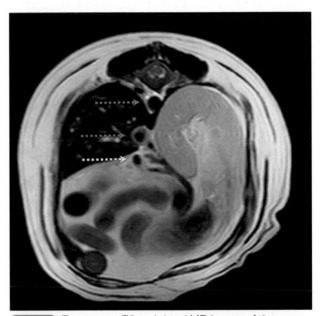

6.1 Transverse T2-weighted MR image of the cranial abdomen of a 5-year-old neutered Dachshund bitch showing the location of the aorta (red arrow), caudal vena cava (blue arrow) and portal vein (yellow arrow). Right is to the left of the image. Vascular anatomy is quite constant: the caudal vena cava is located ventral and to the right of the aorta; the portal vein is located ventral and to the right of the caudal vena cava; the common bile duct is located ventral and to the right of the portal vein; the hepatic artery is located dorsal and to the left of the portal vein.

Plain radiography

Plain radiography is of limited use in the diagnosis of vascular abnormalities. However, plain radiographs should always be obtained before a contrast study is performed. Normal abdominal vessels are rarely seen on plain radiography. If large amounts of intra-abdominal or retroperitoneal fat are present, then the aorta, caudal vena cava, renal vessels and/or circumflex iliac arteries can sometimes be seen on a radiograph (Figure 6.2). Especially in obese patients, the caudal vena cava is seen in the mid-abdomen coursing cranioventrally, diverging from the aorta. The circumflex iliac arteries appear as a single, well

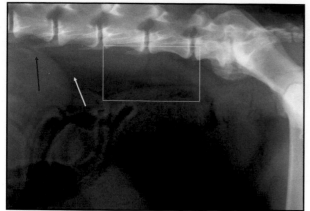

6.2 Lateral abdominal radiograph of an overweight 12-year-old male entire Labrador Retriever. The aorta (red arrow), caudal vena cava (blue arrow) and the circumflex iliac vessels (yellow box) are easily identified against the background of retroperitoneal fat.

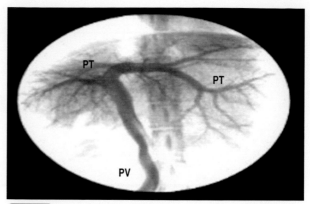

6.3 Image obtained from a normal fluoroscopic IOMP study of a 9-month-old English Springer Spaniel in dorsal recumbency. Note the normal portal tree (PT) opacification. No histopathological abnormalities were found on evaluation of a liver tissue sample. PV = Portal vein.

circumscribed, round, soft tissue opacity in the caudal dorsal retroperitoneal space. This structure should not be misinterpreted as a ureteral calculus.

If the walls of the aorta and caudal vena cava are more clearly visible than normal, two major differential diagnoses should be considered. If the normal soft tissue opacity of the vessels is surrounded by free air, then the cause of the pneumoretroperitoneum should be investigated. Alternatively, pathologically increased opacity of the intra-abdominal vessels may contrast with the normal peritoneal fat. Hypercalcaemia, uraemia and hyperadrenocorticism should be investigated as possible causes of mineralization of the intra-abdominal arteries.

Contrast radiography

Contrast angiographic studies involve the intravascular injection of a water-soluble iodinated contrast medium. Either hyperosmolar (ionic) or iso-osmolar (non-ionic) preparations can be used, although the latter have lower morbidity and are recommended in clinically compromised patients. The choice of vessel, catheterization method and imaging technique (i.e. radiography *versus* fluoroscopy or even more advanced imaging techniques) will depend on:

- The vascular abnormality suspected
- Availability of particular diagnostic imaging techniques
- Personal preference.

Selective contrast studies

Selective contrast studies follow the catheterization of a particular vessel or branch/tributary, usually through interventional radiography. Examples of selective vascular studies include:

- Coeliac artery angiography for hepatic arterioportal (AP) fistulae
- Jejunal vein catheterization (intraoperative mesenteric portography, IOMP; Figure 6.3) for the investigation of portal vein atresia, portosystemic shunts (PSSs) and post-PSS ligation assessment.

Non-selective contrast studies

Non-selective contrast studies involve the injection of contrast medium into a more easily accessible vessel, usually a peripheral vein (e.g. the caudal branch of the lateral saphenous vein). The study allows assessment of the veins in the path of the flow of the contrast medium to the caudal vena cava and right side of the heart. This may be important in the evaluation of adrenal gland neoplasia, particularly right-sided, which commonly invades the caudal vena cava.

Ultrasonography

Ultrasonography is particularly useful as a screening tool and is the only practical method for evaluating abdominal vessels in the conscious patient. Limitations include the need for Doppler technology, a suitable acoustic window for the particular vessel, and operator experience. Vascular ultrasonography is amongst the most technically demanding forms of ultrasonography.

Technique

A lateral and dorsal abdominal approach (ventral to the psoas muscles) is helpful in the evaluation of the aorta and caudal vena cava as they run through the retroperitoneum (Figure 6.4). The vessels are close to the transducer, allowing high-frequency transducers to be used in the majority of cases. Both longitudinal (parallel to the long axis of the body) and transverse (perpendicular to the long axis) images of each vessel should be obtained throughout the length of the vessel. Although possible, a ventral approach to these vessels is not recommended because of the negative effects of interposed gas- or faeces-filled intestinal loops and the presence of marked acoustic enhancement distal to the bladder.

The windows to the portal vein include the ventral midline or slightly right of the midline and the right lateral intercostal approaches.

- The ventral/right ventrolateral approach is particularly helpful in obtaining longitudinal images of the portal vein caudal to the porta

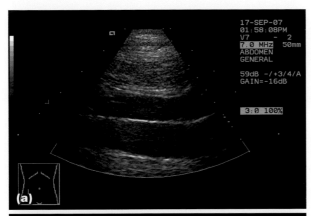

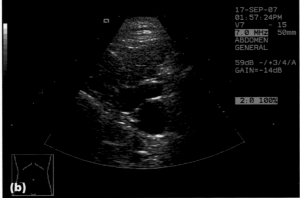

6.4 **(a)** Longitudinal and **(b)** transverse right-sided ultrasonograms of the normal caudal vena cava and aorta of an 8-year-old neutered Labrador Retriever bitch as seen in the caudal retroperitoneum. The transducer was positioned just ventral to the psoas musculature. The caudal vena cava is compressed owing to transducer pressure (yellow arrow in b). The head is to the left in (a). Dorsal is to the left in (b).

hepatis. Images can be obtained with the patient in dorsal recumbency or in right lateral recumbency. With the latter approach, the ultrasonographer may obtain images without intervening gas by sliding the transducer between the examination table and the patient.

- The right lateral intercostal approach is also helpful. With the patient in left lateral recumbency, the right dorsocranial abdominal quadrant can be evaluated. Transverse images obtained using this approach are more easily reproducible. Limitations to this approach include the increased distance to the area of interest compared with a subcostal approach, and possible intervening gastrointestinal gas. This approach is recommended in most cases, especially when portal vein thrombosis and portosystemic shunting are under investigation. However, frequently, a combination of approaches is necessary.

Normal appearance

In the cranial abdomen the caudal vena cava is to the right of midline with the aorta to the left. The aorta is dorsal to the caudal vena cava in the cranial third of the abdomen, but their dorsoventral relationship is variable in the caudal abdomen. The presence of pulsating movements should not be used to differentiate the two vessels, as aortic wall movement can be

transmitted to the caudal vena cava. Transducer pressure can cause the caudal vena cava to collapse, but this is not possible with the aorta. Doppler ultrasonography clearly demonstrates the differing pulse waveform of the arterial aorta compared with the venous flow of the caudal vena cava.

Normal vessels are anechoic tubular structures in longitudinal section, becoming round as the transducer is turned through 90 degrees. The walls should be thin and highly echogenic when perpendicular to the ultrasound beam. It is not unusual to occasionally see moving intraluminal echoes when using modern equipment and high-frequency transducers. Highly echogenic blood (a sign of sludging, agglutination or thrombosis) or turbulence should be investigated further. The routine use of colour and spectral Doppler is crucial in vascular abdominal ultrasonography.

Overview of additional imaging modalities

Computed tomography

The use of computed tomography (CT) angiography is increasing, especially for the detection and characterization of PSS vessels. It can also be used for the investigation of other vascular abnormalities (AP fistulae, thrombosis, pulmonary thromboembolism) or for the assessment of the vascular bed in cases of vascular trauma or neoplasia. Equipment is now more widely available. Automated pressure injectors improve image quality for many studies. There are some substantial benefits of CT angiography over radiography; cross-sectional CT usually provides very detailed anatomical information without superimposed structures and, in addition, the technique is not as operator dependent as ultrasonography. However, cost, availability and familiarity with the technical aspects of CT angiography, as well as the difficulty in interpreting the final images, are often limitations to the use of CT.

Non-selective CT angiography can be performed, using variable time intervals post-injection before obtaining helical angiographic images, but the results can be unreliable. To maximize the advantage that CT technology provides, a low dose test injection is usually recommended to identify the time to peak opacification in the vessel of interest (arterial phase, systemic venous phase or portal phase). Single phase or complex dual phase studies can then be more accurately performed.

Magnetic resonance imaging

Magnetic resonance angiography (MRA) is not routinely used in veterinary medicine, despite improved access to magnetic resonance imaging (MRI) equipment. The more challenging machine-based technical aspects of performing MRA, as well as the duration of a complete MRI examination, make MRA less appealing.

Technique

Several MRA techniques can be used. Images can be obtained with or without the injection of paramagnetic contrast medium into a peripheral vein. The examination can be directed towards the study of fast or slow flowing vessels.

Normal appearance
Vessels are seen as tubular structures of high signal intensity (very bright). Usually the signal from the surrounding soft tissues is minimized or masked/ cropped to allow more detailed assessment of the vascular pattern. Post-processing multiplanar or 3D reconstructions can then be obtained as necessary to better evaluate the vasculature.

Nuclear medicine
Nuclear angiography is mainly used in cases of suspected portosystemic shunting. Access to the radiopharmaceuticals and equipment, as well as appropriate kennelling, are fundamental and may limit widespread use of this technique.

Vascular diseases

Portal vein

Portosystemic shunts
PSSs occur as a result of an abnormal communication between the portal and systemic venous systems. The differentiation between a congenital single (rarely, double) PSS and multiple shunt vessels secondary to portal hypertension is fundamental. The treatment of a single shunting vessel is surgical. However, patients suffering from multiple shunts are not surgical candidates and have a poorer prognosis.

Congenital portosystemic shunts:

- These are usually single (rarely, double) portal–systemic vascular communications in the absence of portal hypertension.
- They are generally extrahepatic in small and medium breeds but more commonly intrahepatic in large breeds of dog.
- The most common extrahepatic shunt in dogs is portocaval, followed by portoazygous. Much less frequently, shunts arise from the left gastric or colonic veins, or, rarely, from the internal thoracic or renal veins. Newer equipment, with improved resolution, may allow more accurate determination of the particular vessels involved. Shunting vessels previously described as portocaval may actually have been of right gastric or splenic origin but with very little distance separating the shunt from the main portal vein.
- The most common origin of the shunting vessel in cats with extrahepatic shunts is the left gastric vein. Portocaval shunts are the next most common.
- Intrahepatic shunts are usually more standardized in their anatomy. There are different opinions in the literature as to the best way to describe them. Classification of intrahepatic

shunts as right, central or left divisional may be helpful. They arise from the left or right main intrahepatic portal branches. A patent ductus venosus is the most common intrahepatic shunt in both dogs and cats.

Acquired portosystemic shunts:

- These are multiple shunts; the shunting vessels are normal non-patent vessels that open because of increased pressure in the portal system (Figure 6.5).
- They usually affect older patients suffering from chronic portal hypertension. Younger patients may also be affected.
- The pattern of shunting will be similar irrespective of the underlying cause of the hypertension.
- The shunting blood usually enters the renal or gonadal veins, the venous sinuses in the vertebral canal or the caudal vena cava itself. Gastrophrenic, pancreaticoduodenal and, rarely, haemorrhoidal PSSs are also sometimes detected.

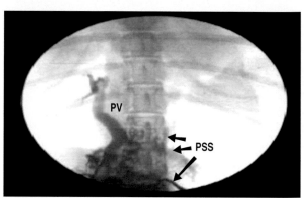

6.5 Image obtained from a fluoroscopic IOMP study of a 6-month-old male Golden Retriever in dorsal recumbency. Multiple acquired PSSs can be seen as irregularly shaped linear opacities. No portal tree opacification was seen at this stage, compatible with the presence of portal hypertension and resistance to flow towards the liver. A liver biopsy confirmed primary hypoplasia of the portal vein (PV).

Hepatic causes of portal hypertension include cirrhosis, severe hepatitis, chronic hepatic congestion resulting in fibrosis, or neoplasia-induced AP fistulae. Prehepatic portal hypertension results from abnormal portal flow secondary to luminal or extraluminal compression of the portal vein, either by a thrombus or an obstructive mass. Portal hypertension may be seen in young patients, secondary to portal vein dysplasia (previously termed idiopathic non-cirrhotic portal hypertension). The liver in these dogs may be similar ultrasonographically to that in dogs with congenital portosystemic shunting: small, smooth in contour and lacking in portal vessels. Post-hepatic portal hypertension is the only type of portal hypertension where shunting will not develop, as the pressure rises equally in both the portal and systemic venous systems.

Choice of imaging technique: A thorough medical assessment of the patient is required prior to imaging. Several factors need to be taken into consideration when deciding which imaging modalities to use:

- If nuclear medicine is available, *per rectal* or trans-splenic portal scintigraphy can be used as an effective non-invasive screening test; however, access to a gamma camera, kennelling and the radiopharmaceuticals is needed, as well as sedation of the patient
- Ultrasonography is more widely available and, in experienced hands, can also be used as a reliable, non-invasive screening technique. An ultrasound examination can help determine whether macroscopic multiple acquired or single shunts exist, and hopefully indicate the path of the shunting vessel. Urolithiasis can be identified and the degree of development of the portal vasculature subjectively assessed. Ultrasonography offers more detailed anatomical information than nuclear medicine
- In the majority of cases, more advanced imaging techniques will be needed to confirm a PSS and to determine the location and path of the shunting vessel. The detailed and global anatomical information offered by IOMP or CT is hard to match with ultrasonography.

Plain radiography: The findings on plain radiography include:

- Microhepatia (more frequent in dogs than in cats)
- Poor or small body condition
- Renomegaly in dogs (but not in all types of PSS)
- Radiopaque uroliths can be found in some cases; uroliths (ammonium urate or biurate urinary calculi) are common but will only be radiopaque if ammonium biurate crystals are combined with struvite or calcium oxalate
- Ascites in patients with marked portal hypertension. This is not as common in cats.

Intraoperative mesenteric portography: IOMP is considered by many to be the definitive method for demonstration of portosystemic shunting. Injection of contrast medium into the spleen or splenic vein under ultrasound guidance constitutes a variation of this study (splenoportography), avoiding the need for coeliotomy, but there are risks associated with the injection, and shunting vessels originating caudal to the splenic vein will go unnoticed.

Following coeliotomy, the technique for IOMP involves injecting a dose of 1 ml/kg bodyweight of a water-soluble, non-ionic iodinated contrast medium (≥300 mg I/ml) through a pre-filled, flexible, polyethylene extension tube into a catheterized jejunal vein. During the injection of contrast medium, radiography or fluoroscopy is performed. The latter technique, when available, allows real-time assessment of the contrast medium flow and a better subjective evaluation of the degree of portal tree opacification. The former can also be useful, but the radiograph should be obtained towards the end of the injection of contrast medium or when considerable resistance to the injection is felt. The contrast medium should be injected quite quickly to obtain good vascular delineation (see Figure 6.3).

When shunting is present, there will be no or limited opacification of the intrahepatic portal vasculature and rapid opacification of the systemic vein receiving the shunting blood (caudal vena cava or azygous vein). One or more shunting vessels will be apparent, and these usually follow a tortuous or looping path (Figure 6.6).

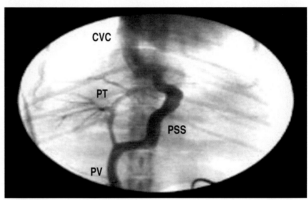

6.6 Image obtained from a fluoroscopic IOMP study of a 15-month-old male neutered Bichon Frisé demonstrating the presence of a single extrahepatic portocaval PSS. Minimal opacification of the portal tree (PT) can be seen (compare with the normal portal tree in Figure 6.3). The patient was in dorsal recumbency; right is to the left. CVC = Caudal vena cava; PV = Portal vein.

If the caudal extent of the loop of the shunt, or where the shunt diverges from the original vessel, is cranial to T13 when viewed on a left lateral recumbent radiograph, then an intrahepatic shunt is likely (Figure 6.7). However, it is important to remember that the location of the shunt may vary from 0.5 to 0.75 times the length of a vertebra, depending on the phase of respiration. A second contrast medium injection with the patient in dorsal recumbency is often helpful to further define the path of the PSS (Figure 6.8) and to establish whether it is left- or right-sided.

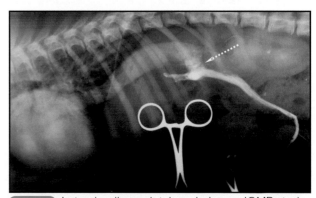

6.7 Lateral radiograph taken during an IOMP study demonstrating a single extrahepatic PSS in a 6-month-old Border Collie. The shunting vessel leaves the portal vein caudal to T13 (arrowed) to reach the caudal vena cava, indicating that it is an extrahepatic shunt. This was confirmed at surgery. (Reproduced from Llabrés-Díaz (2006) with permission from *In Practice*)

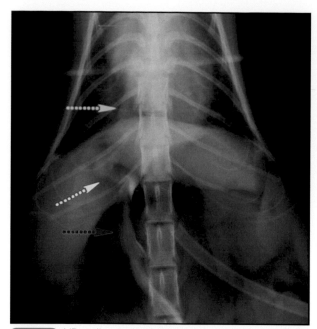

6.8 VD radiograph taken during an IOMP study in a 7-month-old male neutered Domestic Shorthaired cat. ••••••▶ = Portal vein; ••••••▶ = PSS; ••••••▶ = Immediate opacification of the caudal vena cava after injection of contrast medium, without intrahepatic portal vasculature opacification. (Reproduced from Llabrés-Díaz (2006) with permission from *In Practice*)

Ultrasonography: This is considered an accurate tool in the hands of experienced ultrasonographers for the identification and characterization of PSSs, especially single intrahepatic shunts. General ultrasonographic findings correspond with those seen on plain radiography, including microhepatia, renomegaly and cystic calculi. The combined finding of ultrasonographically evident but radiographically occult cystic calculi is supportive of urate stones. Decreased general portal vasculature can be seen in cases of a single congenital PSS and in some cases of microvascular dysplasia. Patients with hepatic microvascular dysplasia or primary hypoplasia of the portal vein may also have a normal sized liver. With acquired multiple shunts there may be accompanying changes, including ascites, pancreatic oedema, urinary calculi, gallbladder wall oedema or gastrointestinal tract oedema.

The overall goal for the identification of an extrahepatic shunt is to find an abnormal extrahepatic vessel entering the caudal vena cava (Figure 6.9), leaving the portal vein or large tributary, or a large aberrant abnormal vessel. It is vital to be familiar with the normal appearance of the vessels and surrounding structures, especially the entrance of the renal veins into the caudal vena cava.

Objective greyscale measurements of the portal vein and aorta have been shown to be quite helpful in the diagnosis of a PSS. In normal cats and dogs, the ratio between the maximum portal vein diameter at the porta hepatis (cranial to the entry of the gastro-duodenal vein) and the maximum aortic diameter (in systole) lies between 0.7 and 1.25. If the ratio is ≥0.8, an extrahepatic PSS can be excluded. Dogs and cats with a ratio ≤0.65 are likely to have an extrahepatic PSS or idiopathic non-cirrhotic portal hypertension.

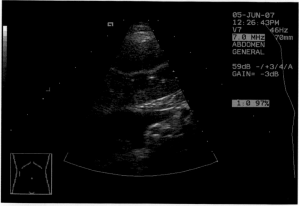

6.9 Longitudinal (head is to the left) ultrasonogram of the cranial retroperitoneum of a 4-year-old male Border Terrier at the level of the right kidney, as seen in the near-field. The entrance point of a single extrahepatic PSS into the caudal vena cava can be clearly seen at this level. A right intercostal approach was used.

An intrahepatic shunt may be easier to identify than an extrahepatic shunt. Patients with smaller and/or short intrahepatic shunts may benefit from using a very cranial intercostal approach, although a ventral approach can also be useful. An abnormal vessel, often quite large, located cranially within the hepatic parenchyma will support the presence of the shunt (Figure 6.10). Rarely, more than one abdominal vessel may be seen.

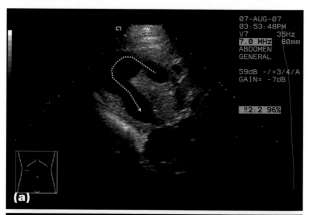

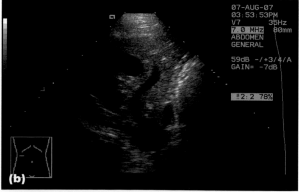

6.10 **(a,b)** Transverse (dorsal to the left) ultrasonograms of the right side of the liver obtained through a right intercostal approach, showing two of the three multiple congenital intrahepatic PSSs found in a 1-year-old Border Collie bitch. The yellow arrow seen in (a) indicates the direction of blood flow into the markedly dilated caudal vena cava. (continues) ▶

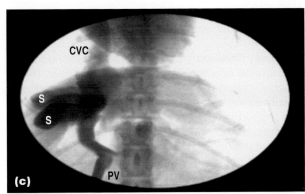

6.10 (continued) **(c)** Image obtained from a fluoroscopic IOMP study with the dog in dorsal recumbency. The multiple shunting vessels (S) are clearly seen to the right of the midline. CVC = Caudal vena cava; PV = Portal vein.

Colour Doppler ultrasonography can detect turbulent flow in the proximity of the shunt, as well as indicating whether the direction of the blood flow is towards (hepatopetal) or away from (hepatofugal) the liver. Spectral pulsed wave Doppler ultrasonography measurements offer similar directional information but more accurate measurements of portal flow velocity. Normal mean portal velocity is 15–20 cm/s in dogs and 10–18 cm/s in cats. With intrahepatic shunts the velocity may be markedly increased, whilst with extrahepatic shunts the velocity is often reduced or reversed.

Computed tomography angiography: Survey CT images should be evaluated before injecting contrast medium via a large gauge catheter into the cephalic or jugular vein (Figure 6.11). Injecting a larger volume of a less concentrated contrast medium will prolong the duration of the vascular phase and reduce the risk of high density streak artefacts.

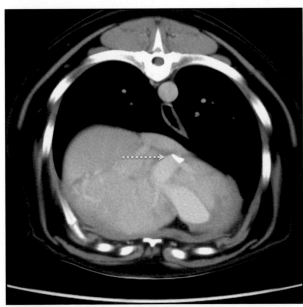

6.11 Non-selective CT angiogram of a 1-year-old male neutered Labrador Retriever showing the exact position (arrowed) where a previous ligation of an intrahepatic PSS had been performed several months earlier. The CT was being performed for the evaluation of a paracostal lesion.

An initial test injection is often very helpful in determining the timing of the subsequent angiographic study. Obtaining sequential images at the site where the portal vein enters the liver after injection of a small (1–3 ml) dose of contrast medium provides the basis for estimating the timing of arterial and portal phases. Obtaining specific patient-based times before performing the helical angiographic study is recommended.

A dual phase CT angiographic technique obtains images of the arterial and portal phases in the same patient. Helical imaging movement is caudal to cranial for the arterial phase and the opposite for the portal phase. The advantage of the dual phase technique is that both the hepatic arteries and the main arterial supply can be visualized; some of them will show increased size, number and tortuosity in patients with PSSs. The hepatic arteries also provide a landmark for assessment of the intrahepatic venous branches. If a dual phase technique is not practicable owing to technical limitations of the equipment, two separate injections, one for the arterial phase and one for the portal phase, may be used.

Nuclear medicine: Nuclear medicine is considered a very good screening test for PSSs, being both sensitive and specific. Unfortunately, it provides little anatomical information, although this is better when trans-splenic portal scintigraphy is used. There are two techniques:

- *Per rectal* portal scintigraphy
- *Trans-splenic* portal scintigraphy

For *per rectal* portal scintigraphy, patients should receive an enema more than 1 hour prior to the study. Sodium pertechnetate (185–740 MBq for dogs and 185–370 MBq for cats, in a final volume of 0.5–1.5 ml) is introduced into the distal colon via a long flexible catheter. The patient must be sedated and positioned in right lateral recumbency. Particular care with radiation safety must be taken to avoid contamination of the environment and/or personnel if isotope leaks from the rectum.

Images are collected by dynamic acquisition at a rate of one image per second for 180 seconds. Lead shielding of the injection site is important to mask the high activity of this area. The location of the radiopharmaceutical deposition is important as very caudal shunting vessels could be missed if the radiopharmaceutical is deposited too cranially. The wrong dose or improper absorption of the radiopharmaceutical because of mixture with faecal material may render the study non-diagnostic.

In simple terms, if the radiopharmaceutical arrives in the heart before the liver a shunt is present. If the radiopharmaceutical arrives in the liver first, followed by the heart, then there is no shunt. Time–activity curves and shunt ratios can be obtained by assigning regions of interest to the heart and liver, and measuring activity in these regions over time. Patients with microvascular dysplasia have a normal nuclear medicine study.

An alternative to the colonic study is trans-splenic portal scintigraphy. A lower dose (74 MBq) of sodium pertechnetate, diluted in a small volume of saline, is injected under ultrasound guidance into the splenic parenchyma, as far as possible from the liver. Dynamic acquisition is then started in the same way as above, and the same calculations performed. The main advantages of this technique are a lower injected dose of the radiopharmaceutical, less radiation exposure of the patient and personnel, higher counts recorded in the liver and the heart than with the previous technique and better anatomical information.

Generally, good results have been obtained using trans-splenic portal scintigraphy. Non-diagnostic studies may be associated with the very rare intraperitoneal injection of the radiopharmaceutical. Importantly, acquired and single or double congenital PSSs can be differentiated, although different types of centrally positioned PSSs cannot be distinguished.

Portal vein thrombosis

Portal vein thrombosis is uncommon but has been described in dogs associated with systemic disease leading to a hypercoagulable state, neoplastic invasion or chronic ehrlichiosis. It is likely that the predisposing factors are similar to those listed below for caval thrombosis.

Caudal vena cava

Thromboembolic disease

Thrombosis is the formation of a blood clot or platelet–fibrin mass within the heart or blood vessels. In small animals, the most common causes of thromboembolism include:

- Vascular endothelial injury associated with infections (e.g. dirofilariasis, sepsis, bacterial endocarditis), indwelling catheters or vascular immune complex deposition
- Endocardial damage and stasis resulting from cardiac disease (e.g. feline hypertrophic cardiomyopathy)
- Primary thrombocytopathies (e.g. myeloproliferative disorders, diabetes mellitus) and disorders associated with hypercoagulability or hypofibrinolysis (e.g. hyperadrenocorticism, disseminated intravascular coagulation, neoplasia and antithrombin-III deficiency secondary to protein-losing nephropathy or enteropathy).

In addition, it is important to recognize the likelihood of caudal vena cava involvement with right adrenal gland neoplasms. The right adrenal gland shares its adventitia with the caudal vena cava, which explains the frequency of vascular invasion by aggressive right adrenal gland masses, as well as the presence of non-neoplastic thrombi due to abnormal flow associated with compression or wall invasion by the mass. The neoplastic process appears to track down the phrenicoabdominal vein to reach the caudal vena cava. Caval thrombi can also be seen with left adrenal gland lesions. Very extensive caudal vena cava thrombosis may cause secondary hindlimb oedema, irrespective of the underlying cause of the thromboembolic episode.

Imaging findings: The general ultrasonographic appearance of a thrombus is that of an intraluminal, variably echogenic lesion; neoplastic thrombi are usually echogenic, whereas aortic thrombi associated with hypertrophic cardiomyopathy are very often anechoic at the time of diagnosis. Selective or non-selective radiographic or CT angiography can also be used; a thrombus will produce filling defects within the vessel lumen.

Congenital anomalies

Several congenital problems have been described that affect the caudal venal cava. These range from duplication of the caudal vena cava, where the common iliac veins combine further cranially than usual, to more extreme cases where a portion of the caudal vena cava fails to develop normally. In the latter, systemic blood returning to the heart will usually find a collateral route, for example via the azygous vein. These congenital problems may be associated with other malformations but are generally accepted to be rare. Concurrent anomalies of the caudal vena cava have been reported in dogs with congenital PSSs, including segmental atresia with azygous drainage of abdominal organs and a double caudal vena cava in the caudal half of the abdomen.

Abdominal aorta

Arterioportal fistula

Arteriovenous (AV) communications can occur anywhere in the body, with the majority of those in the abdomen affecting the liver, involving one or more lobes. Some controversy exists surrounding the most appropriate nomenclature for this condition when the liver is affected. A distinction has been suggested between AV malformations (multiple intrahepatic AV communications) and AP fistula (a single communication between the arterial and portal circulations within the liver) (Figure 6.12). However, the possibility of multiple AP fistulae makes the differentiation more difficult. Cats are even less frequently diagnosed with hepatic AV malformations than dogs. The majority of cases are congenital in origin, although neoplastic and traumatic, including post surgery, causes have been reported.

Imaging findings: The imaging findings are usually associated with portal hypertension, ascites and multiple acquired PSSs.

- IOMP can readily confirm the presence of multiple acquired PSSs, but may not show the AV malformation. It may be demonstrated if the contrast medium is not too diluted by the time it reaches the abnormal communication via the arterial system.
- Ultrasonography is useful in detecting the presence of abnormal vessels (Figure 6.12c). Intrahepatic AV malformations can reach a dramatic size. The very abnormal pulsating blood

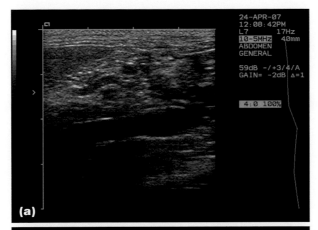

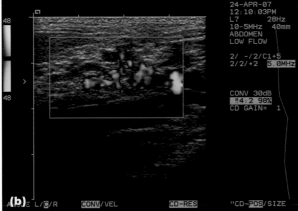

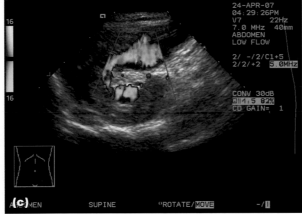

6.12 Longitudinal (head is to the left) **(a)** greyscale and **(b)** colour Doppler ultrasonograms of the retroperitoneum of a 5-month-old male Domestic Shorthaired cat at a level just caudal to the left kidney. Multiple vessels are demonstrated. These were confirmed as multiple acquired PSSs. A large AP fistula was responsible for the sustained portal hypertension in this case. The abnormal communication is demonstrated in **(c)** as a very large intrahepatic vessel with an aliasing artefact on colour Doppler ultrasonography. Pulsating signals were detected using pulsed wave Doppler ultrasonography. These findings were confirmed at surgery, during which the affected liver lobe was removed.

flow, demonstrated by Doppler ultrasonography studies, confirms the diagnosis.
- CT angiography is considered superior to ultrasonography in determining the size and location of the abnormal vessels. With dual phase CT angiography, the early detection of attenuating contrast medium within the portal system during the arterial phase is considered a critical sign for diagnosis. Dual phase CT is clearly superior to single phase CT angiography in this respect, as the arterial phase is not assessed with single phase CT angiography of the portal vessels. Dual phase CT angiography not only allows visualization of the AP fistulae, in the form of tortuous vessels or vessels with aneurysmal dilatations, but also demonstrates the presence of multiple acquired PSSs secondary to portal hypertension. The dual phase technique has to be adapted for the investigation of AP fistulae, as timings to vascular opacification will be slightly different from those of normal patients or patients with congenital PSSs.

Thromboembolic disease
Aortic thromboembolism is common in cats with underlying primary heart disease. A saddle thrombus, where the thrombus affects all components of the major caudal aortic trifurcation, causes sudden onset hindlimb lameness, paresis or paralysis, marked pain, cold extremities, weak pulses and pale or cyanotic pads. More complicated cases have thrombosis of the renal arteries. The condition is less frequent in dogs and more commonly associated with protein-losing diseases. The onset may be less acute, or acute signs may follow a period of lameness. Less frequently, with smaller thrombi, unilateral signs can be seen. Causes of local thromboembolism include neoplastic infiltration of the vessel wall, foreign body or vasculitis.

Imaging findings: Ultrasonography is the imaging modality of choice for large vessels, as it is widely available and permits fast and accurate evaluation of the main arterial abdominal vessels (Figure 6.13) in cooperative patients. The thrombus is usually anechoic, and detection and evaluation of its extent usually requires thorough Doppler or contrast ultrasonography. Selective angiography can also be used, especially if more distal arteries are affected.

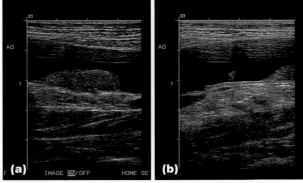

6.13 Left-sided longitudinal ultrasonograms of the distal third of the aorta (dorsal approach) of a 9-year-old neutered Greyhound bitch. Two different intraluminal non-shadowing hyperechoic lesions can be seen. The largest lesion, seen in **(a)**, was slightly caudal to the mobile one seen in **(b)**. A third lesion, not shown here, was seen to be occluding the right external iliac artery. The dog suffered acute onset right hindlimb monoparesis and pain 24 hours prior to the ultrasound examination. Thromboembolic disease secondary to protein-losing nephropathy was diagnosed.

Other abdominal arteries and veins

Volvulus

Intestinal torsion describes the twisting of the bowel on its longitudinal axis, causing luminal obstruction, whilst intestinal volvulus describes a rotation about the mesenteric axis with secondary compromise of blood supply. Both may occur concurrently. Mesenteric volvulus can be suspected from radiographs, where marked and generalized intestinal gaseous dilatation is demonstrated. However, this is a non-specific finding attributable to ischaemia and variable secondary wall necrosis. Deep-chested male large breeds of dog are predisposed. Colonic volvulus causes gaseous dilatation of affected bowel segments. The distension may be progressive and is difficult to distinguish from other causes of megacolon. Doppler ultrasonography is indicated to evaluate the vessels of the affected bowel segment.

Acknowledgements

The author is grateful to Davies Veterinary Specialists and the Animal Health Trust for the figures included in this Chapter.

References and further reading

Bentley AM, O'Toole TE, Kowaleski MP, *et al.* (2005) Volvulus of the colon in four dogs. *Journal of the American Veterinary Medical Association* **227**, 253–257

Bertolini G, Rolla EC, Zotti A, *et al.* (2006) Three-dimensional multislice helical computed tomography techniques for canine extra-hepatic portosystemic shunt assessment. *Veterinary Radiology and Ultrasound* **47**, 439–443

Boswood A, Lamb CR and White RN (2000) Aortic and iliac thrombosis in six dogs. *Journal of Small Animal Practice* **41**, 109–114

Brinkman EL, Biller DS, Armbrust LJ, *et al.* (2007) The clinical utility of the right lateral intercostal ultrasound scan technique in dogs. *Journal of the American Animal Hospital Association* **43**, 179–186

Carlisle CH, Wu JX and Heath TJ (1995) Anatomy of the portal and hepatic veins of the dog: a basis for systematic evaluation of the liver by ultrasonography. *Veterinary Radiology and Ultrasound* **36**, 227–233

Chanoit G, Kyles AE, Weisse C, *et al.* (2007) Surgical and interventional radiographic treatment of dogs with hepatic arteriovenous fistulae. *Veterinary Surgery* **36**, 199–209

Christiansen JS, Hottinger HA, Allen L, *et al.* (2000) Hepatic microvascular dysplasia in dogs: a retrospective study of 24 cases (1987–1995). *Journal of the American Animal Hospital Association* **36**, 385–389

Cole RC, Morandi F, Avenell J, *et al.* (2005) Trans-splenic portal scintigraphy in normal dogs. *Veterinary Radiology and Ultrasound* **46**, 146–152

d'Anjou MA (2007) The sonographic search for portosystemic shunts. *Clinical Techniques in Small Animal Practice* **22**, 104–114

d'Anjou MA, Penninck D, Cornejo L, *et al.* (2004) Ultrasonographic diagnosis of portosystemic shunting in dogs and cats. *Veterinary Radiology and Ultrasound* **45**, 424–437

Finn-Bodner ST and Hudson JA (1998) Abdominal vascular sonography. *Veterinary Clinics of North America: Small Animal Practice* **28**, 887–942

Frank P, Mahaffey M, Egger C, *et al.* (2003) Helical computed tomographic portography in ten normal dogs and ten dogs with a portosystemic shunt. *Veterinary Radiology and Ultrasound* **44**, 392–400

Halfacree ZJ, Beck AL, Lee KC, *et al.* (2006) Torsion and volvulus of the transverse and descending colon in a German shepherd dog. *Journal of Small Animal Practice* **47**, 468–470

Junius G, Appeldoorn AM and Schrauwen E (2004) Mesenteric volvulus in the dog: a retrospective study of 12 cases. *Journal of Small Animal Practice* **45**, 104–107

Lamb C (2005) Doppler ultrasound examination in dogs and cats 2. Abdominal applications. *In Practice* **27**, 238–247

Lamb C and Boswood A (2005) Doppler ultrasound examination in dogs and cats 1. The principles. *In Practice* **27**, 183–189

Lamb CR (1998) Ultrasonography of portosystemic shunts in dogs and cats. *Veterinary Clinics of North America: Small Animal Practice* **28**, 725–753

Lamb CR and Daniel GB (2002) Diagnostic imaging of dogs with suspected portosystemic shunting. *Compendium on Continuing Education for the Practicing Veterinarian* **24**, 626–635

Lamb CR, Foster-Van Hijfte MA, White RN, *et al.* (1996) Ultrasonographic diagnosis of congenital portosystemic shunt in 14 cats. *Journal of Small Animal Practice* **37**, 205–209

Lamb CR and White RN (1998) Morphology of congenital intrahepatic portacaval shunts in dogs and cats. *Veterinary Record* **142**, 55–60

Lamb CR, Wrigley RH, Simpson KW, *et al.* (1996) Ultrasonographic diagnosis of portal vein thrombosis in four dogs. *Veterinary Radiology and Ultrasound* **37**, 121–129

Llabrés-Díaz FJ (2006) Practical contrast radiography 5. Other techniques. *In Practice* **28**, 32–40

Moon ML (1990) Diagnostic imaging of portosystemic shunts. *Seminars in Veterinary Medicine and Surgery (Small Animal)* **5**, 120–126

Morandi F, Cole RC, Tobias KM, *et al.* (2005) Use of 99mTCO4(–) trans-splenic portal scintigraphy for diagnosis of portosystemic shunts in 28 dogs. *Veterinary Radiology and Ultrasound* **46**, 153–161

Seguin B, Tobias KM, Gavin PR, *et al.* (1999) Use of magnetic resonance angiography for diagnosis of portosystemic shunts in dogs. *Veterinary Radiology and Ultrasound* **40**, 251–258

Smith SA and Tobias AH (2004) Feline arterial thromboembolism: an update. *Veterinary Clinics of North America: Small Animal Practice* **34**, 1245–1271

Spaulding KA (1997) A review of sonographic identification of abdominal blood vessels and juxtavascular organs. *Veterinary Radiology and Ultrasound* **38**, 4–23

Sura PA, Tobias KM, Morandi F, *et al.* (2007) Comparison of 99mTcO4(-) trans-splenic portal scintigraphy with per-rectal portal scintigraphy for diagnosis of portosystemic shunts in dogs. *Veterinary Surgery* **36**, 654–660

Szatmari V, Rothuizen J, Van den Ingh TS, *et al.* (2004) Ultrasonographic findings in dogs with hyperammonemia: 90 cases (2000–2002). *Journal of the American Veterinary Medical Association* **224**, 717–727

Szatmari V, Sotonyi P and Voros K (2001) Normal duplex Doppler waveforms of major abdominal blood vessels in dogs: a review. *Veterinary Radiology and Ultrasound* **42**, 93–107

White RN, McDonald NJ and Burton CA (2003) Use of intraoperative mesenteric portovenography in congenital portosystemic shunt surgery. *Veterinary Radiology and Ultrasound* **44**, 514–521

Winkle TJ, Liu SM and Hackner SG (1993) Clinical and pathological features of aortic thromboembolism in 36 dogs. *Journal of Veterinary Emergency and Critical Care* **3**, 13–21

Winter MD, Kinney LM and Kleine LJ (2005) Three-dimensional helical computed tomographic angiography of the liver in five dogs. *Veterinary Radiology and Ultrasound* **46**, 494–499

Zwingenberger AL, McLear RC and Weisse C (2005a) Diagnosis of arterioportal fistulae in four dogs using computed tomographic angiography. *Veterinary Radiology and Ultrasound* **46**, 472–477

Zwingenberger AL and Schwarz T (2004) Dual phase angiography of the normal canine portal and hepatic vasculature. *Veterinary Radiology and Ultrasound* **45**, 117–124

Zwingenberger AL, Schwarz T and Saunders HM (2005b) Helical computed tomographic angiography of canine portosystemic shunts. *Veterinary Radiology and Ultrasound* **46**, 27–32

7

Abdominal lymph nodes

Helena Nyman

Introduction

Lymph nodes are part of the lymphatic system, which acts as a defence system, and are found throughout the body. Lymph nodes may become enlarged as a response to infection, inflammatory stimuli or secondary to invasion by other cells, as seen with primary neoplasia or metastases. An evaluation of the lymph nodes is therefore important for staging in all ongoing disease processes, particularly in cancer patients.

When an abnormal lymph node is encountered it is important to know which anatomical structures it drains to enable a closer evaluation of these regions. It is also important to know which lymph nodes to examine when a particular organ or region is diseased. Lymph nodes are located close to blood vessels and knowledge of the vessel distribution within the abdomen (Figure 7.1) allows the veterinary surgeon to routinely examine the regions where the major lymph nodes are located.

Normal abdominal lymph nodes

Anatomy and function

The main function of the lymph nodes is to filter the interstitial fluid (lymph) before it is returned to the venous blood system. In dogs and cats, they are usually bean-shaped and relatively flattened, solitary nodes. The lymph node parenchyma is divided into poorly defined cortical (paracortical and follicular) and medullary regions. The cortex is made up of lymphoid follicles, which consist of a germinal centre containing B lymphocytes, reticulum cells and histiocytes, and a peripheral area (paracortex) containing T lymphocytes. The paracortex is densely cellular and extends from the capsule to the corticomedullary junction.

Several afferent lymphatic vessels pass through the fibrous capsule surrounding the lymph node and drain into (subcapsular) marginal sinuses. Lymph then circulates through a complex cortical and medullary sinus network and exits through the efferent vessel in the hilar region, where the nodal artery and vein also enter and exit, respectively. The nodal artery gives rise to a rich microvascular network. The structure of a normal node is shown in Figure 7.2.

Tumour cells carried by the lymph may become trapped in the regional lymph nodes, where they will either be phagocytosed and destroyed or initiate metastases. Metastatic foci mainly invade the subcapsular sinus and the medullary sinus regions. In cases where tumour cells have escaped the filter of the lymph nodes and gained access to the blood stream, haematogenous metastases occur.

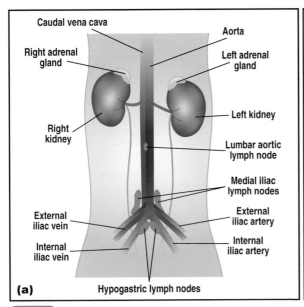

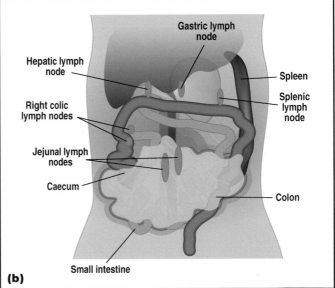

7.1 **(a)** Superficial visceral and **(b)** deep visceral abdominal lymph nodes in the dog.

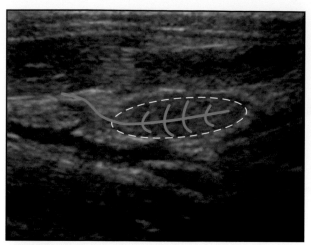

7.2 Ultrasonogram showing the vasculature of a normal lymph node.

Nodal macrophages line the sinus system and are found mostly in the medullary cords. When infectious agents or other noxious substances appear in the area drained by the lymph node, they stimulate hyperplasia of the lymph node with an increase in the size and number of reticular cells and macrophages. Plasma cells appear and lymphocytes and lymphoblasts increase in number. Overall the lymph node enlarges, resulting in stretching of the capsule. Enlargement can result in pain, which may be detected on clinical examination, particularly of the peripheral lymph nodes. The substances which have been phagocytosed in the lymph node are deposited in the reticular cells. The effectiveness of the lymph filter is dependent on the composition and amount of the noxious substance, and the period during which it continues to be present in the node. As more elements are presented, the probability that some of them will escape phagocytosis or binding is increased.

Regional lymph nodes control the 'primary lymph' of an organ or body region. Disease involvement of regional lymph nodes may, therefore, indicate that the preceding organ may be diseased. However, as lymph nodes are placed in chains interconnected by lymphatic vessels, an abdominal lymph node can receive both primary lymph from its own draining area and secondary lymph from a preceding lymph node. Sometimes the afferent vessels bypass the nearest lymph node and enter the node next to it. As there are interconnections between groups of nodes lying at the same level, there may be a bypass of lymph in the horizontal plane as well. This can increase the number of filtration points through which the lymph has to pass, which expands the body's defence capacity, but may also encourage the spread of disease processes along the lymphatic route.

Nomenclature

The nomenclature of lymph nodes is based on location (Figure 7.3). Four lymphocentres drain the abdominal viscera, the dorsal abdominal wall and the organs arising in the lumbar area. In the pelvic cavity, the iliosacral lymphocentre includes all the nodes at the aortic bifurcation and below the pelvic surface of the sacrum. It is responsible for drainage of the pelvic region and is a secondary draining area for all lymphocentres in the hind part of the animal.

Lymphocentre	Number of lymph nodes	Presence	Draining area in dogs	Draining area in cats
Lumbar				
Aortic	2–17 (dogs) 2–12 (cats)	Present	Ribs, last thoracic and all lumbar vertebrae, lumbar and abdominal musculature, mediastinum, pleura, peritoneum, liver, adrenal glands, urogenitalia, aorta, spinal meninges, caudal mesenteric and iliosacral lymph nodes	Diaphragm, adrenal glands, urogenitalia, dorsal abdominal wall, iliofemoral, coeliac, cranial and caudal mesenteric lymph nodes
Coeliac				
Splenic	1–5 (dogs) 1–3 (cats)	Present	Oesophagus, stomach, spleen, pancreas, liver, diaphragm, mediastinum, omentum, gastric lymph node	Spleen, greater curvature of the stomach, left lobe of the pancreas
Gastric	1 (dogs) 1–4 (cats)	Variable	Oesophagus, stomach, liver, diaphragm, mesentery, peritoneum	Oesophagus, stomach, liver
Hepatic	3–8 (dogs) 2–4 (cats)	Present	Liver, gallbladder, stomach, pancreas, duodenum (mediastinum, oesophagus, diaphragm, peritoneum), gastric and pancreaticoduodenal lymph nodes	Oesophagus, diaphragm, liver, greater curvature of the stomach, body and left lobe of the pancreas, duodenum
Pancreaticoduodenal	1–3	Present	Greater omentum, pancreas, duodenum, stomach	Pylorus, duodenum, body and right lobe of the pancreas
Cranial mesenteric				
Jejunal	2 (dogs) 2–20 (cats)	Present	Jejunum, ileum, pancreas	Small intestines, body of the pancreas, caudal mesenteric lymph nodes
Caecal	1–3	Present		Caecum, ileum, colic lymph nodes
Colic	1–2 (dogs) 3–9 (cats)	Present	Ileum, caecum, colon, caudal mesenteric lymph nodes	Ileum, caecum, colon, caudal mesenteric and jejunal lymph nodes

7.3 The different lymphocentres of the abdominal and pelvic cavity and the associated lymph nodes. (continues) ▶

Lymphocentre	Number of lymph nodes	Presence	Draining area in dogs	Draining area in cats
Caudal mesenteric				
Caudal mesenteric	2–5 (dogs) 1–3 (cats)	Present	Colon, rectum	Descending colon, rectum
Iliosacral				
Medial iliac	2–3	Present	Colon, rectum, urogenitalia (excluding kidneys), aorta, spinal meninges, abdominal musculature, as well as skin, musculature and skeleton of the hind part	Colon, rectum, urogenitalia (excluding kidneys), aorta, spinal meninges, abdominal musculature, as well as skin, musculature and skeleton of the hind part
Sacral	1–2	Present	Colon, rectum, urogenitalia (excluding kidneys), spinal meninges, lumbar vertebrae, sacrum, tail, certain areas of the thigh, pelvic bones, femur, deep inguinal lymph nodes	Colon, rectum, urogenitalia (excluding kidneys), spinal meninges, lumbar vertebrae, sacrum, tail, certain areas of the thigh, pelvic bones, femur, deep inguinal lymph nodes

7.3 (continued) The different lymphocentres of the abdominal and pelvic cavity and the associated lymph nodes.

Abdominal and pelvic lymph nodes can be divided into visceral and parietal groups, according to the area they drain. The visceral lymph nodes include the jejunal, hepatic (Figure 7.4), splenic (Figure 7.5), colic and caudal mesenteric, and less consistently the gastric and pancreaticoduodenal (Figure 7.6), nodes. The parietal lymph nodes include the aortic, medial iliac, hypogastric, sacral and iliofemoral nodes.

- The jejunal lymph nodes are the largest of the abdominal nodes, often referred to as the cranial mesenteric lymph nodes. They are variable in length, with an average of about 1 cm in medium sized dogs. These lymph nodes usually occur as two elongated structures along the cranial mesenteric vascular tree, near the root of the mesentery (Figure 7.7ab), but are also seen more peripherally in the omentum (Figure 7.7c).
- The right colic lymph nodes are located at the junction of the ileum and colon (Figure 7.8). They are typically 2–3 mm in diameter and relatively round.

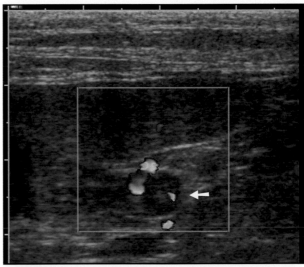

7.5 A normal splenic lymph node (arrowed) next to the splenic vein. Colour Doppler ultrasonography often aids in the detection of lymph nodes as they are always found close to a vessel and also enables distinction of small lymph nodes from vessels and other structures. A small vessel is seen entering the lymph node in the hilar region.

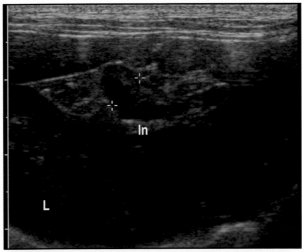

7.4 A normal hepatic lymph node (ln) in a cat, with an oval shape and an echogenic hilus, just caudal to the liver (L).

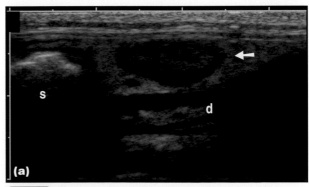

7.6 Normal pancreaticoduodenal lymph nodes (arrowed) in **(a)** a cat. This lymph node is not always visible. The lymph nodes are oval and isoechoic compared with the surrounding organs. d = Duodenum; s = Stomach. (continues) ▶

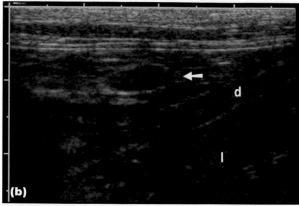

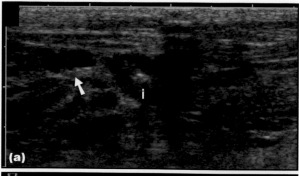

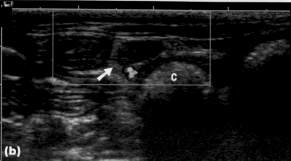

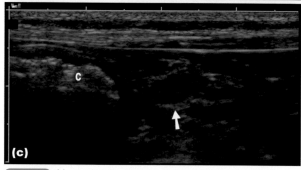

7.6 (continued) Normal pancreaticoduodenal lymph nodes (arrowed) in **(b)** a dog. This lymph node is not always visible. The lymph nodes are oval and isoechoic compared with the surrounding organs. d = Duodenum; l = Liver.

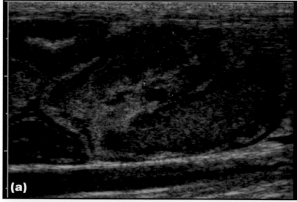

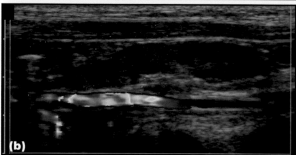

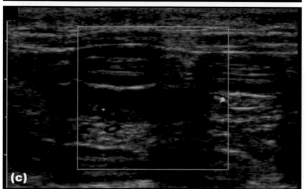

7.7 Normal cranial mesenteric lymph nodes. These nodes are variable in length and the whole node can often not be imaged in one plane due to their elongated, often curving, shape. **(a,b)** These lymph nodes are most commonly located near the root of the mesentery, but **(c)** they may also be seen more peripherally in the omentum. Normal nodes have small amounts of hilar flow or appear avascular.

7.8 Normal colic lymph nodes (arrowed) in **(a)** a cat and **(b,c)** a dog. These lymph nodes are seen next to (a) the ileum and (b, c) the colon. These lymph nodes are small (<4 mm), oval, isoechoic and have an echogenic hilus. Vessels may be used as landmarks to detect the lymph nodes. C = Colon; i = Ileum.

- The left and right medial iliac lymph nodes are similar in appearance but can vary in number. They are located adjacent to the lateral margins of the caudal aorta and corresponding external iliac artery (Figure 7.9). The lymph nodes extend cranially to the deep circumflex iliac vessels and caudally to the level of the branching of the external and internal iliac vessels. The left medial iliac lymph node is often found more ventrally than the right.
- Aortic lymph nodes (Figure 7.10) are located throughout the length of the aorta (cranial to the medial iliac lymph nodes), whilst the hypogastric lymph nodes lie in the angle between the internal iliac vessels and the median sacral artery (caudal to the medial iliac lymph nodes). These lymph nodes are small, round, variably numbered and not always detected unless enlarged. If the lymph nodes are difficult to find, it may be useful to localize the blood vessels in the region of interest and thereafter look for the node as they are usually located close to vessels.

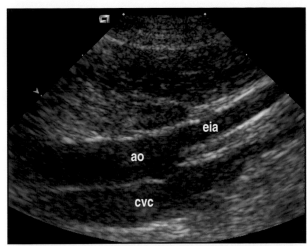

7.9 Normal medial iliac lymph node in a dog, located near the aortic bifurcation of the caudal aorta. These lymph nodes are almost always visible. ao = Aorta; cvc = Caudal vena cava; eia = External iliac artery.

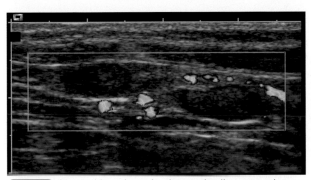

7.10 Normal lymph nodes located adjacent to the aorta. These are variable in number and often small. They may be difficult to detect when normal in size. Colour Doppler ultrasonography may aid in the detection and distinction of normal lymph nodes from vessels and surrounding tissues (e.g. fat).

Size

A difficult diagnostic problem is the question of the 'normal size' of the abdominal lymph nodes. There is great variation in the number and size of lymph nodes both between species, within the same species, and even individual differences between one side of the body and the other. Interpretation of the examination often depends on the personal experience of the examiner.

The accurate identification and characterization of lymph nodes by diagnostic imaging has important therapeutic and prognostic significance in patients with newly diagnosed cancers. The TNM classification, developed by the World Health Organization, is the worldwide accepted and used system for categorizing and staging solid tumours.

- T = tumour size and local tumour invasion.
- N = the extent of metastatic spread to lymph nodes.
- M = solid metastases in distant organs.

The important role of diagnostic imaging is, first, to provide accurate pre-treatment staging of the tumour for planning medical, surgical and radiation interventions and, second, to monitor response to therapy and provide surveillance after curative treatment.

Due to their small size, normal lymph nodes are not visible on abdominal radiographs. Most of the above mentioned lymph nodes can be visualized by ultrasonography with some practice. Computed tomography (CT), magnetic resonance imaging (MRI) and lymphoscintigraphy are other modalities that can be used to detect abdominal lymph nodes.

Radiographic features of abdominal lymph nodes

Normal lymph nodes

Normal lymph nodes are not seen on radiographs. Their small size and opacity make them indistinguishable from the surrounding organs and peritoneal fat.

Abnormal lymph nodes

Enlargement

Enlargement of lymph nodes occurs with a wide spectrum of neoplastic and inflammatory aetiologies (Figure 7.11). The mass effect caused by an enlarged lymph node may be minimal and go undetected. Of the lymph nodes that cause a distinctive radiographic mass effect, only those in the mid-abdomen (visceral group) and caudal retroperitoneum (medial iliac, hypogastric and sacral) are seen commonly. Enlargement of lymph nodes in the visceral group, especially the jejunal lymph nodes, causes a mass effect in the mid-abdomen and centrifugal displacement of the small intestines. This lack of apparent sidedness is classic, although not specific, for jejunal (cranial mesenteric) adenopathy. Other differential diagnoses for a central abdominal mass are covered in Chapter 8. Rarely are the borders of the lymph node accurately detected, even in the most severe cases.

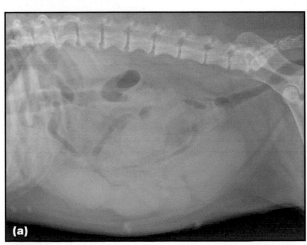

7.11 Enlarged sublumbar lymph nodes due to different disease processes. **(a)** The soft tissue mass in the sublumbar area of this dog is a reactively enlarged lymph node, most likely secondary to pyometra. However, the diagnosis needs to be verified with cytology and/or biopsy. *(continues)* ▶

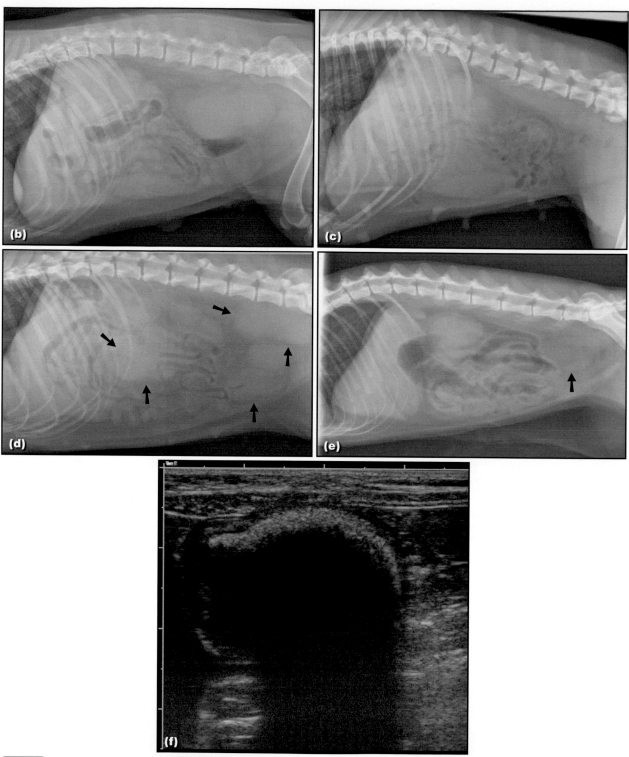

7.11 (continued) Enlarged sublumbar lymph nodes due to different disease processes. **(b)** Ventral displacement of the colon is common with enlarged sublumbar lymph nodes; in this case a metastatic lymph node secondary to an anal gland carcinoma. **(c)** This dog has generalized lymphadenopathy due to multicentric lymphoma. However, the radiograph only shows signs of sublumbar node enlargement, demonstrating the low sensitivity of abdominal radiography in detecting abnormal lymph nodes. **(d)** This dog has three soft tissue masses within the abdomen (arrowed). Firstly, the mass visible in the sublumbar area is a medial iliac lymph node containing metastases of a carcinoma in the colon. Secondly, the colon is displaced ventrally and the soft tissue mass superimposed over it is a carcinoma originating from the wall of the colon. Thirdly, there is a visible mass within the mid-abdomen. Gas-filled small intestinal loops are seen partly superimposed over the soft tissue mass. It is not possible to determine the origin of this mass with radiography alone, but the presence of an enlarged mesenteric lymph node was confirmed by ultrasonography. Cytology confirmed metastatic involvement of this lymph node. **(e)** Soft tissue mass (arrowed) in the caudal abdomen of a cat. The mass is partly superimposed upon the colon. An enlarged sublumbar lymph node may be suspected from this radiograph; however, if this were the case, the colon would be expected to be displaced ventrally. **(f)** Same cat as in (e). Ultrasonography confirmed that the mass was a granuloma, involving the wall of the colon, due to feline infectious peritonitis.

Enlargement of lymph nodes in the caudal dorsal retroperitoneal space (i.e. the parietal group) is detected at an earlier stage as there are fewer organs in this region and the surrounding fat provides contrast. Usually the dorsal border of the enlarged lymph node suffers from border effacement with the adjacent hypaxial musculature, but the remaining borders often are distinct. A mass effect in this region is detected by ventral displacement of the terminal descending colon and border effacement of the adjacent aorta and caudal vena cava. Superimposition of the sartorius and gluteal muscles, localized free fluid and other masses in this region can mimic adenopathy.

The most common cause of radiographically evident adenopathy is neoplasia. Additional imaging and biopsy, most commonly with ultrasonography, are usually indicated to verify suspected adenopathy, provide a pathological diagnosis and to stage underlying disease conditions. Rather than discussing particular organs of origin that cause medial iliac adenopathy, it may be more helpful to consider regions of the body draining to this group of lymph nodes, which include:

- Pelvic canal:
  - Prostate gland
  - Urethra
  - Vagina
  - Rectum.
- Perineum:
  - Anal gland
  - Circumanal glands
  - Perineal skin surface.
- Hindlimbs.

However, adenopathy may also result from multicentric neoplasia, including:

- Lymphoma
- Systemic histiocytic neoplasia
- Other round cell malignancies (mast cell tumour, myeloma).

Although beyond the scope of this Chapter, it is certainly worth commenting on the sternal lymph nodes (Figure 7.12). They are located in the cranial ventral mediastinum and are part of the parietal group of intrathoracic lymph nodes. The sternal lymph nodes drain many organs of the cranial abdomen, including the liver, stomach, pancreas, duodenum and spleen, and the mammary gland tissue. In fact, these lymph nodes may be the most common drainage site for many neoplasms of the organs in the cranial abdomen and the mammary gland tissue, and may also become enlarged with concurrent haemoabdomen. Enlargement of the sternal lymph node may be seen with peritonitis. Ultrasonographic appraisal of the sternal lymph nodes is an important addition to the complete evaluation of the abdomen, especially when concurrent mass lesions are noted in the cranial abdomen.

Mineralization
Changes other than enlargement are rare in the abdominal lymph nodes. However, mineralization may occasionally be seen in association with:

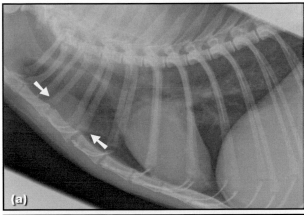

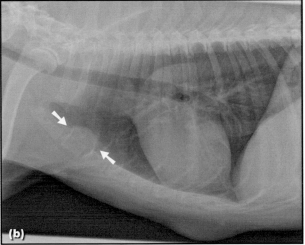

7.12 Lateral thoracic radiographs of **(a)** a cat and **(b)** a dog with sternal lymphadenopathy. The increased soft tissue opacity (arrowed), centred dorsal to S3 in the cat and dorsal to S2 in the dog, represents enlarged sternal lymph nodes. Enlarged sternal lymph nodes may suggest mammary gland disease or disease processes within the abdomen.

- Chronic pyogranulomatous disease
- Atypical fungal and mycobacterial infections, which can cause dystrophic mineralization of the thoracic and abdominal lymph nodes
- Metastatic mineralization, which can occur in any organ of the body with chronic severe hypercalcaemia or uraemia, although most commonly seen in the descending abdominal aorta, kidneys and gastric mucosa
- Metastatic adenopathy, which may be evident histologically but is rarely apparent radiographically
- Prostatic carcinoma, osteosarcoma and other primary neoplasms.

Barium accumulation is uncommon but very opaque in affected lymph nodes. Most commonly this is seen in the tracheobronchial lymph nodes of the thorax following pulmonary aspiration during a positive-contrast study, although any draining visceral abdominal lymph node could accumulate extravasated barium from free peritoneal barium.

Ultrasonographic features of lymph nodes

Ultrasonography is an excellent imaging modality for detection and evaluation of lymph nodes, as it enables real-time evaluation in a non-invasive way. The energy wavelength used to image an object is the fundamental limitation of the spatial resolution. A high-frequency linear transducer is therefore recommended for evaluating small structures such as lymph nodes. Lower frequency transducers have less spatial resolution, but better penetrating properties, and may therefore be required for imaging the more deeply seated abdominal lymph nodes in larger dogs.

Ultrasonography using greyscale, Doppler techniques and contrast media can be used to evaluate characteristics of abdominal lymph nodes such as size, shape, echogenicity, echopattern, margins, acoustic transmission, vascularization and perfusion parameters.

Size and shape

Evaluation of size is usually performed in at least two dimensions. However, due to the variable length of lymph nodes in different locations, the width is more commonly used. There are no published reference values regarding the normal size of abdominal lymph nodes evaluated by ultrasonography in dogs and cats. Normal lymph nodes are usually oval or slender in shape (see Figure 7.7). In the author's experience, most normal lymph nodes are up to a few millimetres wide, depending on the location.

Most inflammatory diseases involve the lymph nodes diffusely, thereby preserving their normal shape. However, neoplastic infiltration of lymph nodes occurs primarily in the cortex, which often results in a greater transverse diameter in these nodes. Eccentric cortical hypertrophy (Figure 7.13) may be a useful sign to indicate focal tumour infiltration. Malignant nodes include metastatic and lymphomatous nodes. A quantitative means of assessing lymph node shape is the short axis to long axis (S/L) ratio. For superficial lymph nodes it has been found that the S/L ratio is usually <0.7 in normal or enlarged benign lymph nodes. An increased S/L ratio is usually seen when lymph nodes are enlarged secondary to malignant disease. However, the diagnostic accuracy of enlarged lymph nodes alone is limited.

Echogenicity

Echogenicity is the subjective evaluation of the greyscale of the tissue of interest compared with the surrounding tissue. Normal echogenicity of lymph nodes is generally described as isoechoic or slightly hypoechoic (Figure 7.14) and with a uniform echopattern or texture. Normal lymph nodes cannot

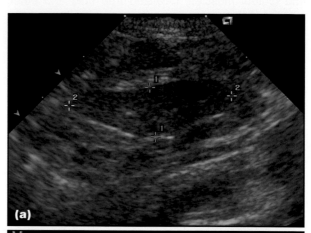

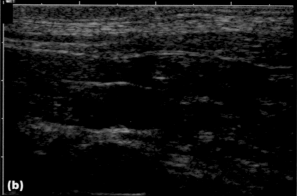

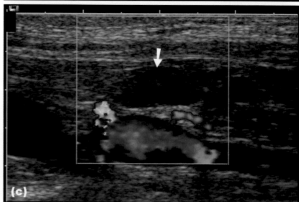

7.14 Normal mesenteric lymph nodes in two dogs. **(a)** This lymph node is almost isoechoic compared with the surrounding fatty tissue, which may make the detection and identification of the lymph node more difficult. **(b)** In cases where the lymph node is similar to the surrounding tissue, it may be helpful to use **(c)** Doppler ultrasonography, as lymph nodes are always found close to vessels. Vascularity may also be detected within the suspicious node, thereby differentiating the lymph node from the surrounding fat. In this case a small hilar signal was seen (arrowed).

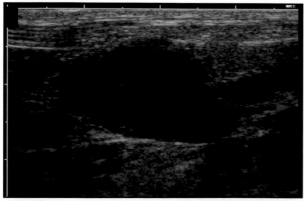

7.13 An enlarged medial iliac lymph node in a dog with a metastatic mammary gland carcinoma. The node is asymmetrically thickened, hypoechoic compared with the surrounding tissue, and without a visible echogenic hilus.

always be detected due to the echogenic similarities with the surrounding fatty tissue. Abnormal lymph nodes are often hypoechoic or anechoic and with a non-uniform echopattern (especially with areas of necrosis that may yield distal acoustic enhancement) (Figures 7.15 to 7.18).

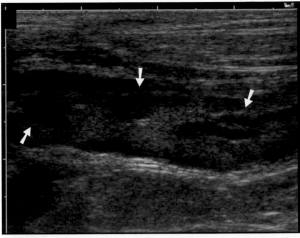

7.17 Lymphadenitis in a mesenteric lymph node of a dog. The node is isoechoic with a hypoechoic rim and has a normal shape. Note the focal hypoechoic areas with echoic bands within them (arrowed). This pattern may be seen with lymphadenitis.

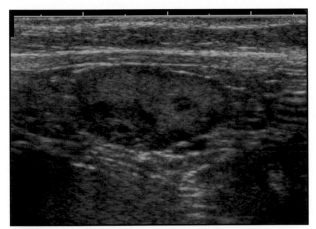

7.15 Enlarged colic lymph node in a cat with feline infectious peritonitis. The lymph node is isoechoic with a hypoechoic rim, and contains a few focal hypoechoic areas that result in a heterogenous echopattern. This appearance is not uncommonly seen, particularly with lymphadenitis. A similar appearance is shown in Figure 7.16.

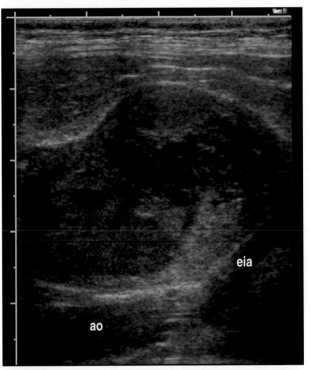

7.18 Enlarged medial iliac lymph node in a dog. The node has a heterogenous echopattern with both hypo- and hyperechoic areas. The hypoechoic area corresponded to necrosis on histopathology. ao = Aorta; eia = External iliac artery.

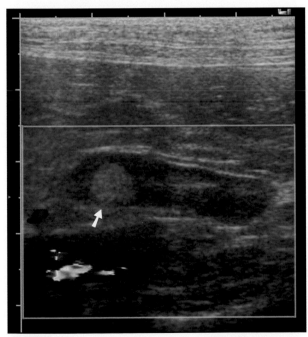

7.16 Medial iliac lymph node in a dog with pyometra. The node is slightly enlarged but has maintained a normal shape. It is hypoechoic compared with the surrounding tissue with an echogenic hilus. An echoic nodule (arrowed) is visible at the cranial pole. There is no detectable blood flow within the node. Fine-needle aspiration of the node showed reactive hyperplasia. It is not certain whether the echoic nodule itself was sampled separately. This appearance may suggest necrosis or an accumulation of fat, but cytology and/or histopathology are required for verification of the diagnosis.

The overall relatively low echogenicity of lymph nodes may be due to the fact that the nodal cortex consists predominantly of homogenous solid tissue with few lymph sinuses. Necrosis can cause both hypo- and hyperechoic areas within the node and may be present in both inflammatory and neoplastic nodes. This may explain why echogenicity on its own cannot be used to differentiate benign from malignant nodes. However, lymph nodes with cystic necrosis are suggestive of malignancy and are not uncommonly seen in metastases from squamous cell carcinomas.

A hyperechoic hilus can be present or absent in both normal and abnormal nodes. It is thought to be the result of reflective surfaces of fat in the hilar region of the node. There is a tendency for this to be more commonly seen in benign rather than malignant nodes. Larger lymphoma nodes are less likely to show a hilus, perhaps due to infiltration by lymphoblasts.

Margins
Border definition can be described as a combination of shape and sharpness of the involved borders. An irregular border may be suggestive of invasive growth and could therefore be interpreted as a sign of malignancy. A sharp border may be seen as a result of a sudden change in acoustic impedance between two tissue structures, whilst a more gradual change in acoustic impedance between two tissue structures would result in a less sharp border definition. Metastatic nodes usually have a sharp border, which may be due to the replacement of normal tissue by the infiltrating tumour cells. Normal nodes often have a less distinct border, which makes them more difficult to delineate.

Acoustic transmission
The transmission of echoes through a lymph node may provide information on tissue composition. Fluid-filled lesions often result in distal acoustic enhancement (Figure 7.19) whilst dense structures, such as bone or mineralization, produce acoustic shadowing. In lesions containing both types of tissue, a mixed acoustic transmission pattern may be seen. Lymph nodes that are fluid-filled or mineralized are considered abnormal. Fluid-filled regions can represent areas of tissue necrosis, abscess or cyst formation. Mineralization is generally dystrophic, insinuating chronicity of either a reactive or metastatic lymph node.

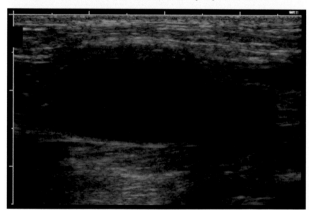

7.19 Medial iliac lymph node in a dog with a metastatic carcinoma. The node is hypoechoic with a slightly asymmetrical enlargement. Note the distal acoustic enhancement, which is often seen in lymph nodes containing necrosis.

Vascularization
Doppler ultrasonography can be used to demonstrate the presence, number, distribution and architecture of blood vessels within lymph nodes. Normal vascular structures within nodes are characterized by an orderly arrangement of branching arteries. Colour Doppler and power Doppler ultrasonography have been shown to be useful in differentiating benign from malignant nodes, primarily based on patterns of vascular distribution within the node. The vascular patterns can be divided into three main groups: hilar; peripheral; and mixed hilar and peripheral. The hilus represents the natural entry site for blood vessels to the lymph node.

- Normal lymph nodes predominantly have a small amount of hilar vascularity (Figure 7.20) or appear avascular.
- Reactive lymph nodes tend to have a prominent hilar vascularity, thought to be due to an increase in vessel diameter and blood flow (Figure 7.21).

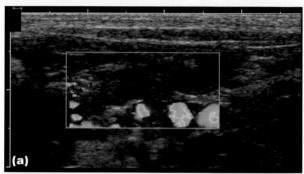

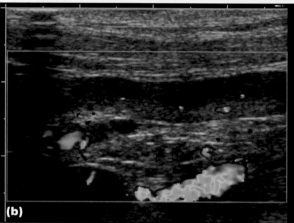

7.20 **(a)** Normal ileocolic lymph node in a cat. **(b)** Normal mesenteric lymph node in a dog. Note that in both cases the lymph nodes are located close to vessels and that a small amount of hilar flow is present in the nodes, which is a typical vascular pattern in normal nodes.

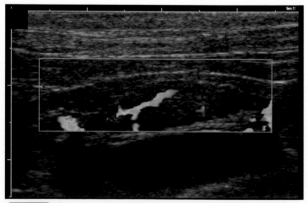

7.21 Reactive hyperplasia in a medial iliac lymph node in a dog with pyometra. The node is oval, slightly hypoechoic and with a moderate amount of primarily hilar flow, which is typically seen with reactive hyperplasia and lymphadenitis.

- Metastatic lymph nodes often have a peripheral perfusion pattern (Figure 7.22). The increase in peripheral nodal vascularity may be due to the initial deposition of tumour cells in the marginal and medullary sinuses, which induces aberrant feeding vessels in the periphery of the tumour nests by tumour angiogenesis.
  Neovascularization is needed to enable growth of tumours or metastases beyond a diameter of a few millimetres.
- As tumour infiltration of the node progresses, increased vascularity is sometimes seen in both the central and peripheral zones of the node (Figure 7.23). A mixed hilar and peripheral perfusion pattern may be seen in both lymphoma nodes and some metastatic nodes, and to a lesser extent with reactive hyperplasia.

Vessel morphology suggestive of malignancy, which may be detected by ultrasonography includes:

- Irregular vessel diameters
- Atypical branching patterns
- Blind-ending vessels
- Focal absence of perfusion (Figure 7.24)
- Displacement of hilar vessels
- Subcapsular vessels (Figure 7.25).

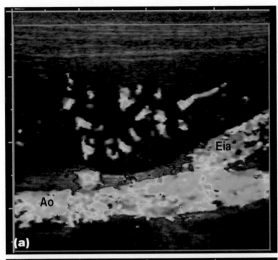

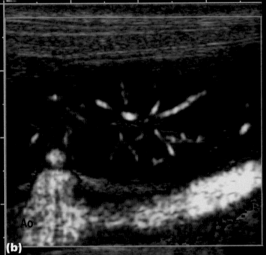

7.23 Medial iliac lymph node in a dog with lymphoma. The node is richly vascularized with a mixed hilar and peripheral pattern, typical of lymphoma nodes. **(a)** Colour Doppler ultrasonogram of the lymph node. **(b)** Power Doppler ultrasonogram of the same node. Power Doppler ultrasonography is more sensitive in detecting flow in small vessels with slow flow, thereby often showing more vessels than seen on colour Doppler ultrasonography. However, the technique is more sensitive to blooming artefacts caused by motion. Therefore, it may often be easier to use colour Doppler ultrasonography, particularly in conscious animals. Ao = Aorta; Eia = External iliac artery.

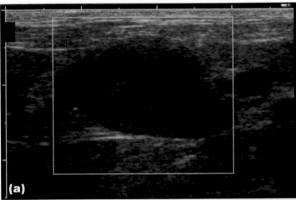

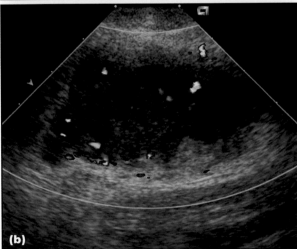

7.22 **(a)** Metastatic medial iliac lymph node in a dog with mammary gland carcinoma. **(b)** Metastatic lymph node within the omentum, secondary to an adenocarcinoma of the small intestine. Both nodes are hypoechoic and show primarily a peripheral vascular pattern, typical of metastatic nodes. Note that some of the smaller blue colour signals in (b) are artefacts (noise).

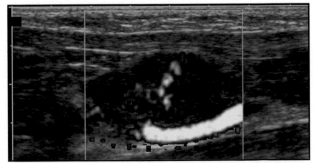

7.24 Metastatic colonic lymph node in a cat with neoplasia. The node is richly vascularized with a mixed vascular pattern. There is no detected vascularity in the caudal pole of the node. It is not uncommon to find areas of hypoperfusion in metastatic nodes. Areas of hypoperfusion may correspond to areas of necrosis.

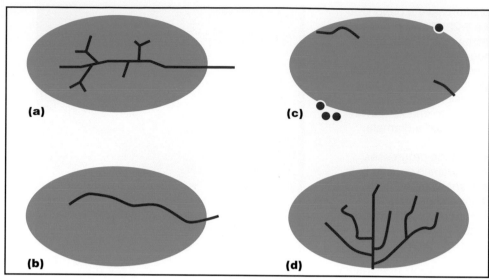

7.25 Different vascular patterns that may be seen in lymph nodes. **(a)** Normal vascularity with a hilar pattern. **(b)** Displacement of the hilar vessel, which may be seen due to deposits of cells within the node secondary to, for example, metastases. **(c)** Peripheral and subcapsular vessels are typical of malignant nodes as metastases are primarily seen in the peripheral areas of the nodes initially. **(d)** Aberrant feeding vessels are also a sign of malignancy.

Spatial resolution of colour Doppler ultrasonography is sufficient to distinguish adjacent extranodal vessels from peripheral intranodal vessels by rotation of the scanning plane in most cases, but when in doubt a vessel has to be regarded as extranodal. If there are only short intranodal vessel segments or single colour spots, Doppler spectral analysis may be used to distinguish between colour artefacts and flow signals.

The pulse repetition frequency and the cut-off frequency of the high-pass filters have to be decreased to the minimum values in order to detect very low flow velocities. Colour Doppler ultrasonography can measure flow in vessels as small as arterioles, depending on depth. Vessels can remain invisible to Doppler ultrasonography if they are too small, too deep, at a suboptimal angle to the beam, or have a blood flow velocity that is too slow to discriminate it from tissue motion.

Vascular flow indices

Spectral waveform analysis of the Doppler shift can be used to determine flow indices within blood vessels (Figure 7.26). The flow indices most commonly used are:

- The resistive index (RI)

  $$RI = \frac{\text{peak systolic velocity} - \text{end diastolic velocity}}{\text{peak systolic velocity}}$$

- The pulsatility index (PI)

  $$PI = \frac{\text{peak systolic velocity} - \text{end diastolic velocity}}{\text{time-averaged maximum velocity}}$$

In combination with other ultrasonography parameters, the use of RI and PI have proven to aid detection of nodal malignancy. This builds on the theory that vascular resistance in vessels of inflamed lymph nodes may be decreased due to vasodilatation, and vascular resistance in the vessels of lymph nodes involved with metastases may be increased due to compression by tumour cells and/or tumour-evoked angiogenesis. Normal nodes and reactively enlarged

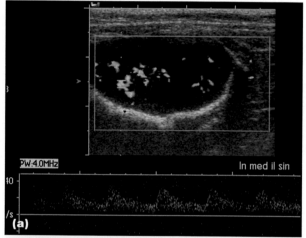

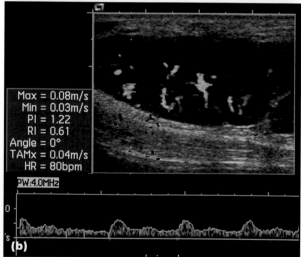

7.26 Spectral Doppler ultrasonography can be used to measure flow velocities in vessels and to calculate the resistive index (RI) and the pulsatility index (PI). **(a)** The actual values for RI and PI are not shown in this image; however, the tracing shows that the velocity within the vessel is high, suggesting that the RI and PI will also be high. This finding is commonly seen with malignancy. **(b)** The RI and PI may vary in a lymphoma node but are often found to be around the same values as benign nodes, as seen here.

nodes often have a RI <0.65 and a PI <1.45, whilst metastatic nodes often have a RI >0.65 and a PI >1.45. Lack of detectable perfusion by Doppler ultrasonography makes the distinction between benign and malignant nodes more difficult as the distribution of blood flow and the PI are two of the more useful parameters in the differentiation of benign and malignant lymph nodes.

As there is an overlap between the presence and absence of the different parameters for benign and malignant lymph nodes, it is necessary to use a combination of criteria when evaluating lymph nodes. If size, distribution of blood flow within the node and the PI are used in combination, it is possible to correctly classify lymph nodes approximately 75% of the time into one of the following four groups:

- Normal
- Reactive
- Lymphoma
- Metastatic.

Ultrasonography is particularly useful for distinguishing normal from reactive lymph nodes, and normal from lymphoma nodes. Metastatic lymph nodes are more difficult to identify, particularly those with early metastases, before the node enlarges and changes in morphology and vascularity can be detected. Ultrasonographic characteristics that can be used to differentiate benign and malignant nodes are summarized in Figure 7.27, and examples of the appearance on ultrasonography are given in Figures 7.28 to 7.33.

Characteristic	Type of lymph node		
	Metastatic	*Lymphoma*	*Benign*
Shape	Round	Round	Oval
Short axis to long axis (S/L) ratio	>0.7	>0.7	<0.7
Hilus	Narrow or absent	Narrow or absent	Usually present
Echogenicity	Often hypoechoic	Hypo(an)echoic	Isoechoic
Border	Sharp	Sharp	Varied
Posterior enhancement	Often present	Often present	Usually absent
Blood flow distribution	Primarily peripheral or mixed	Mixed	Hilar
Resistive index (RI)	High, >0.65	Often low, <0.65	Low, <0.65
Pulsatility index (PI)	High, >1.45	Often low, <1.45	Low, <1.45

7.27 Ultrasonographic characteristics of metastatic, lymphoma and benign lymphadenopathy.

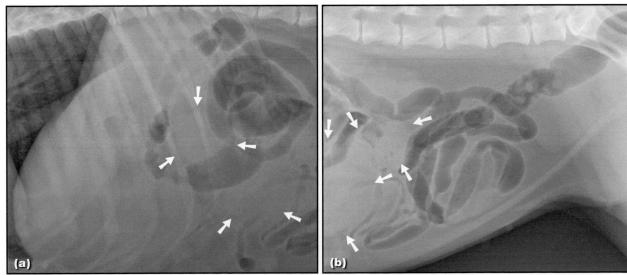

(a) (b)

7.28 Lymph nodes are rarely seen on radiographs unless severely enlarged. **(a,b)** Lateral radiographs of the abdomen of a Great Dane. Note that there are several soft tissue opacities within the abdomen (arrowed).
(continues) ▶

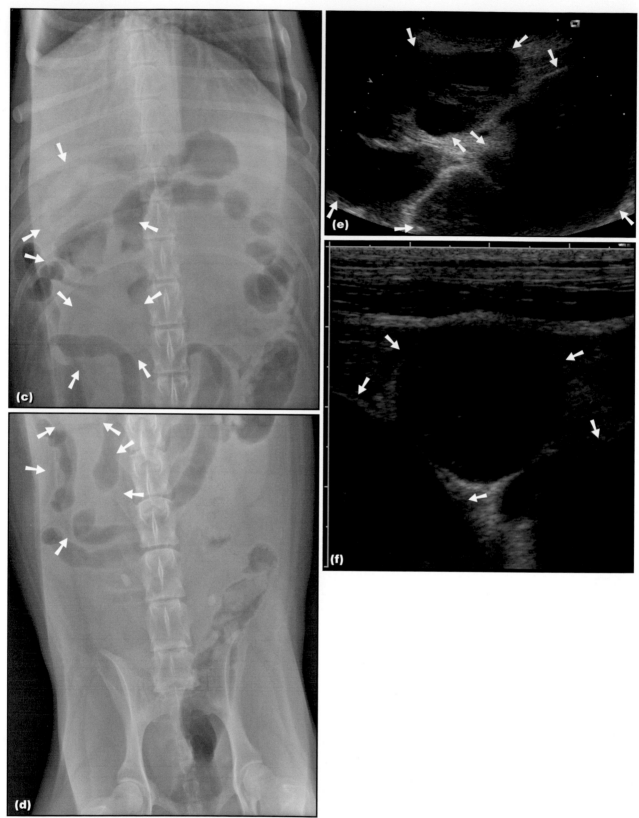

7.28 (continued) Lymph nodes are rarely seen on radiographs unless severely enlarged. **(c,d)** VD radiographs of the abdomen of a Great Dane. The three soft tissue opacities are seen on the right-hand side of the abdomen (arrowed). It is not possible to determine the origin of these opacities by radiography alone, although there was a strong suspicion that one of them would be the right kidney and the other two could be enlarged lymph nodes. This diagnosis was verified by ultrasonography. **(e,f)** Typical ultrasonographic appearance of lymphoma nodes. (e) Two mesenteric nodes (arrowed) and (f) lymph nodes caudal to the liver on the right-hand side (arrowed). The nodes are severely enlarged, asymmetrical in size and outline, markedly hypoechoic, and with clearly defined borders towards the surrounding tissue. As involvement of several lymph nodes is common in animals with lymphoma, it may be helpful to evaluate the surrounding nodes. If several lymph nodes with these characteristics are identified, it is almost certain that lymphoma is present.

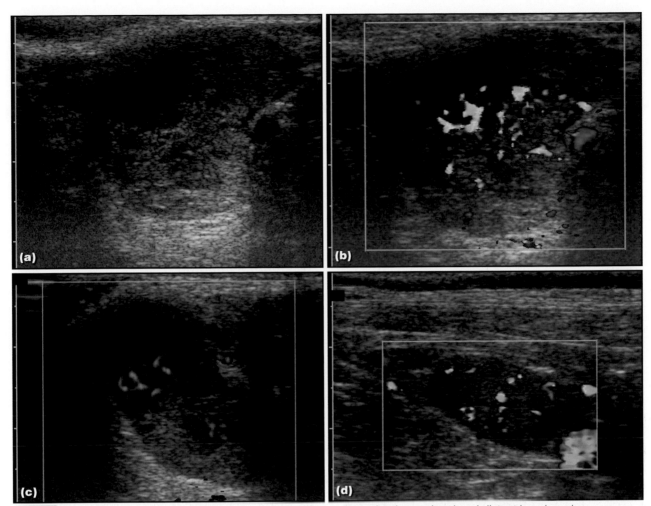

7.29 Dog with a recurring grade II mastocytoma that has metastasized to regional and distant lymph nodes. Metastases were found in **(a–c)** the popliteal lymph node, the inguinal nodes and **(d)** the medial iliac nodes. (a) The popliteal node is severely enlarged, around three times its normal size. It has a heterogenous echogenicity and echopattern. There are ill defined hypoechoic areas, which may represent areas of necrosis or tumour growth. Distal acoustic enhancement is present. (b) Colour Doppler ultrasonographic evaluation of the same node shows rich vascularization. There is an increased amount of vascularity in the periphery of the hypoechoic region. (c) This can be seen even more clearly with the use of power Doppler ultrasonography. This finding suggests that the hypoechoic area may represent an area of growing metastases, which may have induced local angiogenesis. (d) Metastases were also found in the medial iliac nodes. This node is not as enlarged as the popliteal node. It is hypoechoic and well defined, but has an increased amount of flow with a mainly peripheral distribution, which may suggest malignancy. However, the diagnosis should still be verified by cytology and/or pathology.

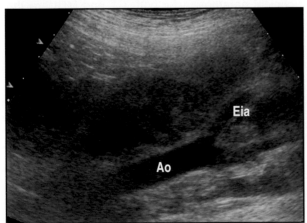

7.30 Medial iliac lymph node in a dog with generalized multiple myeloma. The metastatic node is severely enlarged, hypoechoic and has an irregularly outlined border. It is not possible to distinguish between different types of malignancy based on the results of ultrasonography. Ao = Aorta; Eia = External iliac artery.

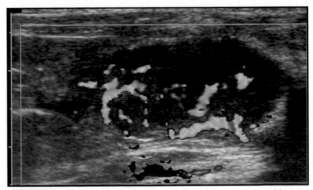

7.31 Caudal mesenteric lymph node in a cat with a metastatic adenocarcinoma in the descending colon. The node is hypoechoic and well delineated from the surrounding tissue. Distal acoustic enhancement is present. The node is richly vascularized with a mixed hilar and peripheral flow. There is no detectable blood flow in the ventral portion of the node and this may represent a region of hypoperfusion, commonly seen in areas of necrosis.

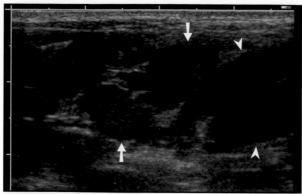

7.32 Normal to slightly prominent colic lymph nodes (arrowed) in a puppy with local inflammation of the caudal part of the ileum (arrowheads). Lymph nodes are often more prominent in young individuals and are therefore considered within normal limits in this case.

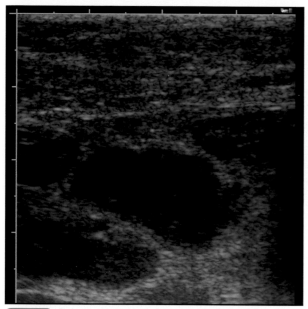

7.33 Enlarged hypoechoic mesenteric lymph nodes in a cat with multicentric lymphoma. The border of the lymph node is slightly irregular and there is no detectable echoic hilus.

Overview of additional imaging modalities

Contrast-enhanced ultrasonography

Contrast media can be used to enhance signals from small vessels, which may lead to better visualization of general vessel topography by showing smaller vessels and perfusion characteristics more clearly. Ultrasonography contrast media are blood pool agents and consist of tiny membrane-stabilized microbubbles containing gas, which scatter the ultrasound wave energy in all directions. This technique allows detection of vessels as small as approximately 40 μm, and enhances sentinel nodes as small as 3 mm. Contrast-specific harmonic imaging doubles the number of secondary and tertiary branching vessels detected within superficial lymph nodes. Areas of hypoperfusion may correspond to areas of ischaemia, necrosis or thromboembolic disease. This technique can also be useful for the evaluation of both peripheral and abdominal lymph nodes. Of particular interest are the canine testes, since the two testicles drain to different sentinel nodes. The right testis drains to lymph nodes within the pelvic canal and adjacent to the aortic bifurcation, whilst the left testis drains to lymph nodes located near the left renal hilus.

Alternatively, contrast medium can be injected into the tissue or organ of interest, rather than intravenously. The contrast medium is subsequently absorbed by the macrophages within the reticuloendothelial system of the lymph node. As this is a new technology and requires dedicated equipment it is not discussed further here.

Computed tomography and magnetic resonance imaging

Abdominal lymph nodes are not routinely imaged by CT or MRI in dogs and cats. They can be detected, although on CT it may be difficult to distinguish lymph nodes from other soft tissue structures due to similar attenuation patterns. Normal mesenteric lymph nodes may be routinely identified at the mesenteric root and throughout the mesentery with the use of multidetector CT. Thin slice imaging reduces partial volume artefacts, and faster scanning times enables better opacification of the mesenteric vessels after contrast medium injection, which improves the distinction between mesenteric nodes and vessels. MRI is comparable with CT for identification of lymph nodes.

With both CT and MRI, abnormal nodes are recognized on the basis of size and shape rather than by any characteristic signal intensity. On cross-sectional imaging, a normal lymph node usually measures <1 cm in size, has a smooth and well defined border, and shows a uniform, homogenous density or signal intensity. Absolute signal intensities of benign nodes cannot be reliably differentiated from those of malignant nodes on either un-enhanced T1- or T2-weighted images.

Optimization of the spatial resolution is essential for evaluation of lymph nodes. The most important technical parameters for both CT and MRI are the field of view and slice thickness. Other important parameters for MRI are matrix size, pulse sequence and number of excitations. As experience and skills improve with these modalities, clinical indications for imaging abdominal lymph nodes will continue to grow.

Lymphoscintigraphy

Lymphoscintigraphy involves the subcutaneous injection of radioactive particles that are then imaged as they pass through the lymphatic vessels to their respective lymph nodal drainage basins. It is usually performed using [99m]Technetium, which is conjugated to sulphur colloid or albumin. Serial gamma scintigrams demonstrate dynamic lymphatic function and the number and location of the sentinel nodes. Lymphoscintigraphy is receiving increasing interest as a tool in staging regional lymph nodes in the early stages of malignancy. The main drawback of lymphoscintigraphy is poor spatial resolution.

Biopsy techniques

Ultrasound-guided fine-needle aspiration cytology is often necessary to determine the definitive status of a lymph node. In patients with known or suspected neoplasia, the lymph nodes most at risk of harbouring metastases are aspirated. It is therefore necessary to have clinical information about the primary tumour and knowledge of the usual patterns of metastases from this tumour type. If the draining node is negative, the likelihood of nodal metastases is very low. Sampling of the medial iliac lymph node is particularly useful for the pelvic area, which may otherwise be difficult to reach.

Although the sampling technique is not difficult, considerable training is required to aspirate lymph nodes as small as 3–5 mm successfully. Fine-needle techniques have advantages compared with core techniques, in most cases, including:

- Decreased pain to the patient
- High cellular yield due to ease of exfoliation of most aetiologies
- Technical ease of the procedure, usually without the need for sedation or anaesthesia
- Decreased likelihood of bleeding.

The advantage of ultrasound-guidance of the needle is the possibility of directing the needle accurately into a very small lymph node, or even to areas of particular suspicion within the lymph node. Fine-needle cytological samples are usually obtained with a 22–23 gauge needle. The length of the needle is chosen based on the region to be sampled. Two or three samples are usually obtained to maximize the chance of diagnostic sampling. To minimize the likelihood of haemodilution, the needle should be rapidly and repeatedly thrust into the node, only using negative pressure (aspiration) when the node is too mobile or firm for the thrusting technique, or when the number of cells harvested is too small. If fine-needle techniques fail to provide a diagnostic sample, then core sampling should be considered. Due to the close association between lymph nodes and blood vessels, Doppler ultrasonography should be utilized prior to biopsy techniques to identify blood vessels and to optimize the appropriate window and needle path.

References and further reading

Kinns J and Mai W (2007) Association between malignancy and sonographic heterogeneity in canine and feline abdominal lymph nodes. *Veterinary Radiology and Ultrasound* **48**, 565–569

Llabres-Diaz FJ (2004) Ultrasonography of the medial iliac lymph nodes in the dog. *Veterinary Radiology and Ultrasound* **45**, 156–165

Lurie DM, Seguin B, Schneider PD, *et al.* (2006) Contrast-assisted ultrasound for sentinel lymph node detection in spontaneously arising canine head and neck tumors. *Investigative Radiology* **41**, 415–421

Nyman HT, Kristensen AT, Flagstad A, *et al.* (2004) A review of the sonographic assessment of tumor metastases in liver and superficial lymph nodes. *Veterinary Radiology and Ultrasound* **45**, 438–449

Nyman HT, Kristensen AT, Skovgaard IM, *et al.* (2005) Characterization of normal and abnormal canine superficial lymph nodes using gray-scale B-mode, color flow mapping, power, and spectral Doppler ultrasonography: a multivariate study. *Veterinary Radiology and Ultrasound* **46**, 404–410

Nyman HT, Lee MH, McEvoy FJ, *et al.* (2006) Comparison of B-mode and Doppler ultrasonographic findings with histologic features of benign and malignant superficial lymph nodes in dogs. *American Journal of Veterinary Research* **67**, 978–984

Nyman HT and O'Brien RT (2007) The sonographic evaluation of lymph nodes. *Clinical Techniques in Small Animal Practice* **22**, 128–137

Pugh CR (1994) Ultrasonographic examination of abdominal lymph nodes in the dog. *Veterinary Radiology and Ultrasound* **35**, 110–115

Salwei RM, O'Brien RT and Matheson JS (2005) Characterization of lymphomatous lymph nodes in dogs using contrast harmonic and Power Doppler ultrasound. *Veterinary Radiology and Ultrasound* **46**, 411–416

Sato AF and Solano M (2004) Ultrasonographic findings in abdominal mast cell disease: a retrospective study of 19 patients. *Veterinary Radiology and Ultrasound* **45**, 51–57

Schreurs E, Vermote K, Barberet V, Daminet S, Rudorf H and Saunders JH (2008) Ultrasonographic anatomy of abdominal lymph nodes in the normal cat. *Veterinary Radiology and Ultrasound* **49**, 68–72

Wisner ER, Ferrara KW, Short RE, *et al.* (2003) Sentinel node detection using contrast-enhanced power Doppler ultrasound lymphography. *Investigative Radiology* **38**, 358–365

8

Abdominal masses

Nicolette Hayward

Introduction

The identification of the origin of abdominal masses depends upon a knowledge of normal radiographic anatomy, as it is often the indirect mass effect on other organs that gives the clue to the principal organ involved. Whilst the origin of the lesion may be obvious in some cases, often it is a case of elimination of normal structures using, most commonly, radiographic and ultrasonographic examination. The normal extent of anatomical variation should also be considered, especially in those structures that are capable of considerable physiological variation, such as the stomach, bladder and uterus.

Radiographic techniques

Positioning

Orthogonal views are necessary to assist in differentiation of masses within the abdomen. The direction of displacement of mobile abdominal structures, such as the intestines, gives vital information about the potential source of the mass. Thus, information gained from routine lateral and ventrodorsal (VD) views can localize pathology to cranial/caudal, dorsal/ventral and left/right aspects of the abdomen.

Furthermore, positional radiography may be performed in order to improve the clarity with which organs may be seen, either normally or pathologically. For instance, the right lateral view results in gas accumulating in the fundus of the stomach, thus delineating the caudodorsal margins of the liver. Meanwhile, the left lateral view highlights the pylorus with gas, and potentially the duodenum. Similarly, the right lateral view often results in the tail of the spleen being more obvious than in the left lateral view.

Horizontal beam radiography allows the effects of gravity on a mass to be seen, as well as the fluid and gas that may be associated with it. Oblique and tangential views may also be useful in localizing peripheral masses.

Compression

Compression techniques have been used to improve visualization of abdominal masses. Application of compression via an abdominal band or paddle/spoon reduces the thickness of the abdomen and thus

enables a lower kV to be used, thereby reducing scatter reaching the film and improving contrast. In addition, this technique may separate overlying structures, thereby making them easier to see.

Compression radiography (Figure 8.1) should not be used where there is a risk of organ rupture, such as in cases of pyometra or splenic haemangiosarcoma. This technique generally requires the presence of personnel within the controlled area during the radiographic exposure, and thus has implications with regard to radiation safety.

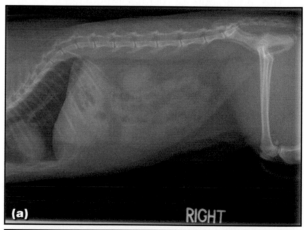

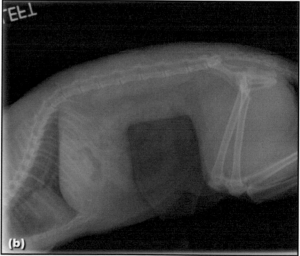

8.1 **(a)** Pre-compression and **(b)** compression radiographs in a cat, demonstrating a linear foreign body. Due care must be taken with radiation safety when applying compression. (Courtesy of R O'Brien)

Contrast medium

Ultrasonography has largely superseded contrast radiography, particularly in the investigation of abdominal masses. However, the latter technique remains useful where ultrasound examination is unavailable or inconclusive.

Positive and negative contrast agents may be useful in isolating the origin of a mass. The diagnosis may be made from the contrast medium becoming incorporated within a mass, thereby implicating it as part of the lesion, or by delineating one of the areas in the differential diagnosis and showing that it is normal. Contrast agents are most commonly used in this way to outline the urinary tract or the gastrointestinal tract. For example, intravenous urography may differentiate a renal mass from other masses (Figure 8.2). Similarly, the presence of a paraprostatic cyst can be ascertained following administration of positive or negative contrast medium to locate the position of the bladder.

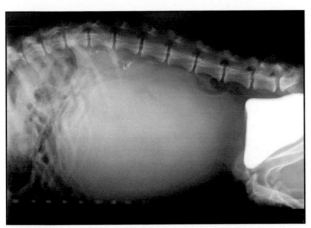

8.2 Intravenous urography used in a dog to differentiate a splenic mass from a retroperitoneal mass, by outlining the position of the kidneys. Contrast medium is seen within the renal pelves ventral to L1 and L2.

Barium may be administered to outline the path of the gastrointestinal tract. Hence, if positive contrast medium can be seen passing centrally through a mass in orthogonal views, then the mass can be confirmed as being of bowel origin. However, barium may also be used to define the course of the normal gastrointestinal tract, for example, when a cranial abdominal mass is present and the caudal margins of the liver are unclear. Thus, contrast medium within the stomach will indicate the position of the caudal border of the liver, and so indicate hepatic enlargement or irregularity.

Normal variants as 'pseudomasses'

Normal structures

Some abdominal structures are seen routinely on survey radiography, such as the liver and bladder, whilst others are less consistently or only partially seen. For instance, the position of the tail of the spleen is highly variable and may lie cranially in apposition to the liver, making definition of its contour unclear, or it may move caudoventrally, adjacent to the bladder. Splenomegaly occurs following sedation and thus the variability in position of the enlarged spleen may result in the misdiagnosis of an abdominal mass.

Some abdominal structures have normal variation in size and contour, in particular the stomach, bladder and uterus. The appearance of the stomach is dependent upon the amount and type of ingesta present, as well as how much gas is present. After a large meal the stomach can enlarge substantially, resulting in caudal displacement of other organs. The urinary bladder can also enlarge to fill the caudoventral abdomen, thereby causing a mass effect from a caudal direction and displacing other organs cranially, in particular the small intestines.

Uterine enlargement is usually not noticeable in the non-pregnant animal, but in pregnancy the uterine body enlarges, separating the colon and the bladder, while the uterine horns displace the other abdominal contents cranially and dorsally. Mineralization of fetuses is observed from approximately 40–45 days' gestation in dogs and cats.

Intra-abdominal fat can also result in a mass effect, particularly in obese cats. This may result in the intestines being pushed laterally and/or ventrally by a large fat opacity. Some animals have an elongated descending colon as a normal variant. This appearance is known as 'redundancy' of the colon and its more tortuous/ventral path may give the impression of being subject to a mass effect originating from the dorsal abdomen. In fat animals, where serosal detail is good, this normal variation may be obvious. However, in thin animals, or where fluid is present, its appearance may be more confusing and result in misdiagnosis of a dorsal abdominal mass. Fluid-filled small intestinal loops can also be misleading when seen end on, or as composite shadows with linear loops of intestine potentially summating as a nodular soft tissue opacity.

In some bitches, the nipples may also give the appearance of small masses as the air surrounding each nipple provides a strong contrast to the soft tissue of the nipple.

Atypical structures

Left limb of the pancreas

The left limb of the pancreas is often not visible ultrasonographically. However, in some animals, particularly in cats, this structure can be quite prominent. It often has a solid, homogenous, hypoechoic appearance, and is located between the greater curvature of the stomach, the spleen and the transverse colon. This prominence may give the appearance of either a pancreatic mass or pancreatitis, but the lack of clinical signs or of any discomfort during the ultrasound examination, together with the lack of adjacent mesenteric hyperechogenicity or fluid, may help in identifying this finding as a normal structure.

Principles of localization

Orthogonal views enable the position of the mass to be established in cranial/caudal, dorsal/ventral and left/right directions, both by direct visualization of the mass and indirectly by the direction of displacement of other organs such as the small intestines. Therefore, a radiograph should be evaluated in a systematic way. Each organ should be assessed in turn on orthogonal views, and thus its influence on, and effects from, other organs can be determined.

The radiographic position of a mass depends on how firmly it is attached and whether it is sessile or pedunculated. The effect it has on adjacent organs may be as a result of pulsion (i.e. the displacement of viscera peripherally) or traction, where the normal organ is attached to the mass and thus pulled out of position.

The small intestines are held within the mesentery and are highly mobile. They are a good marker for the origin of a mass as they are easily displaced. In addition, they can also give crucial information as to the location of a mass. For instance, if the mass is retroperitoneal (e.g. an adrenal gland neoplasm) the intestines will be moved ventrally. Where a large peritoneal mass is present, such as an ovarian tumour, the intestines are able to move dorsally above the mass.

Differential diagnoses

The differential diagnoses of an abdominal mass based on the location of the organ of origin is shown in Figure 8.3. The differential diagnoses based on the pathophysiology of the lesion include:

- Physiological (hypertrophy, hyperplasia, pregnancy, bladder filling)
- Neoplasia
- Infection (abscess, granuloma)
- Haematoma
- Cyst
- Torsion or obstruction.

Liver

The liver lies immediately caudal to the diaphragm and consists of six lobes. Generalized or localized enlargement may occur and the appearance of any focal enlargement depends on which lobes are affected. Hepatic enlargement may be smooth or nodular and irregular, depending on the disease process. For instance, hepatomegaly secondary to right heart failure results in smooth generalized enlargement, whilst primary hepatic neoplasia is more likely to result in an irregular contour. The presence of an abdominal effusion may limit visualization of the liver; however, the presence of gas in the stomach and disturbance of the gastric axis can provide indirect information on the size and position of the liver.

Generalized enlargement
The pylorus is displaced caudally, dorsally and to the left. The duodenum and small intestines are also displaced caudodorsally.

Right-sided liver enlargement
The pylorus, proximal descending duodenum and ascending colon are displaced dorsomedially (Figure 8.4). Caudal displacement of the small intestines also

Location	Section of abdomen	Organ of origin of mass
1	Craniodorsal	Liver; spleen; kidneys; adrenal glands; ovary; stomach
2	Cranioventral	Liver; gallbladder; stomach; pancreas
3	Central	Spleen; lymph nodes; mesenteric masses; gastrointestinal tract; pancreas; uterus; ovary; testis
4	Caudodorsal	Sublumbar lymph nodes; colon/rectum; ureter
5	Caudoventral	Uterus; prostate gland; bladder; testis
A	Left cranial	Liver; stomach; head of spleen; left adrenal gland; left kidney; left ovary
B	Right cranial	Liver; gallbladder; stomach; duodenum; pancreas; right kidney; right adrenal gland; right ovary
C	Central	Spleen; lymph nodes; mesenteric masses; gastrointestinal tract; pancreas; uterus; ovaries; testis
D	Caudal	Sublumbar lymph nodes; colon/rectum; ureter; uterus; prostate gland; bladder; testis

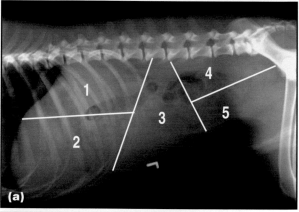

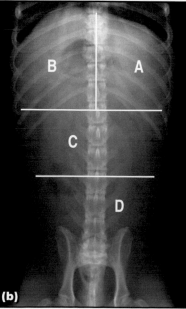

8.3 Differential diagnoses of abdominal masses based on location of the organ of origin. **(a)** Lateral and **(b)** VD radiographs showing abdominal sections.

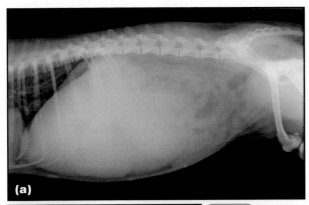

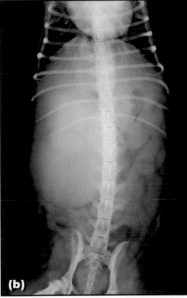

8.4

(a) Lateral and **(b)** VD views of a right-sided liver mass in a dog. The intestines have been displaced caudally and to the left side.

Left-sided liver enlargement
The fundus may be displaced dorsally and medially and the small intestines may move caudally. Entrapment of the stomach can also occur with a pedunculated mass, resulting in it occupying a more craniodorsal position. The head of the spleen may be displaced dorsomedially. Where the margins of the liver are indistinct and ultrasonography is not available, barium may be used to identify the position of the stomach as a landmark.

Spleen
The head of the spleen is fixed in position by the gastrosplenic ligament, while the body and tail are mobile. Therefore, a mass in the body or tail of the spleen is potentially highly variable in position. Sedation will often result in splenomegaly and therefore this finding should not be misinterpreted in the sedated or anaesthetized animal.

Head of the spleen
Enlargement of the head of the spleen results in an increased opacity in the craniodorsal abdomen caudal to the stomach, and the fundic gas shadow may be distorted on a right lateral view. Considerable soft tissue effacement is present in the craniodorsal abdomen owing to the fixed location of the kidneys, liver and stomach. The differential diagnoses for a mass in this area therefore include a mass in one of these organs or in the adrenal glands, which are normally not visible radiographically. On the VD view, the normally crisp triangular shape of the head of the spleen may be missing. The fundus may be dorsally displaced and the left kidney positioned caudally.

Body and tail of the spleen
Depending on the size of the mass, a beak-like appearance may be produced by confluence of the mass with normal spleen (Figure 8.6). The mass may be seen quite far caudally in the abdomen because of the lack of restraint on these parts of the spleen (Figure 8.7). The duration of recumbency before radiography is performed can also influence its position; thus, displacement of other organs is variable. Among the best indicators of the origin of a mass in this situation are the small intestines, which move peripherally around the mass, especially in a dorsal direction.

occurs. If the mass is large and pedunculated, the body of the stomach may be moved craniodorsally. Therefore, the mass may appear caudal to the stomach, which may result in its misinterpretation as a splenic mass from the lateral view (Figure 8.5). Identification of the normal triangular structure of the splenic head on the VD view is useful in differentiating this type of hepatic mass from a splenic mass.

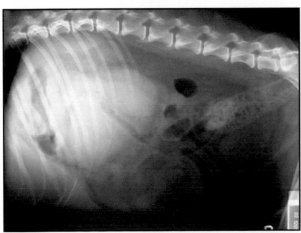

8.5 Lateral view of a pedunculated liver mass in a dog. The gas-filled fundus of the stomach can be seen in a cranially displaced position, whilst the intestines have been displaced caudoventrally.

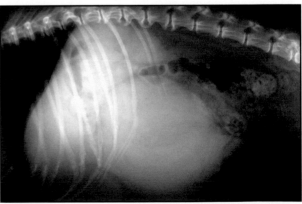

8.6 Lateral view of a mass in the body of the spleen in a dog. A well demarcated 'beak' can be seen at the caudal extent of the mass.

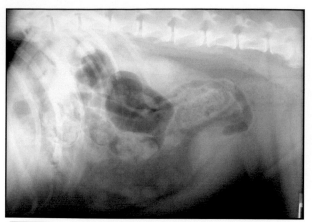

8.7 Lateral view of a mass in the tail of the spleen, illustrating a markedly caudoventral position, with subsequent cranial and dorsal displacement of the small intestines.

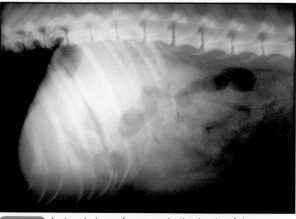

8.8 Lateral view of a mass in the body of the stomach in a dog. Note the increased opacity in the craniodorsal abdomen, with distortion of the fundic gas shadow and caudal displacement of the colon.

Differential diagnoses for a mass in the body or tail of the spleen include an ovarian or testicular mass or torsion, a mesenteric lymph node mass or cyst, or an intestinal mass, although the latter may typically be expected to be associated with gas accumulation proximal to the lesion where luminal occlusion occurs.

Splenic torsion may present as a pronounced mass, which may be associated with gastric torsion, whereupon it has a C-shaped appearance. It may occasionally also be associated with small foci of gas within the parenchyma, and an abdominal effusion may be present making its margins unclear.

Gastrointestinal tract

Stomach
The size of the stomach is variable and depends upon its contents. The thickness of the wall of the gastro-intestinal tract cannot normally be assessed from plain radiographs, as gas–fluid interfaces seen tangentially can mimic wall thickening. Ultrasonography or barium studies should be used for evaluation of the thickness of the wall of the gastrointestinal tract. Radiographically, enlargement of the stomach can be seen as caudal displacement of the small intestines, transverse colon and spleen. The contour of the gas shadow within the stomach may be irregular where masses are present (Figure 8.8). However, stomach wall contractions can alter the shape of the stomach, giving the appearance of 'pseudomasses', which should not be confused with pathological changes.

Intestines
Intestinal masses generally present as mid-abdominal masses, which are difficult to differentiate from circumscribed mesenteric masses, or from splenic, ovarian or testicular masses. They may be seen to cause peripheral displacement of the remaining intestines, although often the effect is unpredictable and may change on serial radiographs. Secondary findings that assist diagnosis of an enteric mass include a gravel sign and/or gas accumulation proximal to an obstruction.

Masses in the large intestine are often quite sizeable by the time they are radiologically detectable,

given the normal wide diameter of this section of the gastrointestinal tract. The small intestines may be ventrally displaced.

Pancreas
Pancreatic masses are often ill defined and vary in appearance according to their position in the pancreas, i.e. whether the right limb, left limb or body is affected. A mass-like effect may also occur with pancreatitis.

Right pancreatic limb masses (Figure 8.9) may result in lateral and ventral displacement of the

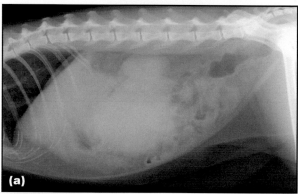

8.9

(a) Lateral and **(b)** VD radiographs of an extensive pancreatic mass in a cat. The duodenum is displaced laterally and the small and large intestines are displaced caudally and ventrally. The mass is poorly defined because of a local peritonitis.

duodenum (best seen in a left lateral view) and displacement of the pylorus to the left side. The transverse colon may be displaced caudally. On the VD view the duodenum is often filled with gas and runs straight down the right body wall; this finding may also be seen with pancreatitis. If the duodenum cannot be visualized, barium may be administered.

Masses in the left limb of the pancreas also result in ventral displacement of the duodenum, with caudal displacement of the transverse colon and small intestines. The body of the stomach may have an indented appearance on the VD view.

Kidneys

The kidneys lie in the retroperitoneal space and, because they are restrained by the retroperitoneal fascia, renal masses have the effect of depressing peritoneal structures ventrally. This is in contrast to peritoneal structures such as the ovary or retained testicle which, when enlarged, can migrate between and minimally displace other peritoneal structures. Renal silhouettes can be difficult to identify, particularly in thin dogs and where gas and fluid are present in the gastrointestinal tract.

Right renal masses (Figure 8.10) may result in medial and ventral displacement of the descending duodenum and ascending colon. Left renal masses produce ventral and medial displacement of the descending colon and small intestines. Comparison

of the retroperitoneal fat with peritoneal fat is useful to identify the presence of fluid or infiltration within either of these compartments.

Adrenal glands

The adrenal glands are not normally identifiable radiographically, although adrenal gland mineralization is recognized as an incidental finding in the older cat. As retroperitoneal structures, adrenal gland masses (Figure 8.11) remain in a craniodorsal position, typically resulting in caudal and lateral displacement of the ipsilateral kidney. The VD view is particularly useful in differentiating adrenal gland masses. Aggressive adrenal gland tumours, such as phaeochromocytomas, may invade the adjacent kidney to produce a confluent shadow.

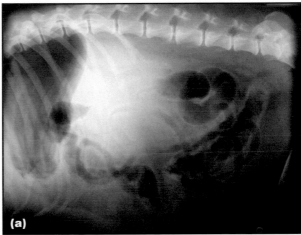

(a)

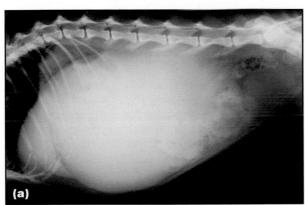

(a)

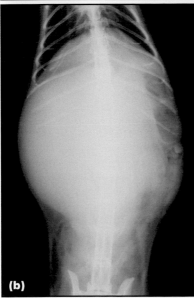

(b)

8.10 **(a)** Lateral and **(b)** VD radiographs of a large mass in the right kidney of a cat. There is marked ventral, caudal and leftward displacement of all peritoneal organs.

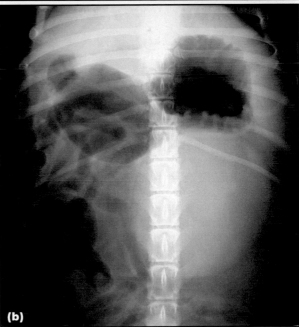

(b)

8.11 **(a)** Lateral and **(b)** VD radiographs of a left adrenal gland mass in a dog. Note the increased opacity in the craniodorsal abdomen with ventral and rightward displacement of the abdominal viscera.

Bladder

The silhouette of the urinary bladder is variable in size, depending upon the degree of fill, and enlargement results in cranial displacement of the small intestines. In the presence of an enlarged prostate gland or paraprostatic cyst it may be difficult to differentiate these structures from the bladder. A bladder mass *per se* is unlikely to produce radiographic change. However, if the mass results in obstruction, the distended bladder may then cause a mass effect. Ultrasonography and/or contrast radiography are most useful in identifying bladder position and associated pathology.

Uterus

The normal uterus is rarely identified radiographically until its diameter exceeds twice that of the small intestines. The uterus lies dorsal to the bladder and ventral to the colon, thus significant uterine enlargement is seen as separation of these two structures (Figure 8.12), and has the effect of displacing the small intestines cranially. Uterine enlargement may present as fluid-filled tortuous soft tissue tubular structures originating from the pelvic inlet. Mineralization of fetuses may be seen at around 40–45 days of pregnancy in dogs and cats.

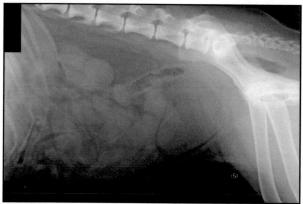

8.12 Lateral radiograph demonstrating a pyometra in a dog. Separation of the colon and bladder can be seen, with coiled distended tubular structures extending cranially.

Ovaries

The ovaries are located within the peritoneal cavity, held by an ovarian ligament caudal to each kidney. As the ovary grows, the ligament is stretched, and therefore enlargement may result in the ovarian mass being variable in position. Small masses may be located caudoventral to the kidneys, whilst larger masses may gravitate to a more ventral abdominal position (Figure 8.13). Ventral deviation of adjacent organs is not seen but medial displacement of the duodenum may be seen with right ovarian masses, or medial displacement of the colon with left-sided masses. Ventral deviation of the ipsilateral kidney may occur with large ovarian masses.

Prostate gland

The prostate gland is often intra-abdominal in older animals and the normal prostate gland may occupy a space equivalent to up to 70% of the distance between the pubis and the sacrum. Prostatomegaly produces cranial displacement of the bladder, and potentially also dorsal deviation or indentation of the rectum. Ill defined mineralization may be present and is most

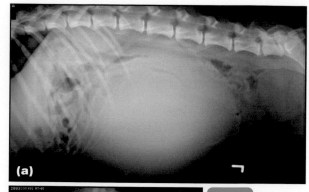

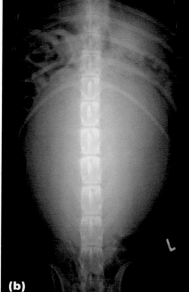

8.13

(a) Lateral and **(b)** VD radiographs of an ovarian cyst in a bitch, which has displaced the intestines dorsally, cranially and caudally. Compare the appearance with that in Figure 8.10, where an equally large renal (i.e. retroperitoneal) mass has displaced the viscera ventrally.

likely to be associated with prostatic neoplasia or prostatitis. Neoplasia may also result in a bony reaction along the ventral bodies of the caudal lumbar vertebrae or pelvis. Paraprostatic cysts may be quite large and give the appearance of a double bladder; they may demonstrate an organized 'eggshell' mineralization (Figure 8.14). Contrast radiography or ultrasonography may be required to clarify the position of the bladder.

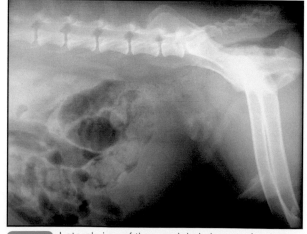

8.14 Lateral view of the caudal abdomen of a dog with a paraprostatic cyst, which has displaced the bladder cranioventrally. Note the 'eggshell' mineralization of the caudoventral part of the cyst.

Sublumbar masses

The normal rectum follows a central path through the pelvis on both lateral and VD views. Depression of the distal colon and rectum occurs when a sublumbar mass (Figure 8.15) is present. These masses may be well circumscribed or diffuse depending on their origin and the presence of adhesions. End-on views of the deep circumflex arteries (seen as small soft tissue nodular opacities) may be seen as a normal finding in the sublumbar region and should not be confused with lymphadenomegaly. Enlargement of the medial iliac lymph nodes is the commonest cause of masses in this area, and often occurs in relation to lymphoma and anal sac adenocarcinoma, although soft tissue sarcoma, granuloma and abscess may also produce this appearance.

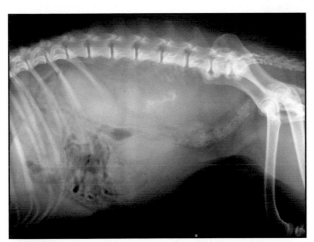

8.15 Aggressive sublumbar carcinoma, displacing the colon ventrally and the bladder and small intestines cranially. There is an extensive periosteal reaction along the ventral surfaces of the vertebrae, with amorphous mineralization within the body of the mass.

Ultrasonography

Ultrasonography is a non-invasive technique that allows structural or parenchymal abnormalities to be identified and thus it is a particularly valuable imaging modality in the investigation of abdominal masses. Masses as small as 2 cm across can be identified by ultrasound examination. In addition, masses that are hidden within the parenchyma of an organ can be identified, despite lack of alteration in the contour, shape or size of the organ (e.g. hepatic metastatic disease).

Where abdominal fluid, peritonitis or lack of fat results in poor contrast on radiography, ultrasonography is an ideal method of evaluating the abdomen. However, ultrasonography should be seen as a complementary technique to radiographic examination. For instance, where a mass involves an entire organ with no normal tissue remaining, it can be difficult to define its origin. In such cases, the mass effect of organ enlargement is often better appreciated radiographically.

Gaining information about the likely origin and degree of malignancy of a mass using ultrasonography can avoid the need for exploratory surgery. Therefore, ultrasound examination aids in surgical planning, both to give an idea of the degree of infiltration or vascularity of a mass with regard to the surgical approach and margins required and, equally, to decide when surgery is not indicated. However, ultrasonography has relatively low tissue specificity, and thus abnormal ultrasonographic findings may have multiple differential diagnoses. Therefore, fine-needle aspiration or tissue core biopsy is indicated to obtain a histological diagnosis of the mass.

A thorough understanding of normal abdominal anatomy, as well as the normal ultrasonographic appearance of intra-abdominal organs, is required in order to identify the origin of abdominal masses. This can prove challenging, even to the experienced ultrasonographer, particularly when the mass is very large or when fluid is present. Where large masses are present, the diagnosis may be made by exclusion (i.e. by the absence of a normal organ).

Approach

Where possible, the ultrasonographer should examine the organs in a routine sequence, so that each normal organ is identified and ruled out as being the source of the mass or masses. Every organ should be fully evaluated, e.g. the spleen should be examined throughout its length, not forgetting the head, which is located cranial to the left kidney. Once a mass has been identified, the remaining abdomen should be thoroughly searched to look for further masses, lymph node involvement and potential invasion of adjacent tissues, e.g. adrenal gland masses invading the caudal vena cava (Figure 8.16).

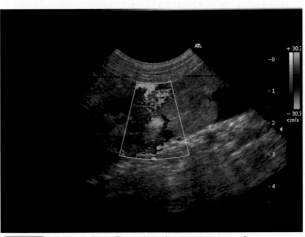

8.16 Colour flow Doppler ultrasonogram of an adrenal gland mass invading the caudal vena cava in a dog.

Mass appearance

Masses may be single or multiple, focal or diffuse, homogenous or heterogenous (Figure 8.17), solid or cavitary. Focal masses are generally easier to identify than diffuse changes, which may be quite subtle (e.g. lymphosarcoma in the liver). The combination of soft tissue, gas, fluid and perhaps mineralization, produces an image that provides information about the structure of the mass, which may be useful for aspiration or biopsy, surgical planning and prognosis.

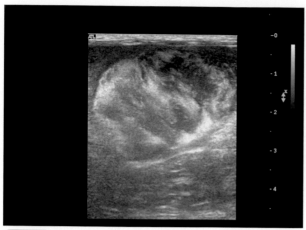

8.17 Ultrasonographic appearance of a heterogenous liver mass in a dog.

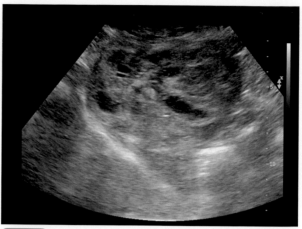

8.19 Ultrasonogram of a cavitary liver mass in a dog.

Cystic masses

Cystic masses are usually anechoic, often with echogenic septae within the fluid, and may be seen as incidental findings. However, these masses may be more significant, for example in polycystic kidney disease (Figure 8.18) where obliteration of the renal parenchyma may be seen. Typically, cystic structures are associated with anechoic content, but echogenic content may be present, e.g. in a paraprostatic cyst, and should not be confused with an abscess.

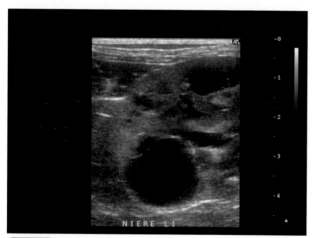

8.18 Ultrasonographic appearance of a polycystic feline kidney. There is loss of the normal kidney architecture due to multiple variably sized cysts.

Cavitary masses

Cavitary masses (Figure 8.19) may contain various echogenicities and echotextures, and are variably well circumscribed. Examples of cavitary lesions include abscesses, haematomas, nodular hyperplasia and neoplasms.

Abscesses: These are variable in appearance. Abscesses are typically irregular with hypoechoic content (Figure 8.20), although the echogenicity of any fluid depends upon its viscosity. Occasionally a foreign body, mineralization or gas may be present. There is minimal acoustic enhancement deep to the abscess. While septation is not a typical feature, abscesses may have a complex internal architecture.

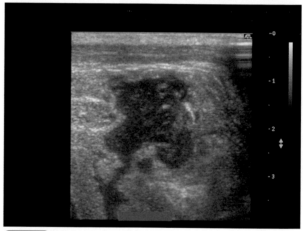

8.20 Ultrasonographic appearance of an encapsulated abscess. Echogenic fluid can be identified centrally.

Haematomas: These also vary in appearance, depending upon how long they have been present, and may range from small hypoechoic focal areas to larger septated masses. In addition, haematomas may contain clumps of echogenic material. Doppler ultrasonography studies show that haematomas are non-vascular and this aids in the differentiation from other types of mass, such as complex neoplasms. The history is useful in making a diagnosis, e.g. recent trauma or surgery, and thus haematomas may be identified that have no association with a specific organ.

Benign nodular hyperplasia: Benign nodular hyperplasia does not have an ultrasonographically unique appearance and is usually seen as hypoechoic and ill defined nodules, although it may present as large mass lesions. Contrast harmonic ultrasonography has been used to differentiate between areas of poor blood supply, such as necrotic hepatic neoplastic nodules, and benign nodular hyperplasia. Therefore, contrast harmonic ultrasonography may be used during ultrasound-guided biopsy procedures to avoid sampling necrotic areas of a mass.

Neoplasms: These may have a similar appearance to haematomas and thus are hard to differentiate, particularly if they are poorly vascularized. However, certain ultrasonographic findings are more likely to be associated with neoplasia, such as target lesions. These masses tend to have a hypoechoic rim with a hyperechoic centre and are most commonly associated with neoplasia, but have also been seen in more benign conditions such as nodular hyperplasia.

Aspiration and biopsy

Ultrasound-guided aspiration and biopsy are under-used diagnostic techniques that can avoid unnecessary exploratory surgery in the investigation of abdominal masses. With practice, fine-needle aspirates and tissue core biopsy samples can be obtained successfully and with minimal risk, saving both time and discomfort to the animal. Complications with ultrasound-guided techniques are rare in comparison with blind methods.

Techniques include 'freehand', more commonly used in practice, or 'guide-assisted', which involves the use of an adaptor that allows accurate placement of the needle. Whichever technique is used, the probe should always be moved towards the needle, rather than blindly moving the needle to find the probe. Practising with water-filled balloons, grapes or olives placed within tofu is useful for the inexperienced ultrasonographer.

Clotting times (prothrombin time (PT) and activated partial thromboplastin time (APTT)), should be obtained prior to biopsy. Obtaining a fine-needle aspirate requires mild to moderate sedation, while tissue core biopsy samples should be obtained under heavy sedation or general anaesthesia.

The choice of fine-needle aspiration *versus* tissue core biopsy (Figure 8.21) depends upon a number of factors. Obtaining a fine-needle aspirate requires less preparation and sedation and is useful for identifying lipidosis or infiltrative neoplasia such as lymphoma, but has a greater risk of producing non-diagnostic samples. Tissue core biopsy samples, on the other hand, are better for identifying the histological type of tissue present, particularly where inflammatory or structural disease is present, but clearly the technique requires more experience and has a slightly higher risk of complications such as bleeding. Following either fine-needle aspiration or biopsy, the area should be rechecked for haemorrhage.

Seeding of tumour cells (e.g. from bladder or prostatic neoplasia) may occur, and suck biopsy using ultrasound-guided catheterization or prostatic washing should be used in place of transabdominal aspiration or biopsy in these cases.

In order to maximize the chances of success, samples should be taken from several representative areas, and cavitary areas should be avoided as dilution with blood is likely. In these cases, areas adjacent to the lesion may produce more successful samples. However, situations remain where laparotomy may be indicated to allow a thorough investigation of the abdomen to be performed and to enable larger biopsy samples to be obtained.

Overview of additional imaging modalities

Magnetic resonance imaging (MRI) has been used in the investigation of abdominal masses. Given its high contrast resolution, MRI is valuable in identifying extension of tumours into bones, the spinal canal, adjacent organs, vessels and lymph nodes. In humans, it has been shown to be the imaging modality of choice in hepatic, pancreatic, renal and adrenal gland disease. Pulmonary metastases may be identified, although MRI is not the most sensitive technique for this assessment and movement artefacts complicate interpretation. In addition, MRI is an expensive imaging modality, and the acquisition of images from both the thorax and the abdomen results in a considerable number of artefacts, which are difficult to eliminate.

Like MRI, computed tomography (CT) can produce multidimensional images of the abdomen. It is used for assessing both primary and metastatic disease, as well as for staging tumours and assessing masses both pre- and postoperatively, and can be used when gas in the abdomen precludes ultrasound examination. In studies of the diagnosis of renal disease in humans, it has been shown to be equal in sensitivity to MRI. CT is also particularly sensitive for detecting early pulmonary metastases. Again, relative to ultrasonography and radiography, CT is a more costly option, but, like MRI, it is likely to be used increasingly, particularly in academic and referral institutions.

References and further reading

Cuccovillo A and Lamb C (2002) Cellular features of sonographic target lesions of the liver and spleen in 21 dogs and a cat. *Veterinary Radiology and Ultrasound* **43**(3), 275–278

Dennis R, Kirberger R, Wrigley R, *et al.* (2001) Abdominal masses. In: *Small Animal Radiological Differential Diagnosis, 1st edn*, ed. R Dennis *et al.*, pp. 226–232. WB Saunders, Philadelphia

Fife W, Samii V, Drost W, *et al.* (2004) Comparison between malignant and non-malignant splenic masses in dogs using contrast-enhanced computed tomography. *Veterinary Radiology and Ultrasound* **45**(4), 289–297

Konde L, Lebel J, Park R, *et al.* (1986) Sonographic application in the diagnosis of intra-abdominal abscess in the dog. *Veterinary Radiology* **27**(4), 151–154

Mattoon J and Nyland T (2001) Abdominal fluid, lymph nodes, masses, peritoneal cavity, and great vessel thrombosis. In: *Small Animal Diagnostic Ultrasound, 2nd edn*, ed. T Nyland and J Mattoon, pp. 82–93. WB Saunders, Philadelphia

Muleya J, Taura Y, Nakaichi M, *et al.* (1997) Appearance of canine

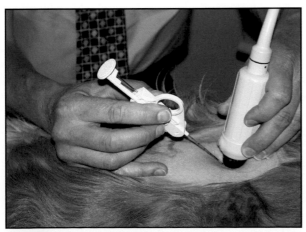

8.21 Ultrasound-guided tissue core biopsy of the left kidney of a dog.

abdominal tumours with magnetic resonance imaging using a low field permanent magnet. *Veterinary Radiology and Ultrasound* **38**(6), 444–447

Noone T, Semelka RC, Chaney DM, *et al.* (2004) Abdominal imaging studies: comparison of diagnostic accuracies resulting from ultrasound, computed tomography, and magnetic resonance imaging in the same individual. *Magnetic Resonance Imaging* **22**(1), 19–24

O'Brien R (2007) Improved detection of metastatic hepatic haemangiosarcoma nodules with contrast ultrasound in three dogs. *Veterinary Radiology and Ultrasound* **48**(2), 146–148

Root C (1974) Abdominal masses: the radiographic differential diagnosis. *Veterinary Radiology* **15**(2), 26–43

Root C (2002) Abdominal masses. In: *Textbook of Veterinary Radiology*, *4th edn*, ed. D Thrall, pp. 493–515. WB Saunders, Philadelphia

Ziegler L and O'Brien R (2002) Harmonic ultrasound: a review. *Veterinary Radiology and Ultrasound* **43**(6), 501–509

9

The stomach

Gabriela Seiler and Wilfried Maï

Normal radiographic anatomy

General anatomy

The stomach is a hollow organ with a musculo-glandular wall. It is located in the cranial part of the abdominal cavity, caudal to the liver. It is divided into several regions from left to right: the gastric fundus; the body; the pyloric antrum; and the pyloric canal. The fundus forms a pouch arising from the left dorsal part of the stomach. The stomach communicates with the oesophagus through the cardia and with the duodenum through the pylorus.

Two gastric curvatures are described (Figure 9.1). The greater curvature is convex and forms the caudoventral border of the stomach, extending from the left side of the cardia to the pylorus. The lesser curvature is concave, and extends from the right side of the cardia to the pylorus. The deep part of the greater omentum inserts on to the greater curvature, and the left lobe of the pancreas is located in this region of insertion. The angular incisure is the point of maximal angulation on the lesser curvature.

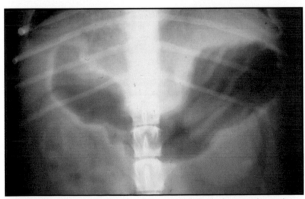

9.1 VD radiograph of the cranial abdomen in a dog. The gastric lumen is clearly visible owing to the presence of air within it. The gastric folds are particularly easily identified in this case, and are oriented parallel to the greater curvature of the stomach. The different compartments of the stomach are visible.

The radiographic opacity of the stomach as well as the ability to see it radiographically depends on its contents. When the stomach is totally empty, or it only contains fluid, it silhouettes cranially with the hepatic shadow (Figure 9.2) and its limits are difficult to determine except for the caudal border. When it is filled with food or gas, it is more easily visible and its contents appear heterogenous and granular (food) or of gaseous opacity (gas-filled) (Figure 9.3).

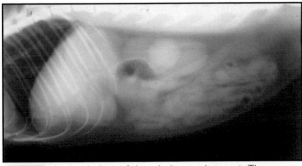

9.2 Lateral view of the abdomen in a cat. The stomach does not contain air and therefore silhouettes with the liver shadow in the cranial abdomen.

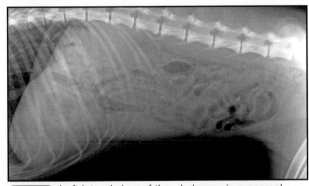

9.3 Left lateral view of the abdomen in a normal dog. Food is present in the fundus of the stomach giving a heterogenous pattern and opacity. Gas is present in the pyloric antrum, which is the non-dependent portion of the stomach on this view. A small amount of gas is also seen in the proximal portion of the descending duodenum. Note the distended caudal oesophagus.

The gastric mucosa has folds that are oriented parallel to the greater curvature of the stomach (see Figure 9.1). These folds are not always visible on survey radiographs. Nevertheless, they are easily visualized on double-contrast studies. They look more tortuous when the stomach is not distended, and are less visible, if not invisible, when the stomach is very distended. In the pyloric region, the folds are thinner and have a spiral course. It is considered that for a moderately dilated stomach, the ratio between the fold height and the inter-fold space is approximately 2:1.

The radiographic aspect of the stomach varies depending on the species and size of the animal, the radiographic view used, the gastric contents, the degree of gastric distension and the possible effects of administered drugs on gastric motility.

Species differences

In the dog, on the ventrodorsal (VD) view the gastric fundus and body are located to the left of the sagittal plane. The pyloric canal and antrum are superimposed on the vertebral column and to the right of the sagittal plane. The pylorus is usually located in the right cranial abdominal quadrant at the level of the 10th or 11th rib. On this view, the great axis of the stomach is often perpendicular to the vertebral column, and the stomach has a transverse orientation within the abdominal cavity (see Figure 9.1). The angular incisure is in this case not well demarcated. In some patients the stomach appears U-shaped, in which case the angular incisure is more clearly visible.

In cats, the stomach is more left-sided than in dogs, and only the pylorus is superimposed on the vertebral column. The great axis of the stomach is much more parallel to the vertebral column than in the dog (Figure 9.4). It is described as J-shaped in this species. In the cat, the gastric mucosal folds are less numerous and thinner than those of the dog.

The gastric axis

On the lateral view, the gastric axis is an imaginary line from the fundus through the body and pylorus (Figure 9.5). In dogs with an intermediate thoracic conformation, this axis should be moderately oblique in a craniodorsal to caudoventral direction. Schematically, this axis is perpendicular to the vertebral column and roughly parallel to the 10th pair of ribs. The pylorus is seen on this view slightly cranial to the gastric body or superimposed on it, and the fundus

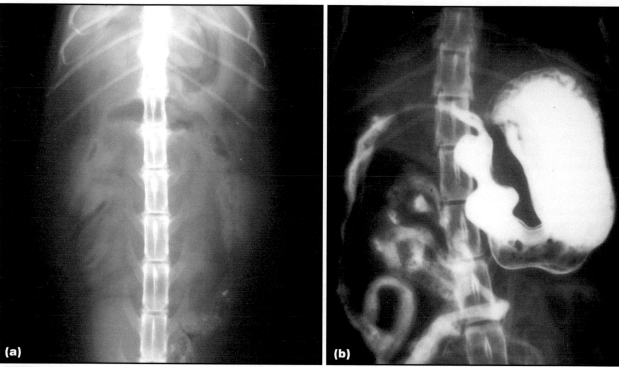

9.4   VD views of the abdomen in a cat. **(a)** The stomach is J-shaped and clearly identified here because it contains gas. Its great axis is parallel to the spine. **(b)** View following administration of barium sulphate. Note the J shape of the stomach filled with barium. In cats the stomach is almost entirely on the left side, with only the pylorus being superimposed on the spine (or slightly to the right if the stomach is distended).

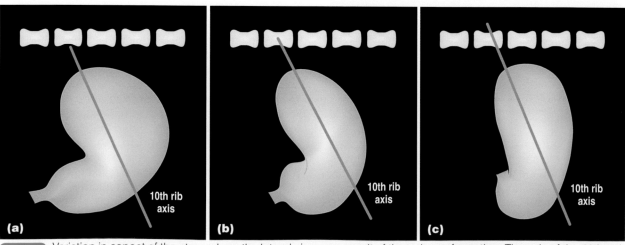

9.5   Variation in aspect of the stomach on the lateral view as a result of thoracic conformation. The axis of the 10th pair of ribs is represented as a grey line. **(a)** Wide, short thorax. **(b)** Intermediate thorax. **(c)** Narrow, long thorax.

corresponds to the most dorsal part of the organ. It is in close association with the left side of the liver and the left crus of the diaphragm.

The shape of the stomach and the orientation of the gastric axis vary depending on the thoracic conformation of the animal. In dogs with long and narrow chests, the stomach appears quite elongated and more perpendicular to the vertebral column than in dogs of medium chest size (Figure 9.5). Sometimes the obliquity can even be reversed (oblique in a caudodorsal to cranioventral direction); this presentation can mimic microhepatia. In contrast, in dogs with a short and wide thorax, the stomach appears more globular with the caudal border being more convex, and the axis being more oblique relative to the vertebral column and more parallel to the 10th pair of ribs (Figure 9.5).

Positional changes and radiography

The most important factor affecting the variation of the radiographic aspect of the stomach is the radiographic view used. Indeed, the view directly influences the way in which gas and fluid contents are positioned relative to each other in the gastric lumen. Owing to gravity, fluids fall into the dependent part of the lumen, whereas gas remains in the non-dependent part, thus modifying the aspect of the gastric gas bubble seen radiographically (Figure 9.6).

In ventral recumbency (dorsoventral (DV) view) the gas is present in the fundus, which is then the most dorsal aspect of the stomach. The gas bubble appears as a round lucent shadow located in the left cranial region of the abdomen. In dorsal recumbency (VD view) the gas is located in the gastric body and pyloric antrum, and the gas bubble appears as a lucent tubular shadow extending on both sides of the vertebral column.

In left lateral recumbency the gas bubble fills the pyloric region and appears as a lucent oval- or triangle-shaped image in the cranioventral part of the abdomen (Figure 9.6c). In right lateral recumbency the gas bubble is located in the fundic region. It appears as a lucent round image in the craniodorsal part of the abdomen, caudal to the left crus of the diaphragm. On a radiograph obtained with the animal in right lateral recumbency, the fluid present in the gastric body/antrum may form a rounded image of tissue opacity that may easily be mistaken for an abdominal mass (Figures 9.6d and Figure 9.7). Veterinary surgeons must be aware of this pitfall, and not mistake the fluid for a mass or a foreign body.

In case of doubt, another view with the animal in left lateral recumbency allows differentiation of the image of the gastric body from a mass because in this case the stomach becomes filled with air and thus appears of gas opacity (Figure 9.8). It is also possible to obtain another view in right lateral recumbency after administering barium sulphate to the animal in order to opacify the gastric lumen.

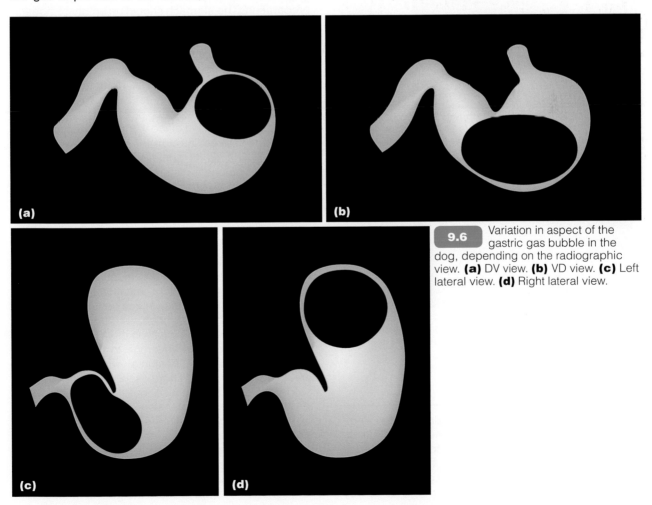

9.6 Variation in aspect of the gastric gas bubble in the dog, depending on the radiographic view. **(a)** DV view. **(b)** VD view. **(c)** Left lateral view. **(d)** Right lateral view.

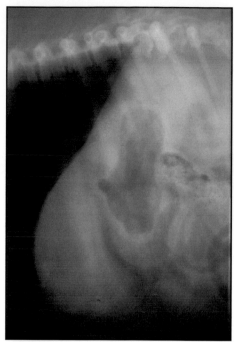

9.7 Right lateral view of the abdomen in a dog. Note the rounded soft tissue opacity caudal to the hepatic shadow in the cranioventral abdomen. This corresponds to the gastric antrum, which in right lateral recumbency is in the dependent portion of the stomach and therefore is filled with fluid.

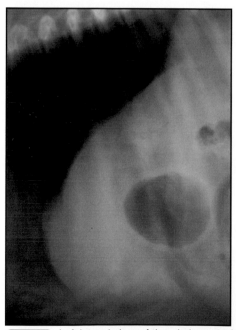

9.8 Left lateral view of the abdomen of the same dog as in Figure 9.7. The gastric antrum is filled with air and forms a rounded image of gas lucency in the cranioventral part of the abdomen.

Contrast radiography

The administration of contrast medium into the stomach allows better identification of the gastric lumen, and the double-contrast technique facilitates the evaluation of the gastric mucosa and the gastric wall. Survey radiographs must be obtained prior to contrast studies to serve as reference images. The survey images are also used to set the radiographic exposure parameters; usually it is necessary to increase the values of these parameters slightly for positive-contrast studies to account for the presence of the highly opaque contrast medium. In addition, survey radiographs may allow the recognition of some lesions that would be masked by the contrast medium, or they may suggest a definitive diagnosis, thus eliminating the need for a time-consuming contrast study.

Contrast studies of the stomach may be used in several circumstances:

- To confirm a suspected gastric abnormality based on clinical suspicion, when survey radiographs are within normal limits
- To confirm a suspected gastric disease based on abnormal radiographic signs on survey radiographs
- To evaluate the size, position and shape of the stomach when these cannot be evaluated on survey radiographs
- To assess gastric motility disorders.

There are different gastrography techniques: simple contrast (negative or positive) and double-contrast gastrography; and the barium meal.

Negative-contrast gastrography

Negative-contrast gastrography (or pneumogastrography) is a simple technique that requires little preparation. The stomach should be empty of ingesta, which may require withholding food from the animal for 12–24 hours. The animal may need to be sedated to allow a nasogastric or orogastric tube to be placed. Drugs that induce gastric hypomotility, such as glucagon, can be administered to induce relaxation and facilitate gastric filling and visualization of the mucosal surface.

Once the tube is in place within the gastric lumen, air is administered through the tube at a volume of 20 ml/kg. The air is administered rapidly until the stomach is palpably distended. If the animal shows discomfort the degree of distension is likely to be sufficient and the injection should be stopped. The tube is kinked and removed rapidly to prevent the escape of air.

Left lateral and VD radiographic views are immediately obtained as these views are often the most diagnostic and are the most likely to reveal pyloric outflow obstruction. Additional views (right lateral, DV and oblique views) can be added if there is still enough air in the stomach.

An alternative to the injection of air is to administer 60 ml of a carbonated beverage to the animal via a syringe (sometimes the animal will spontaneously drink the beverage). There is no need to use an orogastric tube in this case, but this method usually leads to less gastric distension, and the small amount of fluid introduced into the stomach might obscure some gastric structures.

An advantage of pneumogastrography, besides the fact that it is simple to perform, is that there are no complications associated with the technique. In addition, air does not obscure the gastric mucosa and gastric contents, unlike barium, which is useful if endoscopy is subsequently indicated. Ultrasonography should not be performed after pneumogastrography because the air injected into the stomach will prevent ultrasound wave propagation. Ultrasonography should therefore be performed before a pneumogastrogram. Pneumogastrography is a simple technique that allows better delineation of intraluminal foreign bodies when they are relatively radiolucent. It also allows good visualization of intramural gastric masses when they are not clearly seen on survey radiographs (Figure 9.9).

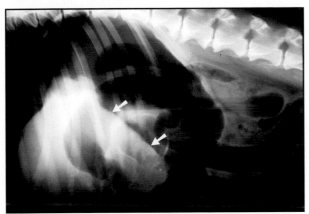

9.9 Pneumogastrography in a dog presented for chronic vomiting. An oblong mass of soft tissue (arrowed) is seen in the cranioventral region of the stomach, outlined by the injected air. An adenocarcinoma was diagnosed.

Positive-contrast gastrography

Positive-contrast gastrography involves the oral administration of a barium sulphate-based contrast medium in order to opacify the gastric lumen. The main goal of this contrast study is to determine the location of the stomach when it is not visible on survey radiographs. The stomach may remain invisible on survey radiographs when it is totally empty of food and does not contain air, or when poor abdominal serosal detail prevents its accurate identification.

The contrast medium used for this study is barium sulphate diluted in order to obtain a 30% weight/volume suspension. If possible, food should be withheld from the animal for 12–24 hours prior to the procedure. Sedation is not usually necessary; however, if the animal is not sufficiently relaxed, light sedation with acepromazine or a light and brief period of ketamine anaesthesia may be used. These drugs have no significant effect on gastric motility. The amount of contrast medium to be used depends on the size of the animal. For large dogs a volume of 7–8 ml/kg may be used, whereas for small dogs and cats relatively higher volumes are used, in the order of 10–15 ml/kg.

A sufficient degree of distension of the stomach must be achieved to obtain a good quality study. Owing to the clinical signs associated with most gastric diseases, it is common for the animal to vomit all or part of the contrast medium just after the ingestion. This is associated with poor quality images because the degree of gastric filling is significantly reduced.

Lateral and VD radiographic views should be obtained immediately after the ingestion of the contrast agent. When the degree of gastric filling is not sufficient, additional views, such as a DV or a contralateral view, may be useful to show the different partitions of the contrast medium in the gastric lumen caused by gravity. The DV view may also better demonstrate lesions in the region of the gastric body and pyloric antrum.

Evaluation of positive-contrast gastrographic images relies on the same criteria as those used when viewing survey radiographs: the size, shape and position of the stomach (see Figure 9.4). The advantage of the contrast technique is that it allows the identification of filling defects, the recognition of the size and shape of the mucosal folds and the evaluation of the mucosal interface, which should normally be smooth and regular in contour.

Double-contrast gastrography

Double-contrast gastrography is technically more complicated and time-consuming than positive-contrast gastrography but it allows a much better evaluation of the gastric wall and mucosal interface of the stomach. This procedure can be performed on anaesthetized animals, although sedation (usually with acepromazine) is adequate, and the anaesthetic drugs used must induce paralysis of the gastric wall (barbiturates, gaseous anaesthetics). If anaesthesia is not performed, glucagon may be used to induce gastric hypomotility (0.10–0.35 mg i.v.). This is absolutely contraindicated in dogs with phaeochromocytoma or uncontrolled diabetes mellitus, as glucagon can cause catecholamine release and hyperglycaemia.

Food must be withheld from the animal for 12 hours prior to the procedure to avoid artefacts caused by food debris within the gastric lumen. After induction of anaesthesia, a gastric tube must be placed in the stomach and a small amount of non-diluted barium sulphate (100% weight/volume) administered through the gastric tube. Generally, a volume of 3–5 ml/kg is sufficient. In order to ensure a good distribution of the contrast medium over the entire mucosal surface, it is worthwhile turning the animal several times. The stomach is subsequently dilated with room air until sufficient dilation is confirmed by transabdominal palpation. Usually, a volume of 10–20 ml/kg is sufficient. Four radiographic views are then obtained: VD; DV; right lateral; and left lateral. The radiographs must be centred on the gastric area. The rationale for obtaining the four radiographic views is to take advantage of the different relative positions of the positive and negative contrast media that result from the effects of gravity. The excellent contrast obtained by the combined use of a positive and a negative contrast agent allows a thorough evaluation of the entire gastric wall.

The appearance of the stomach on double-contrast gastrography varies depending on the radiographic view that is used. The positive contrast agent (fluid) will always fall into the dependent parts of the stomach, whereas gas will be located in the non-dependent parts of the gastric lumen.

- On the left lateral view, the barium sulphate suspension is in the gastric fundus and forms a rounded to oval-shaped opaque image in the craniodorsal part of the abdomen, whilst the air fills the body and pyloric portions of the stomach.
- On the right lateral view, the barium sulphate suspension pools in the pyloric region and the air fills the gastric body and fundus.
- On the VD view, the barium suspension is present in the fundus region on the left, and in the pyloric region on the right, whereas the body is filled with air.
- On the DV view, the barium suspension is present in the body whereas air fills the fundic and pyloric regions.

On all views, a small amount of barium sulphate adheres to the mucosal surface and allows the evaluation of its regularity, as well as the recognition of the mucosal folds. The folds form linear radio-lucencies separated by radiopaque bands, which correspond to the accumulation of positive contrast medium between them. The number of mucosal folds is normally higher in the region of the fundus and the body than in the pyloric region. The size and number of folds can be evaluated on double-contrast studies.

Barium meal

The aforementioned studies involve the use of a liquid contrast medium to opacify the gastric lumen. These studies allow only a qualitative assessment of the gastric wall and contents, and do not provide functional information. The evaluation is static and occurs at a given moment. Gastric emptying disorders are a frequent cause of chronic vomiting and may result from a broad spectrum of pathological conditions. In such cases, the functional disturbances may remain unrecognized by the techniques described earlier. Barium meal studies may overcome the limitations associated with the use of liquid contrast medium. In these studies, a meal mixed with a barium sulphate suspension is administered to the animal, and the gastric emptying is followed over time on successive radiographs. A barium meal study allows evaluation of gastric emptying in a situation that is closer to reality because of the solid nature of the food, compared with the fluid nature of the contrast agent used in barium gastrography. Conventional barium gastrography may not be able to reveal an abnormality of gastric emptying that may become obvious when a barium meal study is performed.

The procedure should be performed after food has been withheld from the animal for 24 hours. If sedation is necessary, acepromazine should be used as it does not interfere with gastric peristalsis. Again, in order to obtain a meaningful result, a sufficient degree of gastric distension is required, which is not always easy with uncooperative animals. A proposed amount to feed is 8 g of wet food mixed with 5–7 ml of barium sulphate per kg bodyweight. Lateral and VD views of the stomach are then obtained every hour until total gastric emptying occurs.

The normal gastric emptying times are <8 hours in the dog and <5 hours in the cat. In addition, emptying should begin <1 hour after the ingestion of the barium meal. When the start of emptying is delayed and/or the total gastric emptying time is prolonged, a gastric emptying disorder may be suspected. Many conditions are associated with such disorders but the most frequent are chronic pyloric obstructive diseases (e.g. hypertrophic pyloric stenosis, pyloric tumours, chronic pyloric hypertrophic gastropathy) or primary disorders of gastric contractility.

In all cases, the interpretation of barium meal studies must be made with caution because many non-pathological causes may lead to abnormal gastric emptying. One of the most frequent pitfalls is the delayed emptying associated with stress and anxiety. Stress can be associated with significant functional gastric disturbances. In addition, the transit times obtained with the barium meal technique are reproducible for a given individual, but in a group of individuals the normal value can vary from 7 to 15 hours. Therefore, the usefulness of this technique for the recognition of minor gastric emptying disorders remains limited.

Ultrasonography

Equipment and patient preparation

For a thorough ultrasonographic examination of the stomach, food should be withheld from the patient for at least 12 hours. Offering water to drink before the examination can be helpful as visibility of the outline of the gastric wall is best in a moderately fluid-distended stomach. A high-frequency transducer of 5–7.5 MHz, or even 10 MHz in small animals such as cats, is needed in order to assess the wall structure and layering appropriately.

Normal ultrasonographic anatomy

The stomach can be visualized by placing the ultrasound probe caudal to the ribcage in a sagittal plane and sweeping it from right to left in a craniodorsal direction. In deep-chested dogs, the stomach is usually tucked under the ribcage and an intercostal window may be needed to evaluate the stomach fully. The stomach can be recognized by its position just caudal to the liver, its size, contents and rugal folds (Figure 9.10). The gastric fundus is seen in the left craniodorsal abdomen and has the most prominent rugal folds when empty. By following the greater curvature of the stomach ventrally and to the right, the body and antrum are examined. Alternatively, to visualize the gastric antrum and pyloric canal, the duodenum can be imaged ventrolateral to the right kidney and followed cranially to the pyloric antrum. A helpful landmark to identify the pylorus is the portal vein at the liver hilus; the pylorus and cranial duodenal flexure are just caudal to the liver hilus and ventral to the portal vein.

Because of the variable gastric contents, altering the position of the animal and using acoustic windows can be useful when imaging the stomach. Gas in the stomach causes deterioration of the image because it reflects a large portion of the ultrasound beam and creates reverberation artefacts, making it impossible

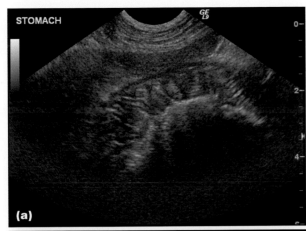

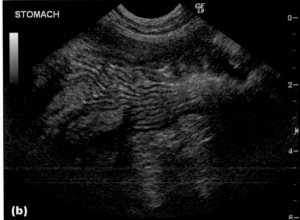

9.10 **(a)** Short axis and **(b)** long axis views of the gastric fundus of a clinically and ultrasonographically normal dog. The stomach is nearly empty and contains only a small amount of gas in some portions. The rugal folds give the stomach wall a striated appearance.

to evaluate deeper structures such as the opposite stomach wall. Given that gas will rise to the non-dependent portion of the stomach, it can be helpful to scan the patient in different positions. For example, in right lateral recumbency the probe can be positioned slightly under the cranial abdomen to examine the now fluid-filled pyloric antrum.

The stomach wall consists of five ultrasono-graphically distinguishable layers: the hyperechoic serosa coating the outside of the stomach; the hypoechoic muscular layer; the submucosa (hyper-echoic); the mucosa (hypoechoic); and the interface between the mucosa and the gastric contents, which is hyperechoic. The ultrasonographic appearance of the stomach wall also depends on the degree of filling of the stomach. In an empty stomach, the gastric wall consists of closely stacked rugal folds, best visualized in a short axis view of the stomach (see Figure 9.10a). It can be difficult to assess the stomach wall correctly in long axis if it is empty and contracted, as an oblique section through a rugal fold can give a false diagnosis of wall thickening and loss of layering. The normal thickness of the stomach wall in dogs is 3–5 mm; the wall tends to be slightly thicker in an empty than a distended stomach. In cats, the normal stomach wall should measure <2 mm between the rugal folds and the rugal folds can measure up to 4.4 mm.

The gastric fundus has the most prominent rugal folds, whereas the wall of the gastric antrum is smoother. The pyloric canal can have the appearance of a hyperechoic mucosal layer, but if it is normal in thickness and the layers are clearly visible, this is a normal finding (Figure 9.11). Gastric motility can be assessed using ultrasonography; a normal stomach containing some food should contract four to five times per minute. However, this depends on the degree of filling and time since the last meal; an empty stomach can be in a resting state and have fewer and weaker contractions.

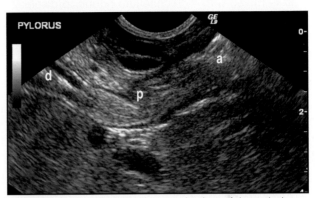

9.11 Normal pylorus. Long axis view of the pyloric antrum (a) on the right, the pyloric canal (p) and the duodenum (d) on the left. The wall of the pyloric canal sometimes has a hyperechoic appearance.

Normal gastric contents are gas, ingesta and fluid. Gas in the stomach appears as a hyperechoic layer outlining the stomach wall and creating multiple reverberation artefacts, so-called 'dirty shadowing', which obscure all deeper structures. The ultrasonographic appearance of ingesta varies with the type of food the animal has been fed. Clumps of hyper-echoic material, sometimes with a rounded (kibble) or linear appearance, are consistent with a recent meal, which should be confirmed by the owner. Fluid in the stomach has a hypo- or anechoic appear-ance, interspersed with bright spots representing gas bubbles (Figure 9.12).

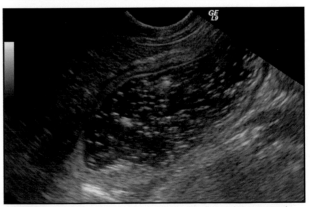

9.12 Normal stomach. Long axis view of the gastric fundus of a clinically and ultrasonographically normal dog. The stomach is moderately distended with hypoechoic fluid containing multiple gas bubbles, seen as hyperechoic specks throughout the gastric contents. The rugal folds are barely visible; note the clear distinction of the wall layers.

Overview of additional imaging methods

Radiography and ultrasonography are the main imaging methods used to assess the stomach in dogs and cats. Other imaging methods are not widely accessible and are used only for specific indications.

Nuclear medicine

Scintigraphy is considered the gold standard for the non-invasive measurement of gastric emptying. With this method, food or water is mixed with a radionuclide; food is mixed with [99m]Technetium bound to disofenin or mebrofenin and water is mixed with [111]Indium bound to DTPA. Transit through the stomach is measured by recording radioactive counts in the area of the stomach over time. Both liquid-phase and solid-phase emptying can be assessed.

Magnetic resonance imaging

In human medicine, magnetic resonance imaging (MRI) is used to monitor gastric emptying and motility simultaneously and non-invasively. Use of MRI in small animals other than for experimental procedures has not been described.

Computed tomography

Computed tomography (CT) is the modality of choice for the preoperative staging and follow-up of gastric cancer in human medicine. Cost, limited availability and the need for general anaesthesia currently prevent the use of this method for gastric imaging in veterinary medicine.

Gastric diseases

Dilatation

Gastric dilatation and gastric dilatation–volvulus

Gastric dilatation–volvulus (GDV) is a condition frequently encountered in emergency practice and usually affects large dogs. This disease must be recognized as soon as possible because it represents a medico-surgical emergency. The radiographic aspect of GDV varies depending on the degree of gastric dilatation, the gastric contents and the degree of rotation of the stomach. Most often the direction of the torsion is clockwise when viewed in a caudocranial direction; although anticlockwise torsion is possible. The degree of torsion varies between 90 degrees and 360 degrees. Volvulus of 360 degrees is difficult to recognize because in this case the different gastric compartments return to their initial positions.

The most constant Röntgen sign associated with GDV is gastric dilatation. Most often, the stomach is distended by large amounts of gas, but fluid and some ingesta may also contribute to the radiographic appearance of the gastric content. In the latter case, the gastric lumen appears to be of mixed opacity and heterogenous. Gastric dilatation is nevertheless not specific for volvulus, and may occur in the absence of volvulus. The recognition of volvulus of more than 90 degrees relies on the displacement of the different gastric compartments (Figures 9.13 and 9.14).

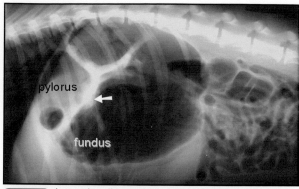

9.13 Lateral radiographic view of the abdomen in a dog presented with a history of acute abdominal distension, tympany and vomiting. A major gaseous distension of the stomach and abnormal positioning of the gastric compartments are visible. The fundus is displaced caudoventrally and the pyloric region is displaced craniodorsally. A line of soft tissue opacity is seen between the compartments (arrowed), and this compartmentalization is an important feature that allows the diagnosis of gastric volvulus to be established.

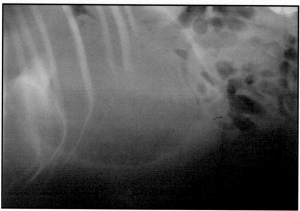

9.14 Lateral radiographic view of the abdomen in a dog presented with abdominal distension, tympany and vomiting of several days duration. A major gastric dilatation is evident in the cranial abdomen and the stomach demonstrates mixed soft tissue and gas opacity. Because of the fluid and gas content, an impression of thickening of the ventral wall of the stomach is present on this radiographic image. This is a false impression and is due to the geometrical arrangement of gas on the one hand and fluid silhouetting with the gastric wall on the other hand. The pyloric region is displaced craniodorsally and the fundus is displaced caudoventrally. In this case a diagnosis of chronic GDV can be established.

During rotation of the stomach, the pylorus moves in a dorsal and cranial direction whereas the fundus and the greater curvature move together in a ventral direction and to the right. The most useful element for recognition of gastric volvulus is probably the pyloric antrum, because this portion when filled with air is more tubular than the rest of the stomach, and therefore more readily identified. In a patient with volvulus, the pylorus is displaced to the left and therefore is filled with air on a right lateral view, which is the opposite of the normal situation. The comparison of both left and right lateral radiographic views is therefore useful to recognize pyloric displacement and, as a result, to differentiate gastric dilatation from GDV (Figure 9.15).

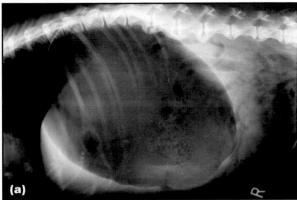

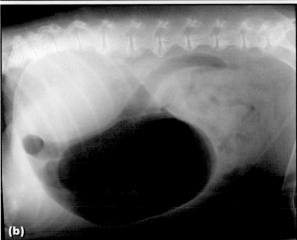

9.15 Dog presented with acute vomiting. **(a)** Right lateral view of the abdomen. There is marked gaseous distension of the stomach. Gas is mostly present in the fundic region in this case, which is expected on the right lateral view if this compartment is in the normal position. **(b)** Left lateral view of the abdomen. There is gaseous dilatation of the pyloric antrum and descending duodenum, whilst the fundic region is dilated by fluid. The pyloric antrum is easily recognized as a triangular lucency and is located in the normal position in the cranioventral abdomen. The fact that it is gas-filled on this view also suggests that it is probably on the right side of the abdomen. The diagnosis was severe gastric dilatation, without volvulus.

Another Röntgen sign frequently encountered in a case of GDV is the compartmentalization sign. This is a line of soft tissue opacity dividing the stomach into two compartments and is attributable to the folding of the gastric wall in on itself. Most often this line is horizontally positioned but it may be obliquely positioned and sometimes vertically, depending on the degree of dilatation and volvulus (see Figure 9.13).

The duodenum may be visible when filled with gas and can help in identifying the displacement because it accompanies the movement of the pylorus as a result of the anatomical relationship between the organs. In a patient with volvulus, the duodenum is visible in the left dorsal part of the abdominal cavity (instead of the right dorsal region). Because of the gastrosplenic ligament, splenic displacement is often observed in cases of gastric volvulus. The spleen can be seen in various locations, most often in the central abdominal region, extending caudally along the left abdominal wall. Splenomegaly is common because

of the torsion of hilar splenic veins at the pedicle and the resulting splenic congestion.

Other radiographic signs can be observed with GDV:

- Paralytic ileus is manifested by a diffuse and moderate to severe intestinal dilatation
- Decreased size of the liver shadow because of the compression by the dilated stomach and also due to the decrease in venous return to the heart associated with the volvulus
- Oesophageal dilatation visible in the caudal thoracic region because of the obstruction in the region of the cardia
- Loss of abdominal contrast due to peritoneal effusion.

In severe cases of GDV, gas lucencies may be seen dissecting between different layers of the gastric wall; this is not commonly observed but is associated with severe necrotic lesions of the gastric wall and a poor prognosis (gastric pneumatosis). Free peritoneal gas can be seen in cases of severe wall necrosis or gastric wall rupture and should be regarded as a bad prognostic sign.

Isolated cases of acute gastric dilatation without volvulus are sometimes seen. The same Röntgen signs of gastric dilatation with gas or fluid/alimentary contents are also seen in these patients. However, displacement of the gastric compartments and a compartmentalization line are not visible in cases of isolated dilatation. Gastric dilatation may result from severe aerophagia or from gastric paralysis or functional disturbances in the motor innervation of the stomach (Figures 9.16 and 9.17). These problems

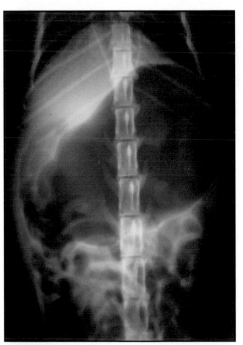

9.16 VD radiograph of the abdomen in a cat with feline dysautonomia. Note the severe gaseous distension of the stomach. The caudal oesophagus is also dilated and its wall is visible in the caudal thoracic region, forming two lines of soft tissue opacity joining at the oesophageal hiatus. Intestinal paralytic ileus is also visible in the rest of the abdominal cavity.

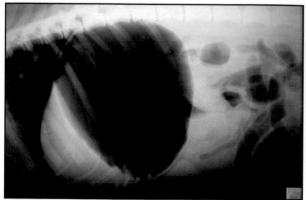

9.17   Marked aerophagia causing gaseous distension of the stomach in a dog.

may be post-surgical complications and may be associated with severe abdominal pain. It is important to differentiate between isolated gastric dilatation and gastric volvulus because a surgical procedure may be contraindicated in cases of isolated dilatation, whereas volvulus usually requires surgical treatment.

Ultrasonographic features: Ultrasonography is not indicated in patients with suspected gastric torsion; the large size and amount of gas within the stomach make it impossible to assess the cranial abdomen. However, ultrasonography can be used to identify a gastropexy site and to assess it for permanent adhesions.

Pyloric outflow obstruction

Chronic pyloric obstruction is a frequent cause of chronic vomiting, especially in dogs. This condition may have various origins, including mechanical or functional disturbances (pyloric spasm). Mechanical causes include any space-occupying lesion located in the region of gastric outflow (pyloric canal or pyloric sphincter), including:

- Neoplastic mass
- Fibrosis
- Inflammation
- Hypertrophic pyloric stenosis
- Chronic hypertrophic pyloric gastropathy.

Depending on the degree and duration of the obstruction, variable stages of gastric dilatation are observed. In severe cases, a substantial degree of gastric dilatation is present, involving all gastric segments (fundus, body, pyloric antrum and canal). The opacity of the stomach is usually mixed (fluid and gas) but the amount of gas is less significant than with cases of acute gastric dilatation. The lack of gas within the stomach makes the identification of the limits of the organ difficult because it silhouettes with surrounding organs, such as the liver. Variable amounts of food and non-digestible ingesta are also frequently present and are responsible for the heterogenous, granular opacity of the gastric contents (Figure 9.18).

When a significant amount of indigestible, opaque material accumulates proximal to the sub-obstruction, it can show up on survey radiographs as a sausage-like granular opacity in the pyloric antrum region: this is called a 'gravel sign' and is suggestive of chronic

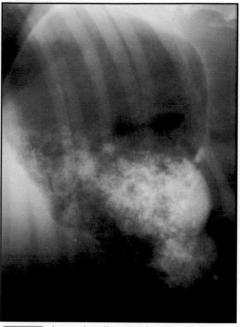

9.18   Lateral radiographic view of the abdomen in a dog presented with a history of chronic vomiting. Gaseous distension of the stomach is evident, and opaque granular material has accumulated in the region of the gastric body and pyloric antrum. These are signs of a chronic gastric obstruction, which in this case was due to a pyloric tumour.

sub-obstructive diseases (Figure 9.19). A barium meal may greatly help the diagnosis of chronic pyloric obstruction. Delay of gastric emptying may also be recognized with the use of a liquid barium sulphate suspension, but this type of contrast study does not reflect exactly what happens from a pathophysiological point of view. Nevertheless, liquid contrast medium suspensions allow better evaluation of the morphology of the pyloric region (Figure 9.20).

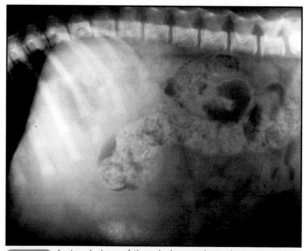

9.19   Lateral view of the abdomen in a dog presented for vomiting. Granular opacities are present in the ventral portion of the stomach, which is distended with a fluid opacity. Its caudal margin is seen at the level of L2–L3. The tubular granular opacity seen in the ventral portion is in the area of the pyloric antrum. It corresponds to the accumulation of indigestible particles cranial to a sub-obstruction of the gastric outflow ('gravel sign'). In this case polypoid gastritis was the cause of the pyloric outflow obstruction.

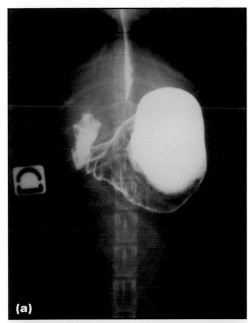

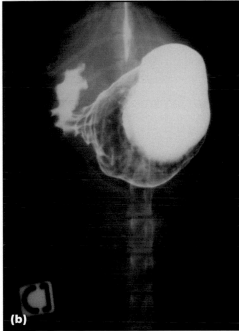

9.20 Positive-contrast gastrography in a dog that presented with a history of chronic vomiting. **(a)** VD view obtained 30 minutes after the administration of barium sulphate suspension. No contrast medium is visible in the duodenum and the mucosal contour in the pyloric region appears to be irregular, with a characteristic 'apple core' aspect. The most distal part of the contrast medium column at the pylorus is teat-shaped on this image. **(b)** VD view obtained 2.5 hours after the administration of barium sulphate suspension. No sign of gastric emptying is visible and the aspect of the contrast medium column in the pyloric region remains the same ('apple core' appearance). The diagnosis was one of markedly delayed gastric emptying and the abnormal aspect of the contrast medium column in the pyloric region was compatible with chronic pyloric stenosis. Infiltrative disease was suspected. In this case pyloric adenocarcinoma was confirmed at surgery.

Different Röntgen signs can be seen on contrast studies in cases of chronic pyloric obstruction, including:

- Intramural filling defect: symmetrical and circumferential
- Intramural filling defect: asymmetrical
- Intraluminal filling defect.

Intramural filling defect – symmetrical and circumferential: Annular thickening in the pyloric region may be caused by hypertrophic pyloric stenosis, pyloric spasm, inflammatory or scar lesions of the pylorus, or some neoplastic lesions involving the pyloric region. A circumferential parietal filling defect is observed in these cases, recognized as an abrupt narrowing of the contrast medium column in the gastric lumen. The contrast medium column may be abruptly interrupted or present several patterns:

- A beak- or teat-shaped end where the contrast medium liquid begins to insinuate into the lumen of the pyloric sphincter (Figure 9.21)
- String-shaped if the contrast medium liquid fills the whole length of the narrowed pyloric segment.

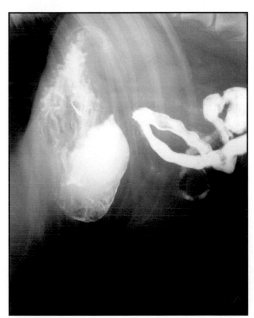

9.21 Pylorospasm in a Dobermann presented for vomiting. On this lateral view taken after barium administration, and on subsequent radiographs, there was a circumferential narrowing of the pyloric canal with a teat-shaped pattern. In this case a spasm associated with severe gastritis was the cause but annular neoplastic infiltrates should also be considered.

Intramural filling defect – asymmetrical: Asymmetrical thickening in the pyloric region can result from inflammation, severe mucosal hypertrophy or some neoplastic diseases. Antropyloric neoplasms can manifest themselves as a localized polypous mass with a centripetal growth and, therefore, are associated with intramural filling defects and may be responsible for an asymmetrical narrowing of the lumen at the pylorus (Figure 9.22).

Intraluminal filling defect: Pyloric foreign bodies are associated with intraluminal filling defects; they are surrounded by the contrast medium and not continuous with the gastric wall on all radiographic views.

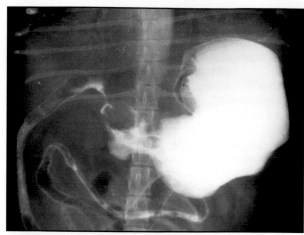

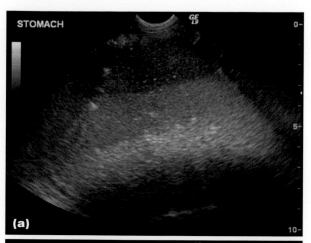

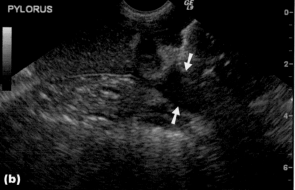

9.22 VD view of the abdomen 60 minutes after barium sulphate administration in a 22-year-old Miniature Poodle presented for chronic vomiting. The mucosal surface of the pyloric antrum is irregular ('apple core' appearance of the contrast medium column) and there is a round filling defect in the most distal portion of the pyloric canal, which is obliterating the lumen and is continuous with the cranial gastric wall. Chronic hypertrophic pyloric gastropathy or a neoplastic disease was suspected. Endoscopy revealed severe lesions of polypoid gastritis and the round filling defect represented a large polyp.

Ultrasonographic features: Pyloric outflow obstruction can be difficult to diagnose ultrasonographically. Secondary signs of chronic outflow obstruction include:

- Distended stomach with an enlarged gastric antrum
- A large amount of ingesta in the lumen, which can have a layered appearance with the solid particles in the dependent part and the liquids and gas in the non-dependent portion (Figure 9.23)
- Antral contractions with minimal propelling of ingesta into the duodenum
- Decreased motility.

The appearance of the obstruction itself depends on its origin:

- Functional obstructions (pylorospasm):
  - Functional obstruction is difficult to diagnose ultrasonographically
  - Pylorospasm may be suspected if the pyloric canal is not seen opening, despite forceful contractions of the pyloric antrum.
- Congenital hypertrophic pyloric stenosis:
  - Circumferential thickening of the pyloric sphincter, mainly of the muscular layer.
- Chronic pyloric hypertrophic gastropathy:
  - Circumferential thickening with mostly preserved layering; the muscular layer can be thickened (Figure 9.24)
  - A thickened gastric wall (>9 mm) and a muscular layer thickness of >4 mm have been described
  - A beak-shaped sign similar to the changes described in positive-contrast gastrography

9.23 Pyloric outflow obstruction. **(a)** Ultrasonogram of an 8-year-old Pug diagnosed with a history of weight loss and vomiting. The stomach is severely distended and contains a large amount of fluid and particulate material, which has a layered distribution: the hyperechoic mineralized particles creating acoustic shadowing in the most dependent portion of the stomach are followed by particulate material without shadowing and then a layer of hypoechoic fluid. This is indicative of a pyloric outflow obstruction; the accumulation of mineralized particles leads to a 'gravel sign' on radiographs. **(b)** Long axis image of the pylorus and proximal duodenum. The hyperechoic lumen of the pyloric canal and proximal duodenum is narrowed and distorted, compressed by a mass in the proximal duodenum (arrowed) causing an outflow obstruction. The mass was surgically removed and a leiomyosarcoma was diagnosed histopathologically.

can sometimes be seen if the thickened portion of the pyloric canal deforms the lumen of the pyloric antrum.
- Focal wall lesions:
  - Neoplasia (see Figure 9.23b), inflammatory polyps, granulomas and focal gastritis
  - Focal asymmetrical thickening of the pyloric canal, usually with loss of layering, can be pedunculated and protrude into the lumen.
- Foreign bodies:
  - The type of foreign body (see below) that tends to be lodged in the pyloric canal is a linear foreign body, where a solid component is anchored in the pylorus and the string component protrudes into the duodenum
  - The gastric component of the linear foreign body can be quite small and requires careful examination of the pylorus.

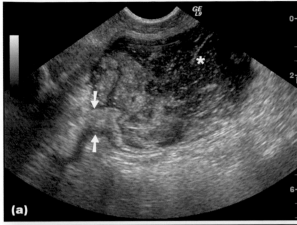

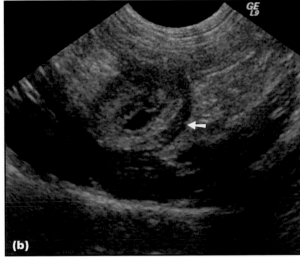

9.24 Hypertrophic pyloric gastropathy. **(a)** Long axis image of the gastric antrum (✱) and pylorus of a 3-year-old neutered Pug bitch, presented with a 2-day history of acute vomiting and abdominal pain. The antrum is distended and filled with fluid and ingesta. The stomach is contracting forcefully; however, the pyloric canal is very narrow and the wall of the pylorus is thickened (arrowed). **(b)** Short axis image showing the mild thickening of the muscular layer (arrowed).

Foreign bodies

Domestic carnivores, especially dogs, are commonly affected by gastric or intestinal foreign bodies because of their habitual feeding behaviour. Gastric foreign bodies may be associated with acute vomiting.

Gastric foreign bodies can be visible on survey abdominal radiographs if they are radiopaque (Figures 9.25 and 9.26). An abnormal shadow of variable shape and opacity (e.g. mineral, metallic) is visible in the regions of the stomach on all radiographic views (VD and lateral). Poorly opaque foreign bodies may be masked by other gastric contents, but can become visible when surrounded by gastric gas, which provides natural contrast. To increase the diagnostic accuracy of survey radiographs, it is recommended that several radiographic views (DV, VD, right lateral and left lateral) are obtained in order to benefit from the gravity-induced changes in the relative positions of gas and fluid within the gastric lumen.

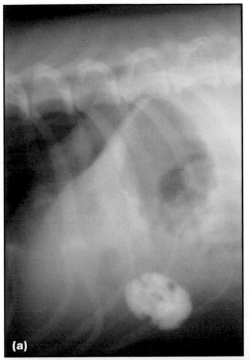

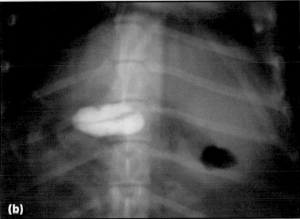

9.25 Dog with a history of acute vomiting. **(a)** Lateral radiographic view of the abdomen. A radiopaque foreign body is visible in the region of the gastric body. **(b)** VD view of the abdomen. The radiopaque foreign body is again clearly visible in the region of the gastric body.

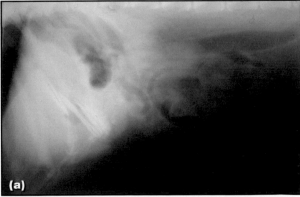

9.26 Dog presented with a history of acute vomiting. **(a)** Lateral radiographic view of the abdomen. Linear opacities are visible in the region of the gastric body. (continues) ▶

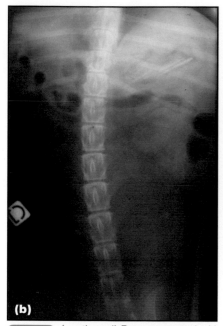

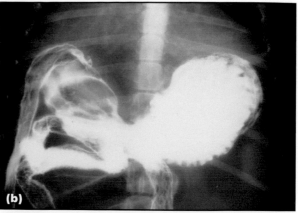

9.27 (continued) Positive-contrast gastrography in a dog presented with a history of acute vomiting. **(b)** VD view of the abdomen. The intraluminal filling defect is visible in the pyloric antrum region and is semi-circular in shape. The foreign body was confirmed as a piece of plastic ball.

9.26 (continued) Dog presented with a history of acute vomiting. **(b)** VD view of the abdomen. The linear opacities are again identified in the region of the gastric fundus and body. They corresponded to gastric foreign bodies.

Non-radiopaque foreign bodies require contrast studies for identification. On contrast studies (simple contrast gastrography or preferably double-contrast gastrography), foreign bodies are associated with filling defects, which have the size and shape of the foreign body (Figure 9.27). These filling defects have the characteristics of intraluminal lesions; they are not continuous with the gastric wall and are mobile within the gastric lumen, depending on the position of the animal. This 'mobility criterion' is not absolute because some foreign bodies may appear fixed within the stomach if they are trapped in the pyloric region.

When following the progression of the contrast medium on a barium series, a delay in gastric emptying caused by the foreign body may be observed. When barium sulphate has evacuated the stomach, the foreign body, especially if it is porous, may remain coated by the contrast medium and be clearly visible as an opaque image in the lumen of the stomach (Figures 9.28, 9.29 and 9.30). This opacity has the size and shape of the foreign body.

The size of the stomach should be evaluated carefully in the case of a gastric foreign body: gastric dilatation reveals that the foreign body has been present for some time before diagnosis. A localized dilatation in the region of the foreign body is more compatible with recent foreign body ingestion, owing to loss of ability of the segment containing the foreign body to collapse.

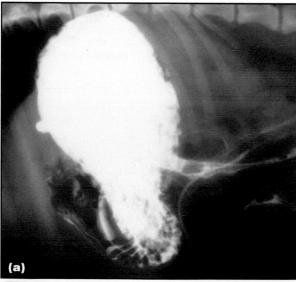

9.27 Positive-contrast gastrography in a dog presented with a history of acute vomiting. **(a)** Lateral view of the abdomen. A filling defect is visible in the region of the gastric body. This filling defect is oval-shaped and seems to be intraluminal in origin because it is surrounded by the contrast medium. (continues) ▶

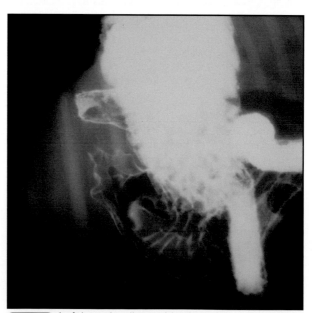

9.28 Left lateral radiographic view of the abdomen of the same dog as in Figure 9.27, after the barium sulphate has partially left the stomach. On this view, the pyloric portion of the stomach does not contain contrast medium but is filled with gas. The new contrast provided by the air allows the barium-coated foreign body to be clearly identified as a crescent-shaped image.

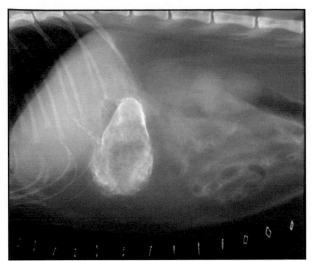

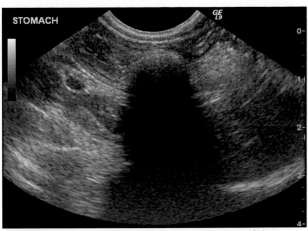

9.31 Gastric foreign body. Long axis view of the stomach of a 4-year-old neutered female Siamese cat with a 1-week history of intermittent vomiting. The stomach contains some fluid and gas. In the gastric fundus there is a round structure with a hyperechoic surface and a strong distal acoustic shadow consistent with a gastric foreign body. A trichobezoar was removed using endoscopic forceps.

9.29 Lateral view of the abdomen of a 9-year-old Domestic Shorthaired cat presented for vomiting. An upper gastrointestinal barium series had been obtained 12 hours before and there is persistent barium in the pyloric antrum with an irregular pattern, suggestive of barium retained within a gastric foreign body. In this case it was a large hair-ball.

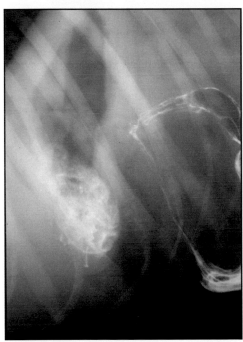

9.30 Lateral view of the abdomen of a 3-year-old Labrador Retriever presented for vomiting, obtained 12 hours after the administration of barium sulphate. There is barium retained in the pyloric antrum, which has an irregular shape and opacity. It was confirmed as a piece of fabric soaked with barium.

Gastric foreign bodies can be recognized ultrasonographically by their shape and acoustic shadowing. In contrast to gas, most foreign bodies cast a uniform, strong and clean shadow with minimal reverberation artefacts (Figure 9.31). Objects with an angular or round shape are also suggestive of foreign material; however, food particles can mimic foreign bodies and the time and type of the last meal should be verified. Foreign bodies typically move within the stomach and can be displaced by repositioning the patient. If foreign material is seen lodged within the pyloric antrum and pyloric canal, the duodenum should be examined for the presence of a linear foreign body component, leading to plication of the bowel.

Thickening

Gastric neoplasms

The most frequent malignant gastric neoplasms in the dog and cat are malignant lymphoma, adenocarcinoma and leiomyosarcoma. Benign neoplasms are occasionally seen, such as leiomyomas or adenomas. Gastric neoplasms are more frequently reported in the dog than in the cat.

Gastric neoplasms can sometimes be identified on survey radiographs of the abdomen, provided the mass is big enough and a natural contrast is provided by gas within the gastric lumen. Furthermore, the gastric mass needs to be tangential to the X-ray beam in order to be seen on the radiograph. In these cases, a parietal mass of soft tissue opacity protruding into the gastric lumen is seen (Figures 9.32 and 9.33).

With the exception of these particular cases, gastric masses or parietal infiltrations require contrast studies for recognition. The sensitivity of double-contrast studies is much greater than that of simple contrast studies in this regard. Indeed, a small mass is often completely obliterated by contrast medium on simple contrast studies (because the contrast medium is much more radiopaque) but often becomes easily visible on double-contrast studies. Nevertheless, the diagnosis is not always straightforward even on double-contrast studies. When an abnormality is seen on one view, the abnormality should be looked for on other views, or on the same view obtained at a different time, in order to be sure that it is not an artefact. It must be kept in mind that the stomach is an elastic organ that undergoes peristaltic activity, and a peristaltic contraction may in some circumstances mimic a parietal lesion.

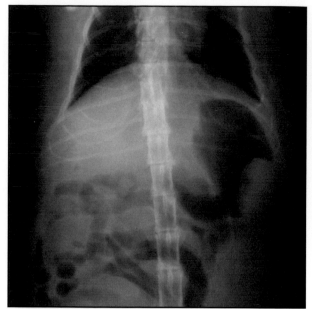

9.32 VD radiographic view of the abdomen of a cat presented with a history of chronic vomiting. The stomach is filled with air, which provides a good natural contrast and allows the identification of a parietal mass arising from the greater curvature of the stomach, protruding into the gastric lumen. This mass is of soft tissue opacity and has a smooth contour. It was confirmed as a gastric lymphoma.

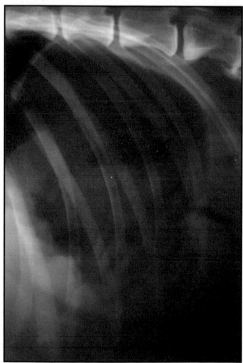

9.33 Lateral radiographic view of the abdomen in a dog presented with a history of chronic vomiting. The stomach is moderately distended by gas, which provides a natural good contrast. Gastric wall thickening is seen in the cranioventral region associated with an irregular, scalloped mucosal contour. This sign is compatible with a parietal infiltration but it may also represent blood clots or mucosal debris adhering to the mucosal surface. Either an endoscopic examination or a contrast study is necessary to confirm the hypothesis of gastric wall infiltration. In this case, it was a localized infiltrative lesion caused by a gastric adenocarcinoma.

The radiographic appearance of gastric neoplasms varies depending on shape, size and location. Some preferential locations are reported, depending on the histopathological type; for instance, adenocarcinoma is frequently encountered in the pyloric region. However, these are only general rules with many exceptions.

Gastric masses are associated with filling defects on contrast studies (Figure 9.34). The continuity between these filling defects and the gastric wall is not always easy to establish with certainty, especially when the lesion is viewed face on and is small. In

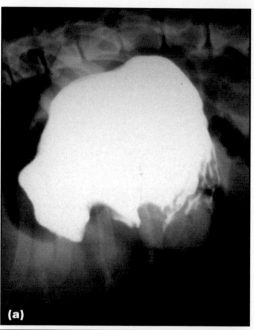

(a)

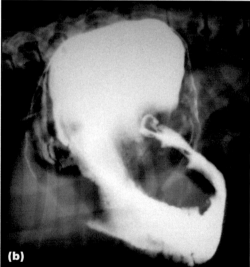

(b)

9.34 Positive-contrast gastrography in a dog presented with a history of chronic vomiting. **(a)** Left lateral view of the abdomen. Barium sulphate fills the region of the gastric fundus. Two filling defects are identified in the ventral region of the stomach, which are continuous with the gastric wall and protrude towards the gastric lumen. **(b)** Right lateral view of the abdomen. On this view there is better filling of the pyloric region by the barium. A filling defect originating from the cranial gastric wall is seen, as well as two other digit-shaped filling defects in the pyloric canal. These multiple filling defects were attributable to multiple masses associated with a gastric adenocarcinoma.

this case, the filling defect may mimic an intraluminal lesion, such as a foreign body. Nevertheless, the continuity with the gastric wall is often seen on at least one view. This stresses how important it is to obtain several radiographic views in order to better understand the origin (intramural or intraluminal) of a filling defect.

Gastric adenocarcinoma (Figure 9.35) often presents as a mass with a centripetal growth pattern and an irregular, moth-eaten contour (more rarely the contour is smooth). This pattern has been referred to as the 'apple core' sign (see Figure 9.20).

In rare cases, malignant lymphoma may have a similar appearance. Gastric leiomyosarcoma tends to have a centrifugal growth pattern, and therefore is rarely associated with filling defects in the column of contrast medium. In some cases, the tumours appear as voluminous masses that may be mistaken for a hepatic mass when they silhouette with the liver.

Secondary signs may be associated with gastric neoplasms. For instance, an abnormal rigidity of the gastric wall can sometimes be identified, or a lack of distensibility. This is better demonstrated on double-contrast studies.

Some neoplasms may be associated with diffuse infiltration of the stomach wall rather than with a mass. This is most often the case with lymphosarcoma (Figure 9.36) and some types of diffuse adeno-carcinoma. In these cases, no filling defects are observed on contrast studies. Double-contrast studies are very rewarding in cases of diffuse infiltration because they easily demonstrate wall thickening and rigidity, as well as the thickening and irregular orientation of the mucosal folds. It is also possible to identify marked irregularities in the mucosal contour as well as the out-pouching of contrast medium corresponding to gastric ulceration, which is frequently associated with gastric neoplasms.

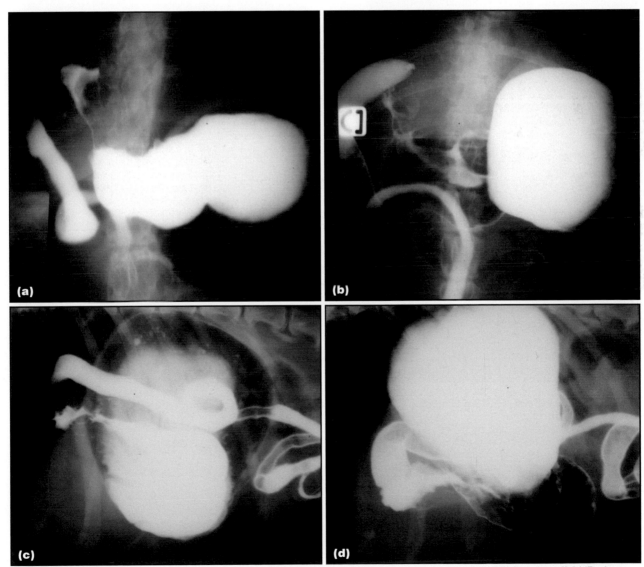

9.35 Double-contrast gastrography in a dog presented with a history of chronic vomiting. **(a)** DV view. **(b)** VD view. **(c)** Right lateral view. **(d)** Left lateral view. The distribution of the contrast medium varies depending on the radiographic view and this allows different parts of the stomach to be evaluated on each image. (a) A narrowing of the gastric lumen can be seen in the pyloric region on the DV view. (b,c) The mucosal contour in this region appears to be irregular on the VD view as well as on the right lateral view. These abnormal images were caused by a pyloric adenocarcinoma. Note in (a) the small out-pouching of contrast medium along the lesser curvature, protruding towards the exterior of the stomach; this corresponds to gastric ulceration associated with chronic gastric disease.

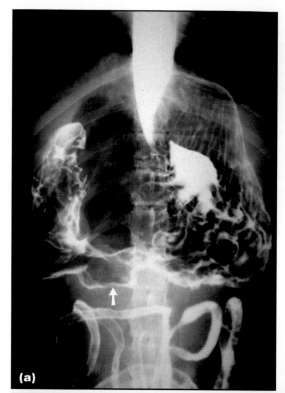

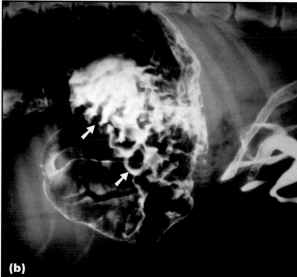

severe inflammatory diseases can mimic gastric neoplasia. Loss of layering, focal thickening and poor motility are commonly observed. Gastric neoplasms can be pedunculated and protrude into the lumen. The lesser curvature and gastric antrum are the most common sites for gastric neoplasia. Regional lymph nodes should be examined for evidence of metastatic spread. The most common gastric neoplasms and their ultrasonographic characteristics are given in Figure 9.37.

Tumour type	Ultrasonography characteristics
Leiomyoma	Focal well defined lesion Hypo- or hyperechoic
Leiomyosarcoma	Large, complex mass Often ulcerated and can lead to wall perforation. (For a description of the ultrasonographic appearance of ulceration and perforation, see below) Most commonly found in the pyloric antrum
Carcinoma	Heteroechoic mass 'Pseudolayering' – layers of hyper- and hypoechoic material not consistent with normal wall layers caused by tumour cell invasion Commonly associated with regional lymphadenopathy
Lymphosarcoma	Most common gastric tumour that leads to diffuse wall thickening, especially in cats The most common appearance of gastric lymphosarcoma is diffuse wall thickening. However, focal, mostly hypoechoic, mass lesions can occur Diffusely hypoechoic wall Circumferential transmural thickening Complete loss of wall layering Decreased motility Almost always associated with regional lymphadenopathy
Histiocytic sarcoma	Has been described to cause diffuse hyper- or hypoechoic wall thickening with loss of layering

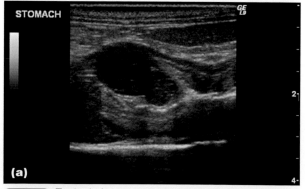

9.36 Double-contrast gastrography in a dog presented with a history of chronic vomiting. **(a)** VD radiograph of the abdomen shows that, although the stomach is well distended by air, the mucosal folds are abnormally prominent, thick and tortuous. A small rectangular out-pouching of contrast medium is also identified along the greater curvature, just to the left of the lumbar spine, corresponding to a gastric ulceration (arrowed). **(b)** Lateral view of the abdomen. The mucosal folds appear to be abnormally thick and tortuous (arrowed). This dog had a diffuse form of gastric lymphosarcoma.

Ultrasonographic features: All gastric neoplasms can have a similar ultrasonographic appearance and cannot be distinguished with certainty; a fine-needle aspirate or biopsy sample is always needed to confirm the diagnosis of neoplasia and to determine the tumour type. This is especially important because

9.37 Typical ultrasonographic characteristics based on tumour type. **(a)** Leiomyoma in a 14-year-old neutered male Shih Tzu with a history of diabetes mellitus. Abdominal ultrasonography was performed to recheck a splenic nodule seen several months previously. In the gastric fundus, there is a well defined hypoechoic mass protruding into the lumen of the stomach. The wall layering is not visible in the area of the mass, which seems to be continuous with the muscular layer of the stomach wall. A biopsy was performed and a leiomyoma was diagnosed. (continues) ▶

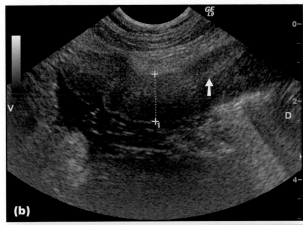

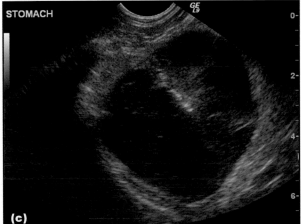

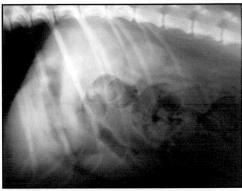

9.38 Lateral view of the abdomen in a dog presented with a history of chronic vomiting. On this survey radiograph, the gastric lumen can be identified by its air content. There is an impression of gastric wall thickening, especially in the caudal aspect, but this sign must be interpreted with caution because of the lack of gastric distension, and also because this image may have been created by mucus adhering to the mucosa and silhouetting with the gastric wall. In this case, the gastric wall was thickened and the dog had severe lesions of chronic gastritis.

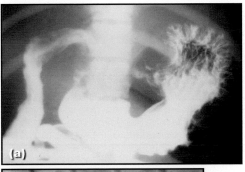

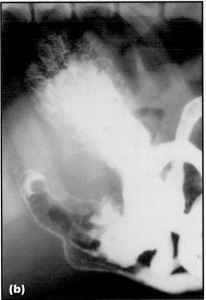

9.37 (continued) Typical ultrasonographic characteristics based on tumour type. **(b)** Gastric carcinoma. Long axis ultrasonogram of the stomach of an 11-year-old neutered Brittany Spaniel bitch with a 1-week history of vomiting. The stomach wall is severely thickened (18 mm) and has lost the normal layering. A hyperechoic layer of tissue (arrowed) is present in the centre of the otherwise very hypoechoic wall, consistent with 'pseudolayering'. **(c)** Gastric lymphosarcoma. A 7-year-old neutered female Domestic Shorthaired cat was presented for vomiting blood and anorexia. A cranial abdominal mass was palpated. On the axial ultrasonogram of the stomach at the level of the fundus, there is severe almost circumferential thickening of the stomach wall with complete loss of wall layering. The stomach wall is uniformly hypoechoic. Gastric and mesenteric lymph nodes were moderately enlarged. Lymphosarcoma was diagnosed on fine-needle aspiration of the stomach wall.

Inflammatory diseases

Gastritis cannot be recognized with certainty on radiographs. Nevertheless, some radiographic signs may increase the index of suspicion. Survey radiographs should be interpreted with caution. Although severe gastric wall thickening may in some cases be suspected from survey radiographs, care should be taken in the interpretation of such images, as it may correspond either to real wall thickening or to mucosal secretions or debris adhering to the wall, mimicking thickening (Figure 9.38). In all suspected cases, a contrast study may provide more specific signs of gastritis, such as gastric wall thickening, thickening of the mucosal rugal folds, or an increase in the number of mucosal rugal folds (Figure 9.39).

9.39 4-month-old Rottweiler presented with a history of acute vomiting. **(a)** VD radiograph of the abdomen obtained 15 minutes after the ingestion of barium sulphate. Gastric emptying has begun and the mucosal rugal folds appear to be markedly thickened in the region of the gastric fundus. **(b)** Lateral radiographic view of the abdomen. Abnormally numerous and thickened rugal folds are identified. Endoscopic examination of the stomach revealed severe lesions of acute gastritis in this dog.

Thickening of the mucosal rugal folds is often particularly clearly visible in the region of the pyloric antrum, where the rugal folds are thin in normal animals. In some forms of atrophic gastritis a decrease in the number and size of the rugal folds may be observed, but this sign is difficult to recognize and should be interpreted with extreme caution. In some cases of uraemic gastritis, linear mineral opacities can be seen within the stomach on survey radiographs that correspond to mineralization of the mucosal layer (Figure 9.40). In all cases, the suspected diagnosis must be supported by the results of other paraclinical examinations (especially endoscopy).

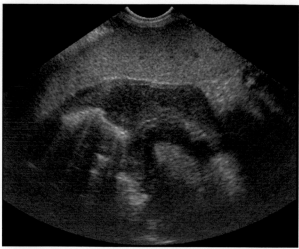

9.41 Gastritis in a 16-year-old neutered Dalmatian bitch with a 1-month history of inappetence, weight loss and chronic intermittent vomiting. The stomach wall is irregularly thickened. In some areas the wall thickening is severe, measuring up to 14 mm. There is almost complete loss of layering. A neoplastic infiltrate was suspected and a biopsy of the stomach wall was performed. Severe lymphoplasmacytic and eosinophilic gastritis was diagnosed.

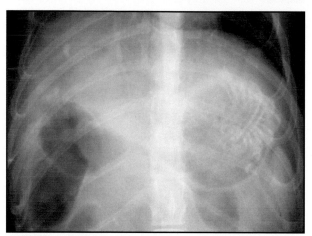

9.40 VD view of the abdomen in a dog with severe chronic renal failure. Fine linear opacities are seen following the mucosal surface of the fundic region of the stomach, consistent with mucosal mineralization seen with uraemic gastritis.

Ultrasonographic features: Ultrasonography is more sensitive than radiography for detecting changes associated with inflammatory diseases of the stomach. Ultrasonographic findings associated with gastritis are diffuse in most cases. Focal polypoid lesions may result from mucosal hypertrophy or gastric gland hyperplasia in patients with chronic hypertrophic gastritis. Severe gastritis (Figure 9.41) cannot always be differentiated from neoplasia or fungal disease associated with pyogranulomatous gastritis, and cytological or histopathological confirmation may be necessary. Underlying diseases, such as pancreatitis, should be ruled out.

Ultrasonographic signs of gastritis are very non-specific and can include:

- Diffuse thickening of the stomach wall
- Increased or decreased echogenicity of the wall
- Fluid accumulation within the gastric lumen
- Enlarged rugal folds
- Decreased definition of the wall layers
- In severe cases, loss of wall layering can be present.

Uraemic gastropathy is characterized by ulceration, oedema, mineralization, submucosal arteriopathy, gastric gland atrophy and necrosis (Figure 9.42). Ultrasonographic changes include:

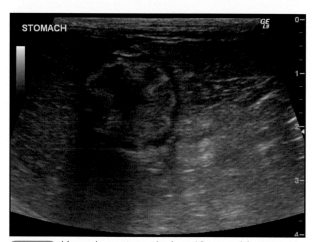

9.42 Uraemic gastropathy in a 16-year-old neutered mixed breed bitch presented for evaluation of recently diagnosed renal disease. Short axis ultrasonogram of the gastric fundus showing the hyperechoic mineralization of the mucosa. Note that an acoustic shadow is cast where the rugal folds are the thickest.

- Poor definition of gastric wall layers
- Mineralization of the gastric mucosa, seen as a hyperechoic line adjacent to the gastric lumen, usually not thick enough to cause acoustic shadowing
- Thickened gastric wall.

Patients with diseases leading to oedema formation, such as hypoproteinaemia, can sometimes develop gastric wall oedema. A very similar ultrasonographic appearance can be seen with gastric wall haemorrhage in patients with a bleeding disorder (Figure 9.43). Ultrasonographic findings associated with gastric wall oedema include:

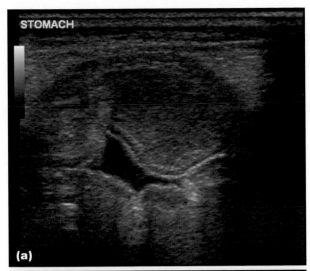

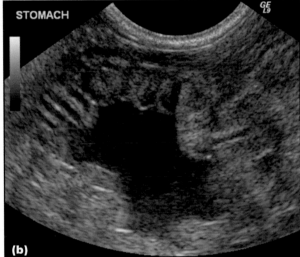

9.43 Rodenticide toxicity in a 1-year-old male
Yorkshire Terrier. **(a)** A short axis view of the
stomach showing severe wall thickening. The wall layers
are indistinct and the main pathology is affecting the
submucosal layer. Haemorrhage due to the rodenticide
toxicity was suspected. **(b)** Repeat ultrasonogram 1 week
after beginning treatment, showing that the stomach wall
has normalized.

- Thickened wall with preserved, but indistinct,
  layering
- The most dependent portion of the stomach is
  the most severely affected by gastric wall
  oedema.

Ulcers

Gastric ulcers cannot be recognized on survey
radiographs but may be identified on contrast studies.
Gastric ulcers may be malignant if they are associated
with a gastric neoplastic disease, but are benign in all
other cases. Benign gastric ulceration is associated
with various causes, including administration of non-
steroidal anti-inflammatory drugs.

Benign ulcers in dogs are more frequently
encountered in the pyloric canal than in the pyloric
antrum, the body or the fundus. Radiographic
identification is not easy and requires high-quality
images. Gastric ulcers are associated with out-
pouching of contrast medium on positive-contrast
studies, which is caused by the accumulation or
adherence of barium sulphate to the crater of the
ulcer. The appearance of an ulcer on radiographs
depends on its position relative to the direction of the
X-ray beam.

When the X-ray beam is tangential to the ulcer,
the lesion appears as a defect in the mucosal contour
within which the contrast medium accumulates. The
shape of this out-pouching of contrast material varies
from a beak-shaped to a square- or oval-shaped
lesion (see Figures 9.35 and 9.36). The margin of the
crater is usually well defined and gastric wall
thickening may be observed at the periphery of the
lesion. The central part of the crater is most often
smooth in contour. When the X-ray beam strikes the
ulceration perpendicularly, the lesion is then seen
face on in radiographs. In this case, the lesion is seen
as a small puddle of contrast medium owing to the
accumulation of contrast medium within the crater,
and a ring-like more lucent region is seen around the
crater that corresponds to the mucosal elevation
associated with the wall thickening. In this region,
there is effacement of the normal rugal folds.

It is very difficult to recognize a gastric ulcer on a
radiograph. Several factors may interfere with the
radiographic identification, including:

- A very narrow orifice may prevent the contrast
  medium from filling up the crater
- A crater filled with cellular debris, mucus, blood
  or food
- Significant oedema of the ulcer margins may
  partially obliterate the orifice and limit access of
  the contrast medium
- Identification of small ulcers may be difficult in
  large patients with radiographs of poor quality
- Marked hypertrophy of the rugal folds may
  obliterate small ulcers.

Malignant ulceration is probably more frequently
recognized than benign because it is usually larger
in area and is associated with prominent gastric wall
thickening or masses. These ulcers often have a
larger width than depth, they are variably shaped
and the central part of the ulcer is most often irregular in contour. The gastric wall at the periphery of the
ulceration is most often markedly modified. Neoplasms that are commonly associated with gastric
ulcers are adenocarcinoma, lymphosarcoma and
mast cell tumour.

When gastric ulceration is associated with gastric
perforation, secondary signs may be identified. Signs
of peritonitis and/or pneumoperitoneum may be
present (Figure 9.44). When such clinical signs are
identified and a gastric perforation is suspected,
barium sulphate **should not** be used for contrast
studies. An iodinated contrast agent may be used.
Barium sulphate induces severe lesions of
granulomatous peritonitis when it penetrates the
peritoneal cavity. Iodinated contrast agents are not
associated with such complications and also allow
the identification of gastric perforation by visualization of leakage of the contrast medium into the
peritoneal cavity after oral administration.

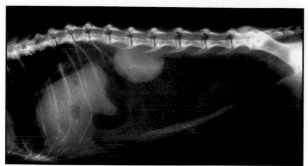

9.44 Lateral radiographic view of the abdomen in a cat presented with a history of chronic vomiting and abdominal tympany associated with acute abdominal syndrome. The overall opacity of the abdominal cavity is markedly decreased owing to the accumulation of free gas. The contrast provided by the free gas is responsible for the abnormally good visualization of the kidneys and margins of the liver, as well as the caudal part of the diaphragm. The diagnosis was pneumoperitoneum caused by perforation of a gastric tumour.

Ultrasonographic features: Small gastric ulcers are difficult to see ultrasonographically as the changes may be subtle. The presence of fluid within the stomach is helpful as it provides a better acoustic window through which to evaluate the stomach wall. Ultrasonographic findings with gastric ulcers (Figure 9.45) include:

* Focal wall thickening with indistinct wall layers or loss of layering
* Disruption of the normal mucosal surface in large ulcers with an ulcer crater
* Focal accumulation of hyperechoic material on the mucosal surface, representing gas bubbles or blood clots
* Decreased motility of the affected wall segment
* Pain associated with transducer pressure.

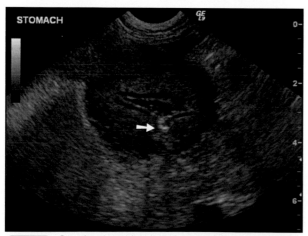

9.45 Gastric ulceration in a 9-year-old neutered male Jack Russell Terrier presented for vomiting and a painful cranial abdomen. Short axis image of the stomach showing that the stomach wall is thickened and that there is decreased definition of the wall layers. The mucosa is interrupted focally (arrowed) and hyperechoic material dissects a short distance into the stomach wall, representing either a gas accumulation or a blood clot. This structure did not move during the examination and the patient exhibited pain on light pressure of the transducer in this area. The findings are consistent with a gastric ulcer.

The patient should be examined carefully for signs of localized peritonitis and perforation, which include:

* Hyperechoic mesenteric fat surrounding the affected segment
* Accumulation of free peritoneal fluid
* Gas dissecting into and through the gastric wall
* Presence of free peritoneal gas.

References and further reading

Agut A, Sanchez-Valverde MA, Lasaosa JM, *et al.* (1993) Use of iohexol as a gastrointestinal contrast medium in the dog. *Veterinary Radiology and Ultrasound* **34**, 171–177

Armbrust LJ, Biller DS and Hoskinson JJ (2000) Case examples demonstrating the clinical utility of obtaining both right and left lateral abdominal radiographs in small animals. *Journal of the American Animal Hospital Association* **36**, 531–536

Baez JL (1999) Radiographic, ultrasonographic, and endoscopic findings in cats with inflammatory bowel disease of the stomach and small intestine: 33 cases (1990–1997) *Journal of the American Veterinary Medical Association* **215**, 349–354

Barber DL (1982) Radiographic aspects of gastric ulcers in dogs. *Veterinary Radiology and Ultrasound* **23**, 109–116

Barber DL and Rowland GN (1979) Radiographically detectable soft tissue calcification in chronic renal failure. *Veterinary Radiology and Ultrasound* **20**, 117–123

Berg P, Rhodes WH and O'Brien JB (1964) Radiographic diagnosis of gastric adenocarcinoma in a dog. *Veterinary Radiology and Ultrasound* **5**, 47–53

Biller DS, Partington BP, Miyabayashi T, *et al.* (1994) Ultrasonographic appearance of chronic hypertrophic pyloric gastropathy in the dog. *Veterinary Radiology and Ultrasound* **35**, 30–33

Bowlus RA, Biller DS, Armbrust LJ, *et al.* (2005) Clinical utility of pneumogastrography in dogs. *Journal of the American Animal Hospital Association* **4**, 171–178

Boysen SR, Tidwell AS and Penninck DG (2003) Ultrasonographic findings in dogs and cats with gastrointestinal perforation. *Veterinary Radiology and Ultrasound* **44**, 556–564

Brawner WR and Bartels JE (1983) Contrast radiography of the digestive tract. Indications, techniques, and complications. *Veterinary Clinics of North America: Small Animal Practice* **13**, 599–626

Burns J and Fox SM (1986) The use of a barium meal to evaluate total gastric emptying time in the dog. *Veterinary Radiology and Ultrasound* **27**, 169–172

Evans SM (1983) Double *versus* single contrast gastrography in the dog and cat. *Veterinary Radiology and Ultrasound* **24**, 6–10

Evans SM and Biery DN (1983) Double contrast gastrography in the cat. *Veterinary Radiology and Ultrasound* **24**, 3–5

Evans SM and De Frate LA (1980) Gastric lymphosarcoma in a dog: a case report. *Veterinary Radiology and Ultrasound* **21**, 55–56

Evans SM and Laufer I (1981) Double contrast gastrography in the normal dog. *Veterinary Radiology and Ultrasound* **22**, 2–9

Fischetti AJ, Saunders HM and Drobatz KJ (2004) Pneumatosis in canine gastric dilatation–volvulus syndrome. *Veterinary Radiology and Ultrasound* **45**, 205–209

Gomez JA (1974) The gastrointestinal contrast study: methods and interpretation. *Veterinary Clinics of North America: Small Animal Practice* **4**, 805–842

Grooters AM, Biller DS, Ward H, *et al.* (1994) Ultrasonographic appearance of feline alimentary lymphoma. *Veterinary Radiology and Ultrasound* **35**, 468–472

Grooters AM, Miyabayashi T, Biller DS, *et al.* (1994) Sonographic appearance of uremic gastropathy in four dogs. *Veterinary Radiology and Ultrasound* **35**, 35–40

Gualtieri M, Monzeglio MG and Scanziani E (1999) Gastric neoplasia. *Veterinary Clinics of North America: Small Animal Practice* **29**, 415–440

Hoffmann KL (2003) Sonographic signs of gastroduodenal linear foreign body in 3 dogs. *Veterinary Radiology and Ultrasound* **44**, 466–469

Kaser-Hotz B, Hauser B and Arnold P (1996) Ultrasonographic findings in canine gastric neoplasia in 13 patients. *Veterinary Radiology and Ultrasound* **37**, 51–56

Kleine LJ and Lamb CR (1999) Comparative organ imaging: the gastrointestinal tract. *Veterinary Radiology and Ultrasound* **30**, 133–141

Kneller SK (1976) Radiographic interpretation of the gastric dilatation–volvulus complex in the dog. *Journal of the American Animal Hospital Association* **12**, 154

Lamb CR (1999) Recent developments in diagnostic imaging of the gastrointestinal tract of the dog and cat. *Veterinary Clinics of North America: Small Animal Practice* **29**, 307–342

Miyabayashi T and Morgan JP (1984) Gastric emptying in the normal dog, a contrast radiographic technique. *Veterinary Radiology and Ultrasound* **25**, 187–191

Myers NC and Penninck DG (1994) Ultrasonographic diagnosis of gastrointestinal smooth muscle tumors in the dog. *Veterinary Radiology and Ultrasound* **35**, 391–397

O'Brien TR (1978) Stomach. In: *Radiographic Diagnosis of Abdominal Disorders in the Dog and Cat,* ed. TR O'Brien, pp. 204–235. WB Saunders, Philadelphia

Patnaik AK, Hurvitz AI and Johnson GE (1978) Canine gastric adenocarcinoma. *Veterinary Pathology* **15**, 600–607

Penninck DG, Moore AS and Gliatto J (1998) Ultrasonography of canine gastric epithelial neoplasia. *Veterinary Radiology and Ultrasound* **39**, 342–348

Penninck DG, Moore AS, Tidwell AS, *et al.* (1994) Ultrasonography of alimentary lymphosarcoma in the cat. *Veterinary Radiology and Ultrasound* **35**, 299–304

Rhodes WH and Brodey RS (1965) The differential diagnosis of pyloric obstructions in the dog. *Journal of the American Veterinary Radiology Society* **6**, 65–74

Scrivani PV, Bednarski RM and Meyer CW (1998) Effects of acepromazine and butorphanol on positive-contrast upper gastrointestinal tract examination in dogs. *American Journal of Veterinary Research* **59**, 1227–1233

Swann HM and Holt DE (2002) Canine gastric adenocarcinoma and leiomyosarcoma: a retrospective study of 21 cases (1986–1999) and literature review. *Journal of the American Animal Hospital Association* **38**, 157–164

Wacker CA, Weber UT, Tanno F, *et al.* (1998) Ultrasonographic evaluation of adhesions induced by incisional gastropexy in 16 dogs. *Journal of Small Animal Practice* **39**, 379–384

Wyse CA, McLellan J, Dickie AM, *et al.* (2003) A review of methods for the assessment of the rate of gastric emptying in the dog and cat: 1898–2002. *Journal of Veterinary Internal Medicine* **17**, 609–621

10

The small intestine

Kate Bradley

Normal radiographic anatomy

The small intestine comprises the duodenum, jejunum and ileum. On a lateral abdominal radiograph, the small intestine occupies most of the mid-ventral abdomen, lying caudal to the stomach and cranial to the bladder. It appears as smoothly curving 'tubes' in long axis views and as circular or ring-shaped opacities in cross section. Peristaltic waves cause transient segmental narrowing, which may be recognized on plain radiographs.

The duodenum runs cranially and laterally from the pylorus and then turns caudally, forming the cranial duodenal flexure. The flexure is held against the caudal surface of the right liver lobes by the hepatoduodenal ligament. The descending duodenum runs dorsally and caudally along the right abdominal wall, before turning medially at the caudal duodenal flexure (Figure 10.1). The ascending duodenum runs cranially and to the left of midline, where it becomes the jejunum at the duodenojejunal junction. The duodenum may occasionally be recognized on a plain radiograph from its characteristic position; it is

relatively fixed compared with the jejunum and ileum, which have a long mesentery and are readily displaced by changes in adjacent structures. The duodenum is also slightly wider then the jejunum and ileum. The terminal ileum may be recognized in some cases at the ileocaecocolic junction, which lies at approximately the level of the fourth lumbar vertebra on a lateral abdominal view. On a ventrodorsal (VD) view, the caecum lies on the right at the level of the second to fourth lumbar vertebrae. The jejunum and ileum are otherwise radiographically indistinguishable.

In an animal that has not eaten, the small intestine contains a mixture of fluid and gas. In the dog, the contents are typically one- to two-thirds gas; in contrast the feline small intestine usually contains very little gas. Loops of intestine should be approximately equal in diameter, although the duodenum is frequently slightly wider than the remainder of the small intestine. There are several useful 'rules of thumb' for normal small intestinal width, including:

- Less than the depth of the endplate of a lumbar vertebral body
- Not exceeding twice the width of other small intestinal loops
- Less than twice the width of the 12th rib
- Not exceeding 1.2 cm wide in the cat.

There is a wide 'normal' range of small intestinal width and it is often difficult to decide from width alone whether the small intestine is normal. Abnormal small intestine needs to be distinguished from normal large intestine; orthogonal views or contrast studies will often be helpful in distinguishing the large intestine.

Most radiologists have different criteria for diagnosing small intestinal dilatation. Small intestine in the dog has been described as being pathologically dilated when it exceeds four times the width of the last rib or is more than 1.6 times the mid-body depth of the fifth lumbar vertebra. If the small intestinal diameter exceeds twice the mid-body depth of L5, there is a high likelihood that an obstruction is present. In the cat, the small intestine is not normally more than 1.2 cm in diameter. The criteria listed above are not definitive and small intestinal width should be interpreted in conjunction with other imaging features and the clinical presentation.

The indications for radiography of the small intestine are summarized in Figure 10.2.

10.1 VD radiograph of the abdomen in a dog following administration of liquid barium, illustrating the position of the duodenum.

Persistent or recurrent vomiting
Diarrhoea (of small intestinal origin)
Abdominal pain or distension
Anorexia
Weight loss
Melaena
Suspected hernia
Suspected ingested foreign body
Palpable mass or bowel wall thickening

10.2 Indications for radiography of the small intestine.

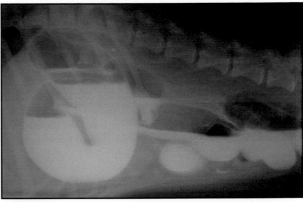

10.3 Horizontal beam lateral radiograph of the abdomen in a dog, following administration of liquid barium. Barium helps to highlight the fluid levels within the stomach and small intestine, which are at a similar level here, making a functional ileus the most likely diagnosis.

Species differences

In the cat, the falciform, peritoneal and retroperitoneal fat is usually more obvious radiographically than in the dog, and gives the small intestine the appearance of being 'bunched' in the mid-abdomen. In many obese cats, all of the small intestine may be to the right of the vertebral bodies on a VD radiograph, as a normal variation. Normal small intestine in the cat also contains less gas than in the dog. The pylorus is positioned further towards the midline and the cranial duodenal flexure forms a sharper angle than in the dog.

Positional changes

Gas will redistribute within the intestine according to the position of the animal. This has less influence on the assessment of the small intestine, compared with the stomach, but does mean that the appearance of the small intestine will vary between right and left lateral, and dorsoventral (DV) and VD views. The duodenum is often easier to identify on left lateral and DV views, as, being located dorsally and on the right, it is more likely to contain gas on these views. Prolonged lateral recumbency may lead to movement of the small intestine towards the dependent side.

Positional radiography

Multiple orthogonal views and, perhaps, all four views can be useful to investigate suspected small intestinal lesions, as the distribution of gas will change on each view. This may outline a lesion on one view but not another. Examples in which two lateral views may aid diagnosis include intussusceptions and foreign bodies.

Standing lateral abdominal radiographs can be useful in some cases to help differentiate between mechanical and functional ileus (Figure 10.3). Where both gas and fluid are present, as with mechanical ileus, there tends to be different 'fluid levels' within the same U-shaped loop. With functional obstructions (e.g. paralytic ileus) the fluid lines within a localized section of intestine tend to be at a similar level. Horizontal beam radiography with the animal in lateral recumbency may also aid in the detection of free abdominal air secondary to intestinal perforation.

Compression techniques involve applying pressure to the abdomen with a radiolucent object, such as a paddle or spoon, to minimize superimposition of other structures. Because the thickness of the area is reduced, exposure factors (kV) should be reduced by 10–15%. Compression is contraindicated if there is a diaphragmatic (or other) rupture, when compression

may increase organ displacement, or if there is suspected organ distension and therefore a risk of inducing rupture. Compression techniques have been reported to be useful in the diagnosis of some pathological conditions of the intestines, such as linear foreign bodies (see Figure 8.1).

Normal variations

In an obese animal, the small intestine may appear bunched and lie more centrally or to the right of the midline within the abdomen. In cats, a large falciform ligament may displace the intestine caudally. Conversely, if there is little abdominal fat, such as in very young or very thin animals, the serosal surfaces will be poorly visible. Subjectively, serosal detail may also seem poor if the intestinal contents are predominantly fluid rather than gas, or if several small intestinal loops are superimposed.

The contents of the small intestine depend on the type of food/other material ingested. Radiopaque objects such as small stones or bone fragments may commonly be seen in 'scavengers', and if aerophagia is present the intestines are likely to contain a higher proportion of gas. Empty, collapsed small intestine may give the impression of fewer loops.

Breed variation

In deep-chested dogs with an empty stomach, the small intestine may occasionally be seen against the dorsal aspect of the diaphragm. Otherwise, although the shape of the abdomen and therefore the distribution of the small intestine may vary slightly, the small intestine does appear very similar between breeds.

Individual variation

The contents of the small intestine in an individual animal will depend on the time post eating, and on the type of diet. Scavenging commonly leads to the presence of small mineral/metallic opacities within the small intestine. Some medications contain radiopaque material, such as calcium, aluminium, silicates, bismuth or magnesium, and can alter the radiopacity of the intestinal contents.

Changes in other organs will alter the position of the small intestine. A full bladder will displace the small intestine cranially, whereas a full stomach will displace the small intestine caudally. In a pregnant animal, an enlarging uterus will displace the small intestine cranially. Prior to radiographic evidence of fetal mineralization, enlarged uterine horns in the mid-abdomen may be difficult to distinguish from the small intestine. However, in most cases the uterus may be followed caudally into the pelvic area, where it lies between the bladder and the descending colon.

Contrast radiography

In most cases, plain radiographs allow assessment of the position of the small intestine, the contour and overall width of the loops, the definition of the serosal surfaces and the nature of the contents. Poor serosal detail may make it difficult to assess the overall diameter of the small intestinal loops, particularly if they are fluid-filled. It is not possible to accurately assess wall thickness or the appearance of the mucosal surface on plain radiographs, owing to summation of the soft tissue of the intestinal wall with any fluid contents (Figure 10.4).

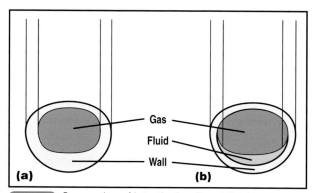

10.4 Summation of intestinal wall and fluid contents can mimic wall thickening on plain radiographs. **(a)** Thickened intestinal wall. **(b)** Normal intestinal wall and fluid contents. These may look identical on plain radiographs; contrast studies and ultrasonography provide information on wall thickness.

Contrast studies may therefore be needed for:

- Accurate assessment of luminal diameter
- Accurate assessment of wall thickness
- Assessment of the mucosal surface
- Identification of radiolucent foreign bodies
- Determination of the position of the small intestine, particularly if serosal detail is poor and the intestines contain little gas
- Measurement of intestinal transit times.

If abnormalities are identified, contrast studies will allow assessment of whether the changes are focal or generalized, and may help to identify which anatomical areas of the intestine are involved. Changes are often non-specific but in some cases it may be possible to make a definitive diagnosis from a contrast study, for example with a foreign body, intussusception or perforation. Clinical indications for contrast studies are summarized in Figure 10.5.

Assuming that plain radiographs are normal or non-diagnostic, contrast radiography is indicated for:

Vomiting (with or without diarrhoea):
- Acute and persistent
- Chronic or recurrent with no response to symptomatic therapy
- Haematemesis.
Palpable abdominal mass
Acute abdominal pain
Suspected linear foreign body
Suspected intestinal foreign body

10.5 Indications for contrast radiography of the small intestine.

Upper gastrointestinal series

For an elective study, food should be withheld from the animal for a minimum of 12 hours and ideally an enema should be administered to remove any opaque faecal material. Under emergency circumstances, a decision should be made as to whether the existing gastric and colonic contents will permit a diagnostic study. Typically, liquid barium sulphate suspension (30% w/w) should be administered either orally or via a stomach tube. Premixed solutions of micro-pulverized barium sulphate are better than hand-mixed suspensions as they tend to show less flocculation and achieve better coating of the mucosa as they pass through the small intestine.

A dose of 13 ml/kg should be used. Underdosing is a common limitation to the usefulness of an upper gastrointestinal series. The stomach has a much greater capacity than 13 ml/kg and the only 'complication' at this dose may be vomition. This can be minimized by prior administration of acepromazine, which provides a substantial antiemetic effect without changing gastric or small intestinal motility.

Lateral and VD radiographs should be taken at regular intervals (every 10–30 minutes), depending on the rate of passage, until the barium reaches the colon. If an abnormality is suspected, it is helpful to repeat the view immediately to confirm that a finding is 'real' and not caused by transient peristaltic waves. A 24-hour radiograph should be taken, unless a definitive diagnosis is reached from the initial study, to assess whether all of the barium has reached the colon normally.

Small intestinal transit time is typically 2–4 hours in the dog, with the small intestine being empty within 5 hours; transit time in the cat is typically shorter at approximately 1 hour. The volume of contrast medium administered and the duration for which food is withheld prior to the procedure do not significantly alter the transit time.

If sedation is used, acepromazine gives reasonable levels of sedation with minimal effects on intestinal motility in dogs. Acepromazine provides less dependable sedation in cats. In cats, a combination of diazepam and ketamine can be used, again with minimal effects on intestinal motility.

Following administration of contrast medium, the small intestine should be assessed for:

- Luminal diameter
- Wall thickening

- Mucosal pattern
- Filling defects
- Transit time
- Leakage of contrast medium.

If a lesion is seen, its location and the length of intestine affected should be assessed. The rule of thumb for upper gastrointestinal radiology is that lesions should be seen 'on multiple views and at multiple times'. An isolated peristaltic contraction may mimic almost any lesion. Verifying a suspected lesion with orthogonal views and determining its persistence through time is an important consideration.

Contraindications

Most contraindications are relative and occur in cases where the diagnosis is already known and an upper gastrointestinal study might delay surgery. An upper gastrointestinal study is contraindicated if there is convincing evidence of small intestinal dilatation on plain films and mechanical obstruction is strongly suspected. Contrast medium will be slow to pass through static, dilated intestine and an upper gastrointestinal study will only delay and possibly complicate any future surgical investigation. Similarly, a series is contraindicated if perforation is strongly suspected, for example if there is pneumoperitoneum and concurrent free fluid with a pointed foreign body evident on plain radiographs. However, if there is any doubt, an upper gastrointestinal study is indicated. Caution should also be used when the patient has demonstrable aspiration pneumonia. Aspiration of barium can 'flood' the lung, whilst aspiration of ionic iodinated contrast medium causes fulminant oedema, which is usually fatal. There is controversy regarding the type of positive contrast medium that should be used with suspected small intestinal rupture; each contrast agent has disadvantages.

A low (3 ml/kg) dose of water-soluble ionic iodinated contrast material (sodium meglumine diatrizoate oral solution) is often diagnostic. Ionic iodinated contrast media should not be used if the animal is very young or debilitated, as fluid drawn into the intestine may lead to dehydration, or if the patient has demonstrable aspiration tendencies. This type of contrast medium becomes very diluted in the intestines and less opaque as the study progresses in both time and distance down the small intestines; this may mean that a distal site of rupture is not readily apparent.

Alternatively, a non-ionic iodinated medium, such as iohexol or iopamidol, can be used. These media have less osmotic effect and are the safest alternatives to barium. Non-ionic iodinated contrast media are cost-prohibitive, except in very small patients, and still suffer from dilution in the small intestines, although to a lesser extent than ionic media. Non-ionic media should be diluted (1:1) with water prior to administration and then used at a similar dose rate to barium (i.e. 13 ml/kg). Transit times are generally shorter with iodine-based contrast media than with barium. Endoscopy or ultrasonography may be performed immediately following administration of iodine-based contrast media, as they are transparent and sonolucent. However, all iodinated contrast media are readily diluted in the gastrointestinal tract and so a diagnosis of perforation is much more difficult to make with diluted iodinated contrast media than with barium suspension.

Iodinated contrast medium is readily absorbed from the peritoneum, whereas barium can lead to granulomatous lesions if not surgically lavaged from the abdomen. However, the use of barium is indicated after negative or equivocal iodine studies. The patient should have surgery immediately after a diagnosis of perforation to minimize barium-associated adhesions and granuloma formation.

Barium-impregnated polyethylene spheres

Barium-impregnated polyethylene spheres (BIPS) are a mixture of small (1.5 mm) and large (5 mm) barium-impregnated spheres, which appear radiographically as radiopaque 'beads'. The theory behind their use is that the smaller spheres move through the intestine at the same speed as ingesta and give an indication of intestinal transit time. The larger spheres can be used for assessment of suspected obstructive lesions, as they may accumulate proximal to a partial obstruction if the luminal diameter is sufficiently narrowed (Figure 10.6). Radiographs taken around 24 hours after administration of BIPS should show all the BIPS in the colon. This technique has limited applications and cannot be recommended as an alternative to a positive-contrast intestinal radiographic study in most cases.

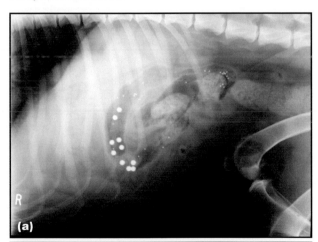

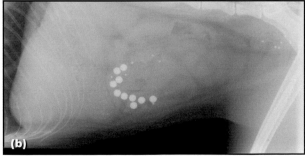

10.6 **(a)** Lateral radiograph of the abdomen in a dog taken 24 hours following administration of BIPS, showing all the BIPS in the colon (i.e. normal transit). **(b)** Lateral radiograph of the abdomen in a cat taken 24 hours following BIPS administration, showing all the large BIPS and some small BIPS accumulating in the small intestine, proximal to a partial obstruction. Some of the small BIPS are seen in the descending colon.

Pneumocolonography

Not a specific contrast study of the small intestines; this contrast study is performed most often to help ascertain which bowel loops are part of the large intestine (see Figure 11.3). This study is usually used when:

- There are clinical signs supportive of small intestinal obstruction
- Most of the small intestine appears normal
- One or two intestinal loops are larger than the rest and they cannot be positively identified as either colon or small intestine.

In cases of suspected small intestinal ileus, a pneumocolonogram will rapidly demonstrate which loops are large intestine, allowing the viewer to identify the small intestines by exclusion. This study is the most rapid means of verifying the identity of the small intestines and is often used in an emergency setting. The only relative contraindication is if an ultrasound examination is planned. An ultrasound study should be performed prior to any negative-contrast gastrointestinal study.

Usually, no patient preparation is necessary. A balloon-tipped catheter is inserted into the rectum and the balloon gently inflated to prevent air reflux. A volume of 8 ml/kg of air is infused into the rectum. A single VD view may be all that is necessary to evaluate the contrast study. The VD view prevents overlap of the ascending and descending segments of the large bowel. More air can be infused as necessary, to effect, to fill the entire colon and caecum. A lateral view may provide supportive information (see also Chapter 11).

Normal variations

With a barium series the small intestinal mucosa should appear uniform. The normal appearance is sometimes described as 'fimbriated' (fringed). The depth of the fringe is typically 1–1.5 mm, which correlates histologically with the length of the villi, with an allowance for radiographic magnification. The degree of fimbriation varies between dogs and is determined by the spatial arrangement of the intestinal villi.

The overall opacity of the contrast medium column within the small intestine varies slightly as the contrast medium mixes with intestinal gas. If iodine-based contrast material is used, dilution will lead to a reduction in opacity as it transits the intestine. This is more severe with ionic than with non-ionic media. Transit time also tends to be faster with iodinated agents as they can induce hyperperistalsis. The diameter of the small intestine will vary slightly because of peristaltic waves; normal narrowing and dilatation should be symmetrical and are unlikely to persist on serial films.

Normal variations (Figure 10.7) include:

- 'Pseudoulcers' (dogs) on the antimesenteric border of the duodenum, mainly in the descending duodenum, although a few may be seen in the ascending limb. They appear as smooth, flat out-pouchings of barium, caused by depressions in the mucosal surface associated

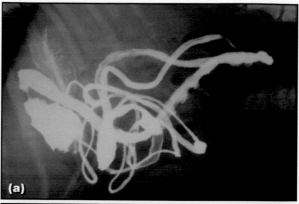

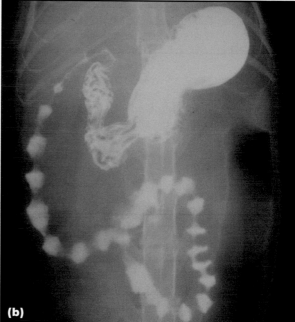

10.7 **(a)** Lateral radiograph of the abdomen in a dog following liquid barium administration, illustrating the normal duodenal out-pouchings or 'pseudoulcers'. **(b)** VD radiograph of the abdomen in a cat following administration of liquid barium, illustrating segmentation of the duodenum and proximal jejunum, sometimes referred to as a 'string of pearls' appearance.

with submucosal lymphoid aggregates. Dimensions of the 'craters' have been reported as 3–9 mm in diameter and up to 2.5 mm deep
- 'String of pearls' (cats); multiple symmetrical segmental peristaltic contractions give a beaded appearance to the small intestine.

Ultrasonography

Anatomy

The normal appearance of the small intestine is shown in Figure 10.8, and normal widths, measured from the lumen to the serosal surface, are given in Figure 10.9.

The descending duodenum can be identified ventral to the right kidney; it is usually the most laterally located loop in this region and appears straight and relatively wide. In cats, owing to the different position of the stomach, the duodenum starts in a more midline position.

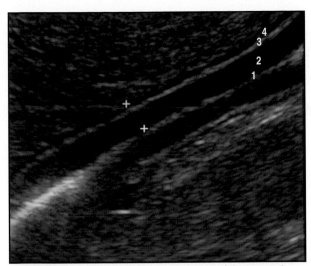

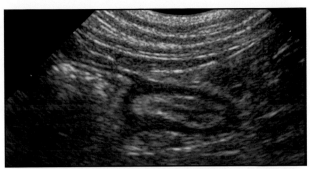

10.8 Ultrasonographic appearance of the normal small intestinal wall. 1 = Lumen (containing mucus); 2 = Mucosa; 3 = Submucosa; 4 = Muscularis.

10.10 Ultrasonogram showing a longitudinal view of the ileocaecocolic junction. Note the prominent submucosal layer of the ileum and the relatively thin wall of the colon compared with the terminal ileum.

Species	Duodenum	Remainder of small intestine
Cat (Newell *et al.*, 1999)	2.4 ± 0.51 mm (range 1.3–3.8 mm)	2.09 ± 0.37 mm (range 1.6–3.6 mm)
Dog (Delaney *et al.*, 2003)	<20 kg: ≤5.1 mm	<20 kg: ≤4.1 mm
	20–30 kg: ≤5.3 mm	20–40 kg: ≤4.4 mm
	>30 kg: ≤6 mm	>40 kg: ≤4.7 mm

10.9 Normal small intestinal widths in the dog and cat.

In some dogs and most cats, it is possible to locate the start of the duodenum at the pylorus and 'follow' the loop of the cranial flexure and descending duodenum. In other cases, particularly in deep-chested dogs, shadowing from the stomach and the depth of the cranial duodenal flexure makes it easier to locate the duodenum by moving the transducer ventral to the right kidney. An intercostal approach can be helpful in deep-chested breeds, as it may not be possible to see the proximal duodenum from a subcostal position.

The jejunum and the proximal ileum are seen throughout the abdomen as continuous loops of small intestine; it is not possible to determine the exact anatomical location of the intestine seen. The terminal ileum can usually be located in the mid-right area of the abdomen, especially in cats, by searching for an area of the small intestine that becomes continuous with the colon (Figure 10.10). The colonic walls are thinner and faeces will typically shadow.

The terminal ileum/ileocolic junction in cats has been described as having a 'wagon-wheel'-like appearance in transverse section. This appearance is caused by a persistently empty lumen and bunching of the mucosa into the lumen. The submucosal layer of the ileum is thicker than in other areas of the small intestine.

Technique

Withholding food from an animal for 12 hours prior to an elective ultrasound examination is helpful to minimize the contents of the gastrointestinal tract. Allowing access to water will not hinder the examination and it may help to outline the mucosal surfaces. If a barium or negative-contrast study is being considered, ultrasonography should be performed prior to administration of the contrast medium. This is less of a concern if iodinated contrast medium is used.

Shadowing and reverberations from the gas within the intestine can be problematic when examining the gastrointestinal tract and other structures deep to the gas-filled loops. These artefacts will preclude examination of the 'far' wall of an intestinal loop unless the gas can be displaced. An alternative acoustic window, such as imaging from the dependent aspect of the dog (i.e. imaging from the right with the patient in right lateral recumbency), may prevent gas artefacts. It may also be possible to prevent gas from obscuring an area of interest either by changing the position of the animal or by altering the position and angulation of the probe; gas will obviously tend to rise whereas fluid contents will settle dependently. Peristaltic waves may clear gas from an area of the intestine and allow a more accurate assessment.

For optimum examination of the wall structure of the small intestine, a transducer with a frequency of at least 7.5 MHz should be used. If a choice of transducer type is available, linear transducers are preferable to sector transducers. Lower frequency transducers will not permit as detailed an assessment of the wall layering, which is one of the most important features to evaluate. Intraoperative ultrasonography can be used to help target biopsy sampling in cases where changes are focal and not evident on gross examination of the serosal surface of the intestine.

Assessment

Ultrasonography and radiography are complementary techniques when it comes to assessment of the small intestine. Radiography is excellent for assessing gas-filled structures. There is good radiographic contrast between the soft tissue structures of interest and the surrounding peritoneal fat. This contrast is the basis for 'serosal detail' within the abdomen. Ultrasonographic images provide more information than radiography in cases where serosal detail is limited; for example, in very young or thin animals, or where an abdominal effusion or peritonitis is present. Ultrasonography is also able to provide information in 'real time', therefore allowing assessment of peristalsis. The main ultrasonographic features to assess are summarized in Figure 10.11 and discussed in more detail below.

Wall thickness
Wall layering
Echogenicity of layers
Luminal contents
Motility: regional and general
Location
Length of intestine affected
Luminal diameter proximal to lesion
Regional mesentery and lymph nodes
Possible metastases, e.g. in the liver or spleen

10.11 Structures of the small intestine which require assessment by ultrasonography.

Normal appearance and layering

In normal intestinal wall (see Figure 10.8), five layers are usually discernible. Working from the lumen outwards, these are:

- Luminal interface – hyperechoic
- Mucosa (widest layer) – hypoechoic
- Submucosa – hyperechoic
- Muscularis – hypoechoic
- Serosal interface – hyperechoic.

The intestine should be assessed for the overall wall thickness, presence of layering, the echogenicity of each layer and the relative width of the each layer. The layers should be visible in both longitudinal and transverse section. However, in transverse section the hypoechoic mucosal layer may not form a complete circle in all loops. Instead, there can be an echogenic stripe on each side of the bowel loop, which has been termed an 'extended mucosal interface' (Figure 10.12). This has been correlated histologically with increased distance between villi at the site of intestinal plication and is only seen in flattened loops of intestine.

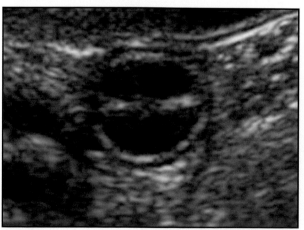

10.12 Transverse ultrasonogram of a section of small intestine illustrating the appearance of an 'extended mucosal interface'.

If changes are present, they should be characterized as focal or generalized, and the area(s) of the small intestine involved should be identified. The length of intestine affected may be difficult to determine accurately if changes extend over more than one field of view, but an estimate can be made. The pattern and distribution of change can be useful in narrowing the list of possible differential diagnoses; however, loss or altering of layering is not pathognomonic for any particular condition.

Thickness of intestinal wall: Ultrasonography provides an accurate means of assessment of wall thickness because the lumen can be identified readily. The width of the small intestinal wall is measured from the lumen to the serosa. Measurements should be made perpendicular to the long axis; oblique measurements may give artificially high values.

The duodenum is usually thicker than the rest of the small intestine, which has been attributed to an increased thickness of the mucosal layer. In the dog, as a general rule, the jejunum should measure no more than 4.7 mm and the duodenum no more than 6.0 mm, but this does vary with the size of the dog (see Figure 10.9). In the cat, the upper limits for normal small intestinal wall thickness are lower, with the duodenum normally measuring <3.0 mm and the jejunum <2.5 mm. The measured wall thickness can vary slightly with the frequency of the transducer used.

Motility: Contractility can be assessed easily by imaging a region of intestine over a short period of time. Normal rates of peristalsis are:

- Proximal duodenum: 4–5 contractions/minute
- Rest of the small intestine: 1–3 contractions/minute.

Luminal diameter: With fluid-filled intestine, the luminal diameter can be measured accurately. The luminal contents can also be assessed over time to see whether they are static or being moved on by peristaltic waves. If the intestine contains gas, shadowing will prevent the far intestinal wall from being assessed and, therefore, the luminal diameter will not be measurable. If the majority of loops are gas-filled, a radiograph should be taken to get an overview of the small intestinal loops.

Luminal contents: In the normal small intestine, four general luminal patterns may be identified (Figure 10.13):

- Mucous pattern: empty bowel, mucus in lumen that is seen as an echogenic line with no shadowing
- Gas: intraluminal, highly reflective interfaces with shadowing/reverberation. Will usually move on with peristalsis or gentle pressure from the ultrasound probe
- Fluid: anechoic luminal pattern. Allows optimal assessment of the bowel wall
- Alimentary: food particles present within the lumen; echogenic, usually no acoustic shadowing, although some food (e.g. bone fragments) will shadow.

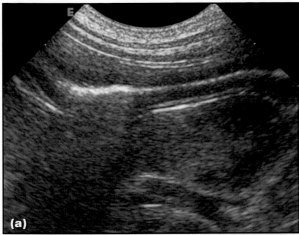

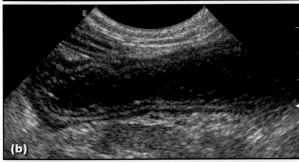

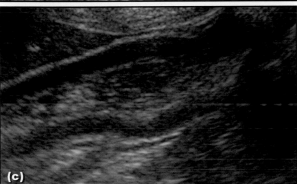

10.13 Ultrasonograms illustrating different intestinal contents. **(a)** Gas on the left, seen as an echogenic line with distal shadowing, and mucus on the right, seen as a thin echogenic line. **(b)** Fluid seen as predominantly anechoic contents. **(c)** Ingesta seen as moderately echoic contents, which may contain 'swirling' echoes when imaged in real time.

Surrounding mesentery: Mesenteric fat is usually hyperechoic to the intestinal wall. However, the echogenicity of the mesentery will increase if it is inflamed, such as with a localized or generalized peritonitis. The mesentery may also appear to increase in size and prominence, leading to separation of the intestinal loops by very echogenic material. The local lymph nodes should also be assessed for enlargement and hypoechogenicity (see Chapter 7).

Overview of additional imaging modalities

Advanced imaging techniques (computed tomography (CT) and magnetic resonance imaging (MRI)) are rarely used in the investigation of small intestinal disease, mainly because of practical issues such as cost and availability of equipment. In humans, CT is used extensively to evaluate the endoluminal and intramural components of the small intestine, as well as the perienteric tissues. It can be helpful for the detection and further evaluation of neoplasia, obstructions, adhesions and ischaemia, as well as any associated peritonitis or extension of disease processes. Barium can be used with CT to help differentiate the small intestine from the surrounding soft tissue, and also to distend the lumen to aid in assessment of the intestinal wall.

A CT image of the abdomen in a dog at the level of the ileocolic junction is shown in Figure 10.14. The thickness and uniformity of the wall and the luminal diameter and contents can be readily evaluated. Assessment of the viability of bowel wall is one possible indication for the use of CT in veterinary patients. Normal bowel wall shows marked contrast enhancement following intravenous administration of an iodinated contrast medium. Any hypoperfused areas resulting from thrombotic incidents or postoperative complications should be detectable. Similar results can be obtained with contrast ultrasonography, although CT provides a more global evaluation.

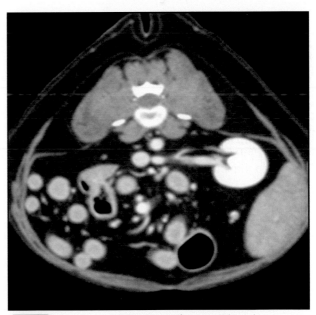

10.14 Transverse CT image of a normal canine abdomen at the level of the ileocolic junction. (Courtesy of T Schwarz)

Intestinal diseases

Displacement
The position of the small intestine can usually be assessed adequately on plain radiographs. Two orthogonal views may be required for a full assessment of intestinal position. If serosal detail is poor and/or the intestines contain little gas, a positive contrast medium or ultrasonography may be helpful for a more accurate assessment of position.

Herniation and rupture

Inguinal: An inguinal hernia may cause caudal displacement of the small intestine. If the hernia contains small intestine, loops may be seen crossing the body wall in the inguinal region and overlying the area of the hernia (Figure 10.15).

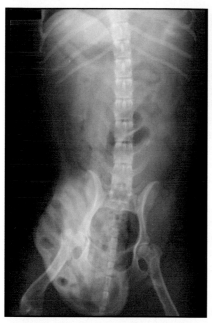

10.15 VD view of a canine abdomen, showing gas-filled loops of small intestine within an inguinal hernia.

Perineal: A perineal rupture may lead to caudal displacement of the small intestine, owing to displacement of the caudal abdominal organs such as the bladder; however, a perineal hernia is unlikely to contain small intestine.

Body wall: Depending on the location of a rupture, the small intestine may be displaced ventrally, to the right or to the left.

Diaphragmatic: Communication between the peritoneal and pleural/pericardial cavities may arise from a peritoneopericardial diaphragmatic hernia (PPDH; Figure 10.16), a diaphragmatic rupture or a

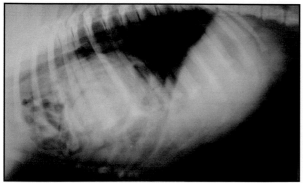

10.16 Lateral view of the thorax and cranial abdomen in a dog, showing gas- and fluid-filled loops of small intestine overlying and cranial to the cardiac silhouette; these loops were contained within a peritoneopericardial diaphragmatic hernia (PPDH). Note the 'empty' appearance of the abdomen and the lack of small intestine in the normal position.

congenital diaphragmatic hernia. The small intestine is usually displaced cranially, either remaining within the abdomen (if the liver/spleen/mesentery/stomach has been displaced) or moving into the thorax.

Paracostal: A paracostal rupture (rupture of the attachment of the abdominal muscles to the ribs) may also cause cranial displacement of the small intestine, which may be seen overlying the diaphragm.

Displacement by masses
The small intestine is relatively mobile within the abdomen and can be displaced by changes in the size of other organs. The direction of displacement may be helpful in determining the origin of abdominal masses (see Chapter 8). Caudoventral displacement of the small intestine caused by a renal mass is shown in Figure 10.17. It should be remembered that a normal variation in obese cats is complete right-sided location of the small intestines.

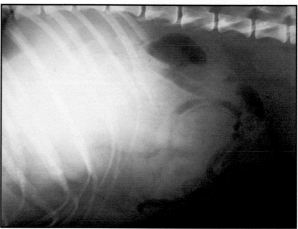

10.17 Lateral radiograph of the abdomen in a dog, showing caudal and ventral displacement of the small intestine by an ill defined dorsal abdominal mass. The mass was confirmed on ultrasound examination to be of renal origin.

Functional disease without ileus
One of the most common clinical presentations of small intestinal disease is diarrhoea resulting from enteritis. Plain radiographs are often unrewarding in these cases. The intestines are usually relatively devoid of ingesta and may contain a higher than normal ratio of fluid to gas. Small bubbles of air may be present within the small intestinal lumen.

In many patients with enteritis, upper gastro-intestinal studies may also be normal. In some acute cases, small intestinal transit time may be increased; however, in other cases the intestine may be hypermotile, leading to a decrease in transit time. In chronic cases of enteritis, transit time is usually normal. The small intestinal wall may be diffusely thickened. In severe cases, 'corrugation' of the intestines may be seen (Figure 10.18a) and there may be adherence of contrast medium to any areas of ulceration. If ulceration is present, lymphosarcoma should be considered as a differential diagnosis (see below).

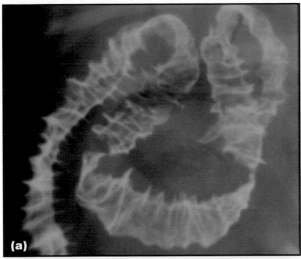

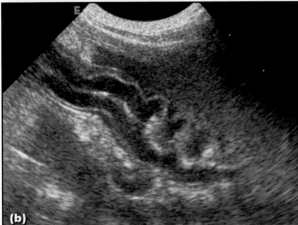

10.18 **(a)** Close-up view of a VD radiograph of the abdomen in a dog following barium administration. Obvious corrugation of the small intestine is visible. **(b)** Ultrasonogram of corrugated small intestine. Note the undulating appearance of the hyperechoic luminal and submucosal layers.

Changes seen ultrasonographically, as with radiography, are non-specific and can be associated with other types of underlying pathology. Mild thickening of the small intestinal wall may be present. Wall layering is usually preserved, although the relative thickness and echogenicity of the layers may be altered. Corrugation of the intestine may be present, and is easier to recognize ultrasonographically than radiographically, by following the hyperechoic, undulating line of the mucosa/luminal interface (Figure 10.18b). Corrugated intestine needs to be distinguished from plication caused by a linear foreign body. Corrugation may be functional (spasticity) or structural, whereas plication is always structural and is an indication for surgery (see below).

In addition to enteritis, other conditions in which corrugation of the small intestine may be seen include:

- Pancreatitis
- Peritonitis
- Neoplasia:
  - Pancreatic tumours
  - Lymphoma
  - Carcinomatosis.

- Bowel wall ischaemia
- Lymphangiectasia.

Ileus

Ileus is defined as distension of the small intestine. The changes are usually readily recognized in survey radiographs, although the underlying cause may be harder to determine.

Radiographic changes

In all cases there will be increased width of small intestinal loops; these will be dilated with fluid, gas or a combination of the two (Figure 10.19). As fluid and soft tissue are of the same radiographic opacity, fluid-filled distension of the small intestine cannot be

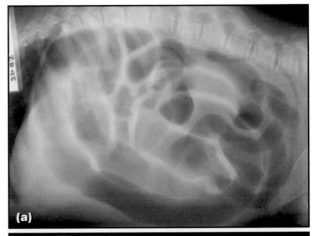

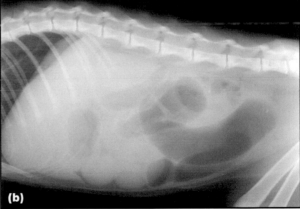

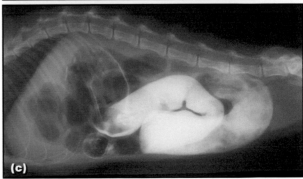

10.19 Ileus. **(a)** Lateral radiograph of a dog showing generalized gaseous distension of the small intestine. **(b)** Lateral radiograph of a cat showing distension of the small intestine by a mixture of gas and fluid. **(c)** Lateral radiograph of a cat showing small intestinal distension; administration of barium has highlighted the areas of fluid distension.

distinguished from wall thickening on plain radiographs alone (see Figure 10.4). If the cause of dilatation is obstructive, the dilatation will be mainly gaseous in the early stages. Over time, the proportion of fluid will increase as more fluid is produced and sequestrated. If the intestine is mainly gas-filled, it may be possible to get an idea of wall thickness from plain radiographs. However, upper gastrointestinal studies or ultrasonography are necessary to accurately differentiate whether the intestines are thickened, distended with fluid, or a combination of the two.

There is a wide range of normal small intestinal widths, and deciding whether a loop of intestine is normal is not always easy; however, there are some objective measurements that can be applied. In the dog, normal loops will not usually exceed the height of an endplate of a lumbar vertebral body, or twice the width of the 12th rib, and an upper limit of 12 mm is useful in the cat.

An assessment should be made as to whether the dilatation is generalized or localized. Generalized distension is consistent with a functional (adynamic or paralytic) ileus or a distal mechanical obstruction. In most cases, localized severe distension will be the result of a mechanical obstruction, although milder localized functional ileus can occur, particularly secondary to localized peritonitis, pancreatitis, surgery or trauma. Prolonged ileus caused by a mechanical obstruction will lead over time to a functional, paralytic ileus and, in these cases, the original underlying cause may be hard to ascertain.

As well as the width of the intestinal loops, the position may also change. As intestinal loops increase in diameter, they may be seen to 'stack' and curve abnormally, giving a 'hairpin'-like appearance. An accumulation of particulate material of mineral opacity ('gravel sign') confined to a segment of small intestine is abnormal. Additional orthogonal views or a contrast study (pneumocolonography) may help to determine whether particulate material is present within the large intestine (and therefore normal) or within the small intestine. A 'gravel sign' is usually seen with distal small intestinal ('low') chronic partial obstruction (Figure 10.20). An upper gastrointestinal or BIPS

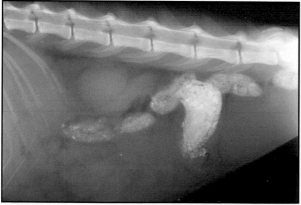

10.20 Lateral radiograph of a cat showing a moderately distended loop of small intestine filled with particulate mineral material, running vertically across the caudal abdomen. This is a 'gravel sign' and consistent with a chronic partial obstruction. Normal faecal boluses can be seen in the descending colon.

study may be useful in cases in which the plain radiographic findings are equivocal, as long as the clinical condition of the animal permits a further 6–24 hours of conservative treatment.

An upper gastrointestinal series may be able to provide more information about the site and cause of a chronic partial obstruction. Contrast medium will be seen to stop abruptly with a complete obstruction. With partial obstructions, localized or generalized dilatation may be seen, possibly with dilution of contrast medium if there are areas of fluid sequestration.

Ultrasonographic changes

An ultrasonographic examination allows assessment of the motility of the small intestine, which can be useful in differentiating mechanical from functional ileus. With functional ileus, motility will be decreased or absent. Intestinal contents may be seen to 'slosh' backwards and forwards with little net forward movement. With mechanical ileus, motility may be decreased, normal or increased, depending on the duration and site of obstruction.

Luminal dilatation may be assessed readily with ultrasonography if the intestines contain fluid. If the distension is due to gas, the deeper intestinal wall will not be seen ultrasonographically and radiographs should be taken to give a better overview of the location and extent of the intestinal dilatation. With high obstructions or localized functional ileus, luminal dilatation will be focal. Luminal dilatation is likely to be more generalized with low acute obstructions/partial obstructions, diffuse functional ileus and diffuse neoplasia.

Classification of ileus

Classification of ileus may be based on:

- The number of distended loops, i.e. whether the dilatation is localized or generalized
- Whether peristalsis is present (dynamic) or absent (adynamic).

Number of loops: The number of distended loops may be assessed using either radiography or ultrasonography, although radiography provides a better overview of the whole abdomen and permits an accurate assessment of the diameter of the gas-filled loops. Ultrasonography is more useful in cases where loops are distended with fluid and allows differentiation between wall thickness and luminal diameter.

Presence of peristalsis: The uniformity of width of the intestine may be assessed radiographically. With dynamic ileus, peristaltic waves will cause some variation in the width of the small intestine, whereas in adynamic cases, loops will tend to be of a more uniform diameter.

However, peristaltic activity is more reliably assessed by ultrasonography, where the nature and frequency of the peristaltic waves can be observed. The use of pulsed-wave Doppler ultrasonography to assess small intestinal contractions has been described but is not a widely used clinical technique. A caveat to the evaluation of peristalsis with either upper gastrointestinal radiography or ultrasonography is seen with the cat, in which high sympathetic tone may lead to intestinal stasis, with or without ileus.

Differential diagnosis

Differential diagnoses for ileus are summarized in Figure 10.21. Foreign bodies and neoplasia are discussed in detail later. Some of the other differential diagnoses of ileus are discussed briefly below.

Type of ileus	Functional causes	Mechanical causes
Generalized	Gastric dilatation–volvulus (GDV) Severe enteritis Peritonitis Volvulus Electrolyte imbalance Recent surgery Dysautonomia Parasympatholytic drugs	Distally located: • Foreign body • Intussusception • Neoplasia • Adhesions • Granuloma • Polyps • Strangulation with herniation
Localized	Enteritis Recent surgery Pancreatitis Localized peritonitis	As above but more proximal location

10.21 Differential diagnoses for ileus.

Vascular compromise: Blood supply to the small intestine may be compromised by volvulus (twisting of the root of the mesentery), thromboembolic disease, or entrapment in a hernia or within a mesenteric tear. Entrapment or volvulus will lead to a fixed and possibly displaced intestinal position with proximal dilatation; these features may be recognized radiographically (Figure 10.22).

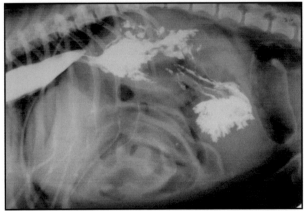

10.22 Lateral radiograph of a dog taken following administration of barium. The stomach and transverse colon are displaced caudally by moderately dilated small intestine. The oesophagus is also dilated. Free gas can be seen between the liver and diaphragm, consistent with intestinal rupture. The surgical diagnosis was small intestinal entrapment in a mesenteric tear.

With volvulus, compromised loops become turgid and permeable, leading to the accumulation of free fluid. Most affected bowel loops will be severely dilated with gas. Oedema of the intestinal wall will lead to thickening of the loops and may cause loss or alteration of the intestinal layering.

Infarction of the small intestine secondary to thromboembolism results in loss of motility, progressive thickening and loss of layering, and hyperechogenicity of the surrounding mesentery with a small amount of free fluid, consistent with localized peritonitis.

Toxic: Anything that results in intestinal stasis can lead to bacterial overgrowth and an imbalance in the normal flora. Production of endotoxins, enterotoxins and gas can result in ileus. Viral infections may also cause ileus, in particular canine parvovirus, which can lead to a pronounced paralytic ileus. Exogenous toxins and certain drugs can also cause intestinal stasis and ileus, for example botulinum toxin, anticholinergics and opioids.

Neurological: Dysautonomia is very regional in its occurrence and causes adynamic ileus. In humans, visceral neuropathies can cause 'pseudo-obstruction'; this is a term used when clinical and radiographic features are suggestive of an intestinal obstruction, but where no cause of obstruction is found at exploratory laparotomy. It can manifest as an acute or chronic condition and can be either primary (idiopathic) or secondary to an underlying disorder. Anything leading to disorders of the myenteric plexus, smooth muscle or endocrine control of gastrointestinal motility could cause a pseudo-obstructive condition, which is effectively a functional ileus.

Plain radiographs show intestinal, oesophageal, gastric or urinary bladder dilatation, and barium studies show variably delayed transit of contrast medium through the bowel. In reported veterinary cases, there have been histological changes in the tunica muscularis, including hypoplasia and atrophy, fibrosis and a mononuclear cell infiltrate. Ileus has also been reported in a dog secondary to neuronal degeneration and necrosis of the myenteric plexuses throughout the small intestine.

Metabolic: Electrolyte imbalances can cause a functional ileus. In many cases, hypokalaemia is the underlying cause and can occur as a result of diarrhoea, vomiting, gastric dilatation and volvulus, diuretic therapy, hyperaldosteronism or iatrogenic overhydration. Other signs that may be seen with hypokalaemia include skeletal muscle weakness, arrhythmias and renal failure. Ileus can also occur secondary to uraemia.

Guidelines for surgical versus medical therapy

Imaging findings can be helpful when making a decision whether to intervene surgically or whether conservative management is indicated, at least in the short term.

Surgery is indicated in patients in which there is evidence of mechanical obstruction. The typical radiographic appearance is of a severely dilated group of small intestinal loops and a concurrent normal appearing group ('regional ileus' or 'two populations of bowel'). Additional features supportive of surgical intervention include ileus with a palpable abdominal mass or opaque foreign body of appropriate size. In general, gas dilatation is more severe than fluid, and regional ileus is more severe than generalized, although there are exceptions to these guidelines.

If free abdominal air is present, with no history of recent abdominal surgery or abdominocentesis, then a rupture is likely and makes surgery the treatment of choice.

The location of changes can also be important. Duodenal lesions may be amenable to endoscopic biopsy (or retrieval of foreign material), whereas for localized jejunal and ileal changes, a laparotomy (or laparoscopy) may be needed. The nature of the lesion is also important, as endoscopic biopsy specimens will only sample the mucosa and will not obtain representative samples of deeper lesions. Ultrasonographic assessment may help to determine whether some or all of the intestinal wall is involved, and whether a mucosal or full-thickness biopsy sample would be most appropriate.

Foreign bodies

Foreign bodies are one of the most common causes of mechanical ileus. In many cases, foreign bodies are incidental radiographic findings; common objects include stones and fragments of bone. If they are not causing an obstruction, the intestine (in the absence of other pathology) should appear normal in terms of the diameter and relative distribution of fluid and/or gas. If foreign bodies do become lodged in the small intestine, the clinical signs seen will vary according to the extent of the obstruction (complete/partial) and the site of obstruction within the small intestine. Proximal duodenal lesions may be difficult to identify on plain radiographs. Localized jejunal and ileal changes result in more dramatic regional ileus. Imaging features of radiopaque and radiolucent foreign bodies are discussed below.

Radiopaque foreign bodies

Radiopaque foreign bodies are readily identifiable on plain radiographs (Figure 10.23).

The significance of any foreign material seen should be assessed in the context of the following findings:

- *Clinical presenting signs:* complete proximal small intestinal obstruction is usually associated with vomiting and severe fluid and electrolyte loss. Distal obstruction is typically associated with less severe signs, including anorexia and intermittent vomiting. Partial obstructions can also cause intermittent vomiting and diarrhoea
- *Size:* smaller foreign bodies are more likely to be incidental findings
- *Position:* a foreign body in the proximal duodenum may cause little or no intestinal distension. More distally located foreign bodies will cause progressive dilatation of loops proximal to the obstruction
- *Loss of serosal detail:* weight loss associated with chronic vomiting and/or diarrhoea can lead to a reduction in abdominal serosal detail. If body condition is reasonable, reduction in serosal detail may be the result of perforation and a localized peritonitis. A significant reduction in serosal detail may lead to an underestimation of the diameter of fluid-filled intestine

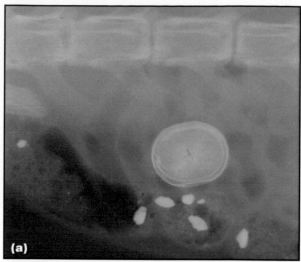

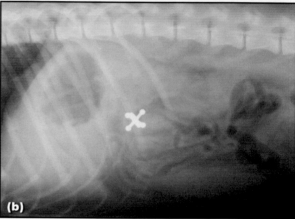

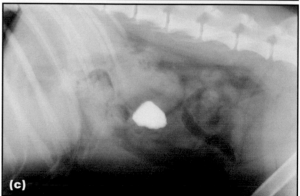

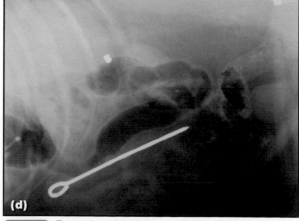

10.23 Examples of radiopaque foreign bodies. **(a)** Button. **(b)** Jack. **(c)** Stone. **(d)** Skewer (with incidental shotgun pellet).

- *Free peritoneal gas:* the presence of free gas in the absence of recent surgery or abdominocentesis makes perforation very likely and is an indication for exploratory surgery. Free gas is easiest to recognize in the craniodorsal abdomen, immediately behind the diaphragm.

Coexisting pathology should also be ruled out, as foreign material may be retained secondary to another cause of intestinal narrowing (e.g. neoplasia) and may mimic a primary obstruction. Ultrasonography is helpful for further assessment of the degree and extent of intestinal dilatation, the appearance of the intestinal wall at the site of the obstruction, and for assessment of the surrounding area.

Radiolucent foreign bodies
Some radiolucent foreign bodies may have a characteristic gas pattern that allows them to be recognized on a plain radiograph, such as corn-on-the-cob, nut kernels and peach stones (Figure 10.24). Fabric foreign bodies may also be recognized in some cases from the characteristic pattern of gas trapped within the material (Figure 10.25).

However, in many cases, radiographic findings are non-specific and relate to the presence of a complete or partial mechanical obstruction (i.e. localized or generalized intestinal distension). The degree of distension seen is usually greater with distal obstructions than with proximal ones. Partial obstructions may cause little or no intestinal distension. The amount of distension caused by fluid accumulation tends to increase over time; early in the course of obstruction there is usually more gas than fluid, and this balance shifts over time as more fluid is produced and sequestrated. The presence of a 'gravel sign' makes a chronic partial obstruction very likely, but is non-specific for the cause of the obstruction.

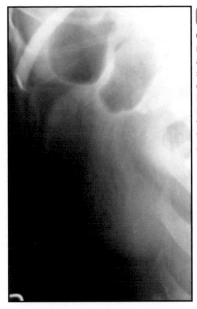

10.25 Close-up of a VD radiograph of the abdomen in a dog showing a characteristic striated lucent pattern, resulting from gas trapped within a fabric foreign body (in this case a sock).

If foreign bodies cause small intestinal perforation, there may be free gas and/or a reduction in serosal detail (see Figure 10.22). In some cases, particularly with very proximal or acute obstructions, plain radiographs may be normal.

An upper gastrointestinal study can be helpful for further investigation of a suspected mechanical obstruction and may confirm the presence and nature of a radiolucent foreign body. Localized intestinal dilatation may be easier to recognize with an upper gastrointestinal series, and barium in and around the foreign body can create abnormalities in the luminal contrast medium pool. For example, intestinal nematodes are commonly seen as linear filling defects. A radiograph obtained 24 hours after the administration of barium can be helpful, as some

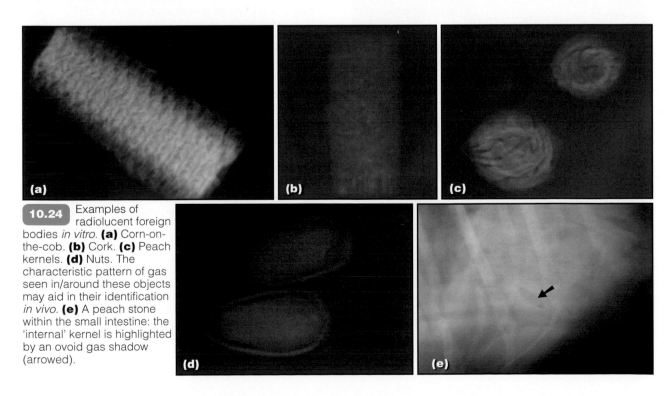

10.24 Examples of radiolucent foreign bodies *in vitro.* **(a)** Corn-on-the-cob. **(b)** Cork. **(c)** Peach kernels. **(d)** Nuts. The characteristic pattern of gas seen in/around these objects may aid in their identification *in vivo.* **(e)** A peach stone within the small intestine: the 'internal' kernel is highlighted by an ovoid gas shadow (arrowed).

foreign bodies, particularly fabric, can retain contrast medium once the majority of it has transited the small intestine and entered the colon (Figure 10.26). If a perforation is present, contrast medium may be seen leaking into the peritoneal cavity (Figure 10.27); if perforation is suspected prior to the upper gastrointestinal study, use of a water-soluble contrast agent may be preferable to barium (see above).

Ultrasonography is a very sensitive technique for the detection of intestinal foreign bodies, and will often lead to detection of foreign bodies that are not visible radiographically. The foreign body itself is usually recognizable from its surface reflection of sound, leading to an echogenic interface with very well defined distal acoustic shadowing (Figure 10.28). In addition, intestinal wall changes are frequently seen in the area of the foreign body, most commonly localized thickening and loss of layering. Usually the proximal small intestinal segment is distended with fluid whilst the distal segment is empty. Lack of

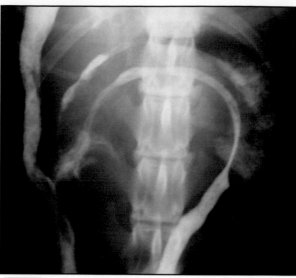

10.27 VD radiograph of the abdomen in a dog. Contrast material can be seen leaking out of the jejunum, just medial to the descending duodenum.

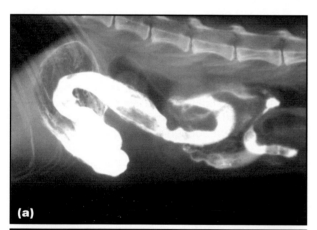

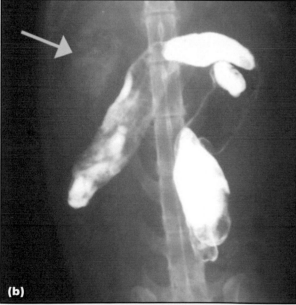

10.26 **(a)** Lateral abdominal radiograph of a cat following liquid barium administration. Note the duodenal distension and the ill defined filling defect. **(b)** VD radiograph taken 24 hours after barium administration. Most of the barium is in the colon; however a small amount is retained within the duodenal foreign body (arrowed).

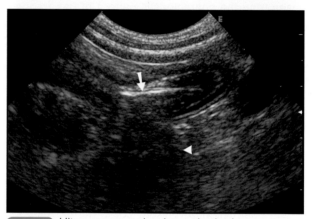

10.28 Ultrasonogram showing a shadowing, echogenic linear structure (arrowed) within the lumen of a distended area of small intestine. This appearance is consistent with an intestinal foreign body. Note also the shadowing artefact (arrowhead).

ileus in the proximal segment and a foreign body of small diameter, relative to the diameter of the small intestine, questions the clinical relevance of the foreign body. Intestinal motility can also be assessed.

Ultrasonography can also be used to detect any perforation of the intestine by the foreign body, particularly in cases where there is no free gas detectable radiographically. Changes that may be seen on ultrasound examination in cases where perforation has occurred include:

- Changes to the affected area of intestine:
  - Wall thickening
  - Loss of layering
  - Fluid distension
  - Reduced motility
  - Corrugation.
- Peritoneal fluid (localized or generalized)
- Localized increased echogenicity of the mesenteric fat
- Regional lymphadenopathy

- Free air, recognized as reverberation artefacts between the non-dependent abdominal wall and organs such as the liver and stomach, or trapped adjacent to the site of perforation. Air may not always be radiographically apparent in cases of perforation.

Linear foreign bodies

Linear foreign bodies can be found in both dogs and cats, although they have been reported more frequently in cats. The type of materials ingested include thread (possibly still attached to a needle), fabric, carpet, string, plastic and tights. This is an important surgical condition. For a linear foreign body to cause clinical signs, one end (the proximal portion) must be 'fixed', with the remaining (distal) portion loose, to cause the plication. Most linear foreign bodies in dogs lodge in the pylorus and subsequently extend into the small intestine, where peristaltic waves will cause plication of the intestine around the linear foreign body. Cats are more likely than dogs to have a linear foreign body starting from under the tongue.

Diagnosis may be aided by plain and upper gastrointestinal radiography and ultrasonography. On plain radiographs, any radiopaque areas within or attached to the linear foreign body will be visible. The intestine may have a bunched and plicated appearance and may be moderately dilated with fluid and gas. Small intestinal ileus is seen more commonly in dogs than in cats with linear foreign bodies. Many cats will have plicated intestines without small intestinal dilatation. The affected portion of intestine is typically located within the central region of the abdomen on a lateral radiograph and may subjectively appear shorter than normal. 'Teardrop', crescent-shaped, triangular or irregularly shaped gas bubbles are commonly seen (Figure 10.29a), rather than the normal smooth tubular gas pattern. A similar pattern of gas distribution may sometimes be seen if adhesions are present secondary to peritonitis. Similarly, the bunched, plicated appearance may transiently persist following passage of a linear foreign body. Perforation of the small intestine is a relatively common sequel to a chronic linear foreign body, occurring more frequently in dogs than in cats. This may be due to the types of foreign body ingested; perforation is most commonly associated with fabric and plastic. These are uncommonly eaten by cats, which are more likely to ingest string or cord. The abdomen should therefore be carefully assessed for loss of serosal detail and the presence of any free peritoneal air (see Figure 10.22).

An upper gastrointestinal barium series will allow a better overview of the position and diameter of the small intestine and may highlight the bunching and plication pattern (Figure 10.29b). Occasionally a linear foreign body may be recognized as an intraluminal filling defect.

On ultrasonography, the same abnormal plicated path of the small intestine may be seen. This may be particularly obvious with the duodenum, which will adopt a very spastic, undulating course rather than its normal straight course along the right abdominal wall. A hyperechoic, shadowing linear structure may be

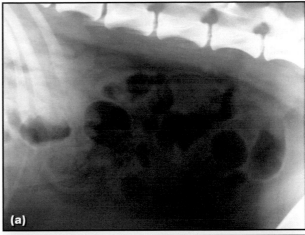

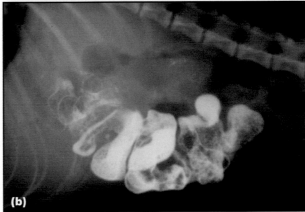

10.29 Linear foreign bodies. **(a)** Plain lateral radiograph of the abdomen in a dog showing variably sized and shaped gas bubbles within the small intestine. **(b)** Lateral radiograph of the abdomen in a cat following contrast medium administration, highlighting the 'bunched' appearance of the small intestine.

seen within the lumen of the intestine. Shadowing of the linear foreign body depends on the diameter of the foreign body; very thin foreign bodies (tinsel, thread) may not have a distinct shadow. The course of the linear luminal lesion should be followed proximally to its origin (often within the pylorus) and distally along the small intestine, often through several 'hairpin' bends. The layering of the intestine is usually preserved, until there is necrosis of the bowel. A common concurrent finding is an intussusception, caused by the abnormal intestinal motility of the plicated segment. A small adjacent region of hyperechoic peritoneum and a small amount of free peritoneal fluid may be seen secondary to inflammation, vascular compromise or perforation. In rare cases, intestinal perforation caused by a linear foreign body may not produce detectable free fluid on ultrasound examination.

Focal small intestinal thickening

Although plain radiographs may be suggestive of small intestinal thickening, a combination of normal intestinal wall with adjacent fluid contents cannot be differentiated from genuine wall thickening, as fluid and soft tissue have identical radiographic opacities (see Figure 10.4). Focal thickening is particularly difficult to recognize and plain radiographs are often normal unless there are secondary consequences of the thickening.

If focal thickening is severe enough to cause a chronic partial obstruction, a 'gravel sign' may be seen on a plain radiograph, which although non-specific does indicate chronic small intestinal pathology.

An upper gastrointestinal study or ultrasonography is therefore necessary for an accurate assessment of intestinal wall diameter and can also help to distinguish intraluminal lesions, with no point of attachment to the intestinal wall, from asymmetrical mural lesions.

Focal thickening associated with neoplasia
The most common causes of small intestinal neoplasia, together with their main characteristics, are summarized in Figure 10.30.

Species	Distribution	Typical appearance
Dog		
Adenocarcinoma	Focal	Thick wall, asymmetrical, loss of layering, decreased/mixed echogenicity
Lymphoma	Focal or diffuse	Symmetrical transmural thickening, loss of layers, hypoechoic appearance
Leiomyosarcoma	Focal	Large eccentric masses, may contain hypo- or anechoic foci
Cat		
Lymphoma	Focal or diffuse	Thick wall, loss of layering, hypoechoic
Mast cell tumour	Focal	Eccentric thickening, loss of layering, hypoechoic
Adenocarcinoma	Focal	Annular or mural thickening, loss of layering

10.30   Common causes of small intestinal neoplasia.

In dogs, the most common tumour types are adenocarcinoma, lymphoma and tumours of smooth muscle origin. In cats, lymphoma, adenocarcinoma and mast cell tumour are most frequently seen. Other less frequently reported intestinal neoplasms include osteosarcoma, fibrosarcoma, haemangiosarcoma, round cell tumour, spindle cell tumour, malignant histiocytosis and undifferentiated sarcoma.

Benign lesions are less common than malignant ones; examples include leiomyomas and polyps. Benign lesions usually appear smooth and well marginated. Leiomyomas are typically small (<3 cm) and homogenous, although they can contain hypoechoic foci, as can leiomyosarcomas. Polyps are also smoothly marginated and may be pedunculated in appearance. The majority of neoplasms tend to cause focal intestinal thickening; the notable exception is lymphoma, which can be focal or diffuse (see below).

In many cases, plain radiographs are unremarkable. In reported case series, around half of the cases have changes visible on plain films; more masses are usually palpable than are visible on plain radiographs. It is not always possible to be sure of the organ of origin of a mass, unless the mass contains gas continuous with that in other loops of bowel. Small intestinal masses are usually quite centrally located within the abdomen on lateral views, with peripheral displacement of the remainder of the intestine. Dystrophic calcification may occasionally be seen within the thickened mass. If the mass is causing a partial obstruction, a 'gravel sign' may be seen. Neoplastic infiltration of the intestinal wall may cause perforation, which can be recognized on plain films if there is evidence of free peritoneal fluid and free gas.

Lesions are best assessed using either upper gastrointestinal studies or ultrasonography. Upper gastrointestinal studies will lead to the detection of lesions in some cases where plain radiographs are normal, but will still be unremarkable in a significant number of cases. Findings may be non-specific, with the upper gastrointestinal study only confirming a complete or partial obstruction. If a mass lesion is visible, it typically appears either as an irregular filling defect originating from one side of the intestinal wall, or as an annular constriction with luminal narrowing over a length of a few centimetres. Multifocal lesions can occur and are usually asymmetrical, in contrast with peristaltic narrowing, which should be smooth and symmetrical. Contrast medium adherence to the mucosa is indicative of mucosal ulceration. Patterns of thickening are shown in Figure 10.31.

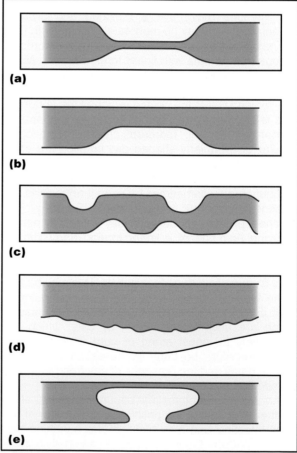

10.31   Different patterns of intestinal wall thickening, frequently associated with neoplasia, which may be recognized with ultrasonography or contrast radiography. **(a)** Annular. Luminal narrowing giving an 'apple-core' appearance. **(b)** Mural. Eccentric narrowing of lumen. **(c)** Multifocal. Asymmetrical areas of thickening along intestinal wall. **(d)** Ulceration. Irregular wall thickening, barium may remain adherent to ulcerated areas. **(e)** Pedunculated mass.

Ultrasonography is more sensitive than radiography for the detection of small intestinal neoplasms. On ultrasound examination the intestine should be assessed for the following:

- Wall thickness and symmetry
- Wall layering
- Motility
- Location of lesion
- Length of intestine affected
- Regional lymph nodes
- Distant metastatic spread.

Wall thickness and symmetry: In the dog, intestinal wall thickening is defined as a width of >5 mm (>6 mm for the duodenum). In the cat, both duodenum and jejunum should be <4 mm (see Figure 10.9). Smooth muscle neoplasms may cause eccentric thickening of the affected bowel segment. In some cases, the thickening may be so pronounced as to appear mass-like rather than tubular. In these cases, gas within the mass and the associated shadowing or reverberation artefacts can be helpful in identifying the intestinal origin of the mass.

Wall layering: Layering of the wall is usually lost with neoplastic infiltrates (Figure 10.32). However, this is a non-specific finding as wall layering may be preserved with some neoplastic lesions and lost with some inflammatory and necrotic conditions. In some cases, it may be possible to determine the layer of origin of the lesion; for example, leiomyosarcomas arise from the tunica muscularis and grow in a centrifugal manner (exophytic).

Motility: The motility of affected intestinal segments is typically reduced, although in some cases it can be increased. The combination of altered motility with a focal mass can lead in some cases to a secondary intussusception.

Location of lesion: The location of the lesion may be determined ultrasonographically to be duodenal, jejunal or ileal. The duodenum is more frequently involved in dogs than in cats. The ileum is more commonly affected in cats than in dogs and is a predilection site for lymphoma. The intestine proximal to the lesion should be assessed for the presence of obstructive ileus.

Length of intestine affected: The length of affected intestine can be gauged with ultrasonography by following the lesion proximally and distally until normal intestine is seen.

Regional lymph nodes: Small intestinal neoplasia typically metastasizes to the mesenteric lymph nodes and mesentery. Enlarged mesenteric lymph nodes are usually rounded in shape and hypoechoic (see Chapter 7).

Distant metastatic spread: If intestinal neoplasia is suspected, the entire abdomen should be examined for any evidence of distant metastases. The lymph nodes are the most common site of metastasis, followed by the liver.

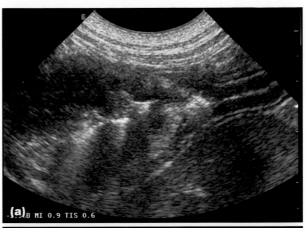

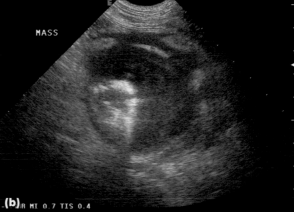

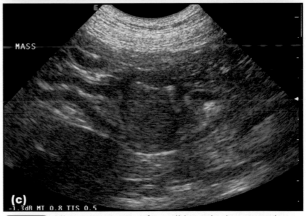

10.32 Ultrasonograms of small intestinal masses in three different patients. **(a)** Longitudinal image showing symmetrical wall thickening with loss of layering and an irregular lumen. **(b)** Transverse image showing loss of layering and eccentric wall thickening. **(c)** Longitudinal image showing localized intestinal dilatation associated with an intraluminal mass. In all cases reverberation artefacts from luminal gas help to identify the mass as being of intestinal origin.

Carcinomatosis can occur secondary to primary intestinal neoplasms. It is defined as the widespread dissemination of tumours of epithelial origin to the peritoneal lining. All three components of the peritoneum may be affected: parietal (lining the inner body wall); visceral (covering the organs of the abdomen); and connecting peritoneum (the omental and mesenteric layer). The ultrasonographic appearance is variable; indistinct hypoechoic peritoneal fat or more distinct rounded masses within the mesentery may be seen.

Findings very suspicious for neoplastic infiltration are therefore focal thickening, loss of layering and involvement of the mesenteric lymph nodes. Characteristic features of neoplastic compared with inflammatory disease are summarized in Figure 10.33. However, there are always cases that do not have the 'typical' appearance, and cytology is needed for a definitive diagnosis.

Assessment	Neoplasia	Enteritis
Localization	Usually focal	Usually diffuse
Thickness	Moderate to severe increase	Mild to moderate increase, greatest with haemorrhagic, necrotizing or suppurative enteritis
Wall layering	Lost	Preserved May be lost with severe necrotizing, haemorrhagic or granulomatous enteritis
Motility	Mainly decreased Some cases normal or increased	Mainly decreased Some cases normal or increased
Lymph node involvement	Common (>80% of cases)	Approximately 40% of cases

10.33 Ultrasonographic assessment of neoplasia and enteritis.

It is usually possible to obtain cytological samples from thickened intestinal wall or enlarged regional lymph nodes using ultrasound-guided fine-needle aspiration. Histological biopsy specimens may be obtained by automatic or manual biopsy devices if the lesions are large (>2 cm diameter). Ultrasound-guided biopsy techniques have the advantage of being quick and relatively non-invasive, but care must be taken to avoid vascular structures, which are usually closely associated with the lymph nodes. Tumour seeding is a potential risk if a neoplastic lesion is aspirated or biopsied, although this has only been documented with transitional cell carcinoma. Another potential complication is penetration of the intestinal lumen, which may lead to leakage and peritonitis; the risk of this can be minimized by using a fairly shallow needle angle, and not attempting to aspirate a lesion unless the wall is markedly thickened. Ultrasound-guided aspirates and biopsy samples tend to be more sensitive for the diagnosis of malignant than benign lesions.

Focal non-neoplastic thickening

Non-neoplastic causes of focal thickening are less common than neoplastic causes. However, granulomas, abscesses, cysts, scar tissue/adhesions and haematomas are all differential diagnoses for focal thickening of the intestine. Thickening is usually less marked with non-neoplastic than with neoplastic processes, but changes seen on both radiography and ultrasonography are non-specific and biopsy is needed for a definitive diagnosis.

Ulceration of the small intestine may cause focal or diffuse changes on an upper gastrointestinal study; these are often associated with small intestinal thickening, although in some cases thickness may be normal. The ulcerated area may be recognized as linear or crater-like out-pouching(s) of the contrast medium column. Non-neoplastic causes of small intestinal ulceration include administration of non-steroidal anti-inflammatory drugs (NSAIDs) and Zollinger–Ellison syndrome, which is associated with hypergastrinaemia produced by a pancreatic neoplasm. The presence or absence of ulceration is therefore not particularly helpful in distinguishing neoplastic from inflammatory causes of focal intestinal thickening.

Intussusception

Intussusception is a 'telescoping' or 'inversion' of the bowel, where one segment (the 'intussusceptum') ends up inside another segment (the 'intussuscipiens'). Intussusception causes a mechanical obstruction (usually partial) and hence, in the first instance, a localized ileus. The condition may be primary or secondary to any underlying pathology that affects peristalsis. Coexisting pathology in animals with reported intussusception includes intestinal parasites, focal neoplastic lesions, linear foreign bodies and systemic diseases including distemper, parvovirus infection, histoplasmosis and toxoplasmosis. Intussusceptions are common in neonates with pre-existing intestinal motility disorders.

A common location for an intussusception is adjacent to a primary lesion, e.g. a neoplastic mass or a linear foreign body. Historically, the most common site was the ileocolic junction and such cases were thought to be secondary to hookworm parasitism. However, intussusception can occur in any location within the gastrointestinal tract.

On plain radiographs, the intussusception may be visible in some cases as an elongated, sausage-shaped soft tissue opacity (Figure 10.34a). Ileocolic intussusceptions are located in the mid-abdomen, caudal to the stomach, and displace the remainder of the small intestine caudally. In ileocolic intussusceptions, a gas opacity may outline the crescenteric end of the intussuscepted bowel segment (Figure 10.34b). If the intussusception causes a chronic partial obstruction, a variable degree of intestinal distension and a 'gravel sign' may be seen.

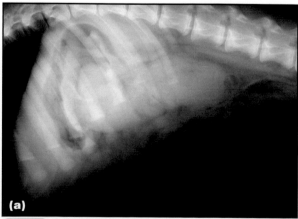

(a)

10.34 Radiographic features of intussusception. **(a)** Plain lateral abdominal radiograph showing a sausage-shaped soft tissue opacity in the mid-abdomen. (continues) ▶

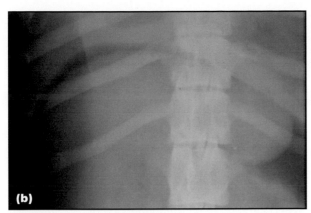

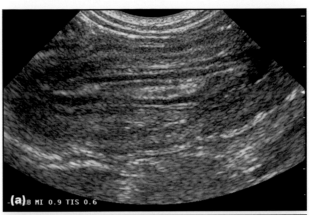

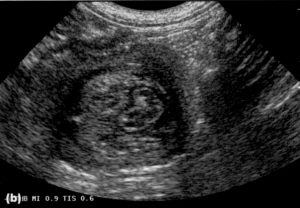

10.34 (continued) Radiographic features of intussusception. **(b)** A gas lucency highlights the crescenteric end of the intussuscipiens in an ileocolic intussusception.

10.35 Ultrasonograms of an intussusception in **(a)** longitudinal and **(b)** transverse section. Note the multilayered appearance.

An upper gastrointestinal series can be helpful in the diagnosis of a small intestinal intussusception; a sharply demarcated narrowing of the intestinal lumen is typically seen. Barium may also enter the space between the intussusceptum and intussuscipiens, and has been described as having a 'corkscrew' or 'coiled spring' appearance. Intussusceptions involving the large intestine benefit from a large intestinal contrast study, rather than an upper gastrointestinal series.

Regardless of location, most intussusceptions can be diagnosed more quickly and staged more completely with an ultrasound examination performed by an experienced ultrasonographer. Intussusceptions have a very typical ultrasonographic appearance; they are seen as multiple concentric rings in transverse section, and multiple layers in longitudinal section (Figure 10.35). These rings or layers represent the wall layers of the intussusceptum and intussuscipiens; the appearance may become confused if other structures (e.g. fat, lymph nodes, tumours, pseudocysts) are associated with the invaginated bowel. Mesenteric fat commonly invaginates together with the section of intestine and appears as an eccentric, semilunar or G-shaped hyperechoic area interspersed between the layers. Intussusceptions always cause some degree of obstructive ileus, resulting in the proximal (orad) intestinal segment becoming distended with fluid and the downstream (aborad) segment empty.

Treatment of an intussusception usually involves surgical reduction, with or without resection of the affected segment.

Diffuse small intestinal thickening

Diffuse thickening associated with neoplasia
Lymphosarcoma is the most common neoplasm that causes diffuse small intestinal change. In many cases the entire small intestine is affected. Plain radiographs are normal in most cases. Infrequently, particularly in cats, a mass may be seen associated with the intestine and/or mesentery. The lesions tend not to be obstructive, therefore, intestinal dilatation is not a common feature. Generalized mesenteric lymphadenopathy can cause loss of serosal detail. On an upper gastrointestinal study, multiple areas of ulceration or constrictions produce an irregular appearance to the small intestine, with multiple 'apple-core' like areas (Figure 10.36). Corrugation of the intestinal wall may be seen on both radiography and ultrasonography.

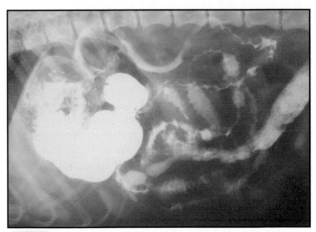

10.36 Lateral abdominal radiograph of a dog with intestinal lymphoma, taken following administration of barium. The small intestine has a chewed out, 'apple-core' appearance with multiple asymmetrical areas of luminal narrowing.

On ultrasound examination, the small intestine is usually thickened. The thickening can be symmetrical or asymmetrical. The wall tends to appear hypoechoic, with loss of layering (Figure 10.37). A common manifestation of lymphoma in cats is intact layering but

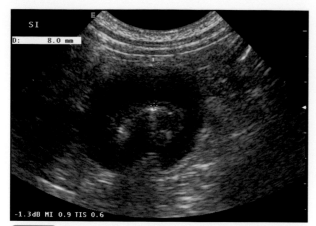

10.37 Transverse ultrasonogram showing a thickened loop of intestine with complete loss of layering. This appearance is typical of, but not specific for, intestinal lymphoma.

selective thickening of the outer hypoechoic layer (muscularis propria). Regional motility is usually reduced. Regional lymph nodes are often enlarged, rounded and hypoechoic. Another common presentation of lymphoma in cats is a mass lesion associated with the intestine and/or mesentery.

Fine-needle aspirates are often diagnostic in cases of lymphoma; sampling the mesenteric lymph nodes is an alternative to sampling the intestinal wall, and may be safer if the intestine is not markedly thickened.

Diffuse non-neoplastic thickening

Causes of non-neoplastic diffuse wall thickening include severe chronic enteritis (for example, secondary to inflammatory bowel disease), acute ulcerative enteritis and lymphangiectasia. In many cases imaging changes are either absent or non-specific.

Inflammatory bowel disease: The term inflammatory bowel disease describes a group of gastrointestinal disorders that are characterized histologically by inflammatory infiltrates in the mucosa, with no known inciting cause. Plain and upper gastrointestinal study radiographs are normal in most cases of inflammatory bowel disease. Abnormalities that may be seen on upper gastrointestinal studies include rapid passage of barium through the small intestine and a slightly irregular mucosal surface. Wall thickness usually appears normal, although in a minority of cases the intestinal walls may be thickened enough to be evident radiographically.

On ultrasonographic examination, many cases will appear normal. However, ultrasonography will detect abnormalities in a higher proportion of cases than radiography. Severe cases are more likely to have abnormalities than cases of mild or moderate severity. Wall layering is usually preserved with non-neoplastic disease, although layers may occasionally be lost with inflammatory bowel disease, as well as with other inflammatory conditions such as severe necrotizing enteritis and fungal infections.

Wall thickness may be normal or increased, and in some cases changes may be focal rather than diffuse.

Selective thickening of the muscularis layer has also been reported in cats, causing overlap with the previous description of diffuse lymphoma. In many cases there will be enlargement of the local lymph nodes (see Chapter 7); lymph node involvement is more common in severe cases.

Granulomatous enteritis: Granulomatous enteritis is rare in the UK but more common elsewhere, for example in subtropical areas where it can occur secondary to infestation with parasites such as *Pythium insidiosum*. Ultrasonographic changes include extensive, marked wall thickening with loss of layering and regional lymphadenopathy.

Lymphangiectasia: This is a term applied to the pathological dilatation and rupture of lymphatic vessels, leading to leakage of contents into the intestinal wall and lumen. It can be a primary condition, or it may occur secondary to other conditions, including lymphatic obstruction, pericarditis, congestive heart failure and infiltrative diseases of the small intestine. Lymphangiectasia usually causes mild diffuse changes in the small intestine. In most cases, there are no detectable radiographic changes. Ultrasonographic features that may be seen include:

* Hyperechogenic striations of the mucosal layer
* Increased wall thickness
* Altered layering: the submucosal layer may be thickened
* Altered motility: the intestines may be hypermotile
* Luminal dilatation
* Corrugation
* Free fluid, secondary to a protein-losing enteropathy.

The changes do not always correlate with the severity of the condition, although, as with inflammatory bowel disease, more severe cases are more likely to show abnormalities. There is a strong correlation between the echogenic mucosal striations seen ultrasonographically (Figure 10.38) and lacteal dilatation observed on histopathology.

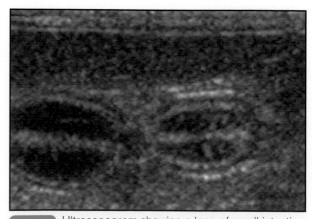

10.38 Ultrasonogram showing a loop of small intestine deep to the spleen. Transversely oriented echogenic striations can be seen within the mucosal layer, which are characteristic of lacteal dilatation.

References and further reading

Baez JL, Hendrick MJ, Walker LM, *et al.* (1999) Radiographic, ultrasonographic, and endoscopic findings in cats with inflammatory bowel disease of the stomach and small intestine: 33 cases (1990–1997). *Journal of the American Veterinary Medical Association* **215(3),** 349–354

Boysen SR, Tidwell AS and Penninck DG (2003) Ultrasonographic findings in dogs and cats with gastrointestinal perforation. *Veterinary Radiology and Ultrasound* **44(5),** 556–564

Delaney F, O'Brien RT and Waller K (2003) Ultrasound evaluation of small bowel thickness compared to weight in normal dogs. *Veterinary Radiology and Ultrasound* **44(5),** 577–580

Evans KL, Smeak DD and Biller DS (1994) Gastrointestinal linear foreign bodies in 32 dogs: a retrospective evaluation and feline comparison. *Journal of the American Animal Hospital Association* **30,** 445–450

Goggin JM, Biller DS, Debey DM, *et al.* (2000) Ultrasonographic measurement of gastrointestinal wall thickness and the ultrasonographic appearance of the ileocolic region in healthy cats. *Journal of the American Animal Hospital Association* **36,** 224–228

Graham JP, Lord PF and Harrison JM (1998) Quantitative estimation of intestinal dilation as a predictor of obstruction in the dog. *Journal of Small Animal Practice* **39(11),** 521–524

Kull PA, Hess RS, Craig LE, *et al.* (2001) Clinical, clinicopathologic, radiographic, and ultrasonographic characteristics of intestinal lymphangiectasia in dogs: 17 cases (1996–1998). *Journal of the American Veterinary Medical Association* **219(2),** 197–202

Moon ML, Biller DS and Armbrust LJ (2003) Ultrasonographic appearance and etiology of corrugated small intestine. *Veterinary Radiology and Ultrasound* **44(2),** 199–203

Morgan JP (1981) The upper gastrointestinal examination in the cat: normal radiographic appearance using positive-contrast medium. *Veterinary Radiology* **22,** 159

Myers NC and Penninck DG (1994) Ultrasonographic diagnosis of gastrointestinal smooth muscle tumors in the dog. *Veterinary Radiology and Ultrasound* **35(5),** 391–397

Newell SM, Graham JP, Roberts GD, *et al.* (1999) Sonography of the normal feline gastrointestinal tract. *Veterinary Radiology and Ultrasound* **40(1),** 40–43

Nyland TG, Wallack ST and Wisner ER (2002) Needle-tract implantation following US-guided fine-needle aspiration biopsy of transitional cell carcinoma of the bladder, urethra and prostate. *Veterinary Radiology and Ultrasound* **43(1),** 50–53

Paoloni MC, Penninck DG and Moore AS (2002) Ultrasonographic and clinicopathologic findings in 21 dogs with intestinal adenocarcinoma. *Veterinary Radiology and Ultrasound* **43(6),** 562–567

Penninck DG, Nyland T, Fisher P, *et al.* (1989) Ultrasonography of normal canine gastrointestinal tract. *Veterinary Radiology* **30,** 272–276

Penninck D, Smyers B, Webster CR, *et al.* (2003) Diagnostic value of ultrasonography in differentiating enteritis from intestinal neoplasia in dogs. *Veterinary Radiology and Ultrasound* **44(5),** 570–575

Rudorf H, Van Schaik G, O'Brien RT, *et al.* (2005) Ultrasonographic evaluation of the thickness of the small intestinal wall in dogs with inflammatory bowel disease. *Journal of Small Animal Practice* **46,** 322–326

Sutherland-Smith J, Penninck DG, Keating JH, *et al.* (2007) Ultrasonographic intestinal hyperechoic mucosal striations in dogs are associated with lacteal dilation. *Veterinary Radiology and Ultrasound* **48(1),** 51–57

Tyrrell D and Beck C (2006) Survey of the use of radiography *versus* ultrasonography in the investigation of gastrointestinal foreign bodies in small animals. *Veterinary Radiology and Ultrasound* **47(4),** 404–408

11

The large intestine and perianal region

Lorrie Gaschen

Introduction

Constipation and diarrhoea are the most common signs of large intestinal disease. Dietary, infectious and parasitic diseases are the most common causes of large bowel diarrhoea in dogs. Inflammatory bowel disease caused by lymphocytic–plasmacytic colitis is diagnosed by ruling out other causes of diarrhoea and by performing a histological examination. Colonoscopy using a flexible endoscope has become a common follow-up procedure to survey radiography for imaging the large intestine. Survey radiographs are still important for recognizing situations in which endoscopy may not be feasible, such as obstipation. Strictures may also prevent passage of the endoscope, and contrast radiography may be the only means of diagnosing the extent and nature of disease.

Ultrasonography has also replaced much of the use of contrast radiography and should be considered complementary to survey radiography. Artefacts produced by the contents of the colon can prevent observation of much of the wall using ultrasonography. However, the wall thickness and layering of the colon can be assessed in the near-field of the transducer. The regional lymph nodes and neighbouring organs can also be examined, which can be important for determining the extent of some lesions.

Ultrasound-guided tissue sampling of masses or wall infiltrations can also be performed. Cross-sectional imaging of the large intestine can be advantageous, especially for the intrapelvic portion. Perianal masses or rectal lesions can be examined with computed tomography (CT) and magnetic resonance imaging (MRI) because superimposition of the pelvis is no longer a concern. Dogs and cats with faecal incontinence may also benefit from cross-sectional imaging, either using CT or MRI, in order to examine the spinal cord and cauda equina.

Normal radiographic anatomy

To examine the large intestine, lateral and ventrodorsal (VD) radiographs of the abdomen are performed to include the pelvis and perianal region. This may require additional views in large dogs. The normal colon has a shape similar to the number '7' on VD radiographs, although this varies with positioning, colonic content and species. Species differences are mainly associated with the appearance of the caecum. The caecum is generally located in the mid-abdomen and to the right of the midline in dogs. It is compartmentalized and is often filled with gas (Figure 11.1ab). The gas-filled caecum should not be confused with focal small intestinal dilatation. The shape of the caecum may resemble a comma or 'C' shape in both the lateral and VD views. In cats, the caecum is smaller and not compartmentalized or gas-filled (Figure 11.1c); therefore, it is generally not visible radiographically.

From the caecum, the large intestine continues cranially as the ascending colon for a short distance on the right side of the abdomen. Caudal to the stomach, in both dogs and cats, the ascending colon turns to the left at the right colonic flexure to become the transverse colon. The stomach is an important

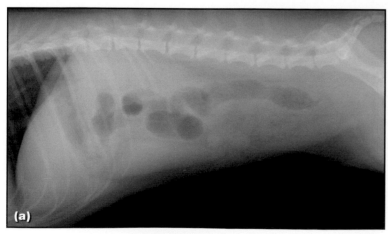

11.1 Radiographs of the abdomen showing the normal appearance of the colon and caecum. **(a)** Lateral radiograph of the gas-filled colon. The caecum is located in the right mid-ventral abdomen and appears as a gas-filled compartmentalized structure. (continues) ▶

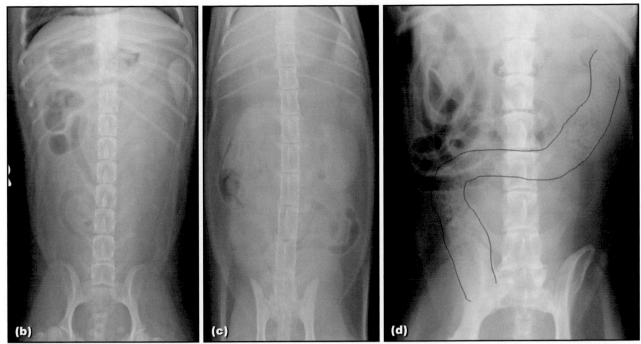

11.1 (continued) Radiographs of the abdomen showing the normal appearance of the colon and caecum. **(b)** VD view of the canine abdomen showing the 'C' shape of the gas-filled caecum. **(c)** VD view of the normal feline abdomen. There are some normal appearing faeces in the colon. The caecum is not generally visualized in the cat. **(d)** VD view of the abdomen in a dog. The course of the descending colon is tortuous and shifts from the left side to the right at the mid-abdomen. This is a normal variation in dogs and cats, especially when the colon is distended.

landmark for identifying the transverse colon. At the right colonic junction, the descending colon continues caudally to the left of the spine. The rectum is the entire intrapelvic portion of the large intestine and has a more midline position. The colonic segments are best identified when they are filled with gas or faeces. However, empty sections of the colon can also be detected in dogs and cats because they have excellent serosal detail.

Variations in the position of the colon occur in normal dogs and cats. The descending colon may be located to the right of the midline when distended with gas or faeces. It may also have a more tortuous course, switching from the left to the right side of the midline between the transverse colon and the rectum. A large urinary bladder can also cause displacement of the descending colon. The ascending colon is more consistently positioned on the right side of the abdomen because of its involvement with the mesoduodenum.

The content, position and size of the large intestine are variable in normal animals. When empty, the colon appears as an opaque tubular soft tissue structure. Its normal faeces-filled width should not be greater than three times the width of the small intestines or the length of the seventh lumbar vertebra (L7). Normal faeces have a granular appearance attributable to mixed soft tissue, gas and mineral opacities (Figure 11.2). This appearance helps to differentiate small from large intestinal segments in fasted patients. The colonic wall may have a corrugated appearance in normal cats and dogs owing to peristalsis. This finding should not be interpreted as abnormal unless it is static and also detected on subsequent radiographs.

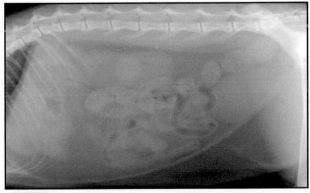

11.2 Lateral view of a normal feline abdomen showing the normal appearance of faecal balls. The colon is not dilated and the faecal balls have a mixed soft tissue and gas opacity, and are not desiccated as seen with obstipation.

Positional radiography can be used to take advantage of the gravitation of the solid, fluid and gas content of the large intestine. Large gas bubbles in the large intestine can help to outline the wall or soft tissue lesions. Since gas moves to the non-dependent portion of the abdomen, the patient's position can be changed from right to left lateral recumbency, for example, to observe different regions of the colonic wall.

Air may be present in the anal sacs and is a normal variation. On the VD view of the pelvis, the anal sacs may be observed as small oval lucencies superimposed on the ischial tuberosity and should not be confused with focal bony lysis. This finding can be uni- or bilateral.

Contrast radiography

Prior to performing contrast procedures of the colon, food should be withheld from the animal for 24 hours and a cleansing enema administered. In addition, survey radiographs should be taken just prior to the procedure. These are to ensure that the colon is empty and can be used for comparison with the contrast radiographs. Any remaining faecal material can mimic lesions in the contrast examination and complicate interpretation. The procedures are performed with the patient in lateral recumbency and usually require sedation or general anaesthesia, especially if the animal is anxious or appears to be experiencing pain. Negative-, positive- and double-contrast procedures can be performed. It should also be noted that although 8 ml/kg bodyweight of contrast medium is recommended, an additional 4 ml/kg bodyweight should be considered as necessary to completely distend the colon.

Pneumocolonography

Pneumocolonography is indicated for detecting intraluminal, mural and extramural lesions of the colon. It can also be used simply to identify the location of the colon and differentiate it from distended small intestinal segments (Figure 11.3). A catheter, preferably balloon-tipped, is placed into the rectum. Most dogs tolerate this without the need for additional sedation. Air (8 ml/kg bodyweight) should be slowly infused to avoid discomfort to the patient. Lateral and VD radiographs of the entire abdomen should be obtained immediately, preferably with the catheter in place to avoid air leakage. Oblique views may also be necessary to demonstrate a lesion.

Barium enema

The indications for performing a barium enema include:

- Strictures
- Irregular mucosal surfaces
- Diverticula
- Herniation
- Displacement
- Intussusception.

The barium enema is a technically challenging procedure. The patient should be prepared by withholding food for at least 24 hours and then administering cleansing enemas. Even a small amount of faeces creates irregularities that mimic lesions and render the study non-diagnostic. The patient should then be placed under general anaesthesia. A 20% w/v barium suspension (1 part barium to 2 parts water) at a dose of 8 ml/kg can be slowly infused into the colon via a cuffed tube inserted into the rectum, to prevent leakage. Alternatively, the barium can be introduced via a gravity system. In either case, the administration of barium should be slow, and radiographs can be obtained in order to check the state of filling.

Iodinated contrast media can be used to perform a barium enema but will not result in adequate mucosal detail. Their main indication is in instances of suspected large intestinal rupture and peritonitis. Barium is absolutely contraindicated in patients with suspected colonic perforation, which has been described following corticosteroid therapy in dogs. There is a synergistic relationship between colonic

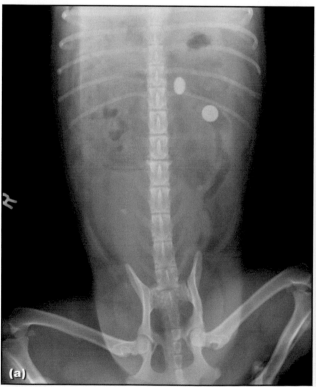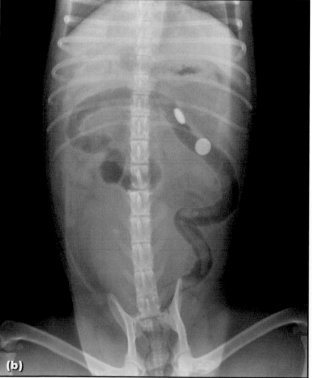

11.3 VD radiographs taken **(a)** before and **(b)** after administration of 8 ml/kg bodyweight of air by rectal tube in a dog with Pepto-Bismol tablets in the descending colon. Radiography was instrumental in differentiating between a small and large bowel location of the foreign body. (Courtesy of R O'Brien) (continues) ▶

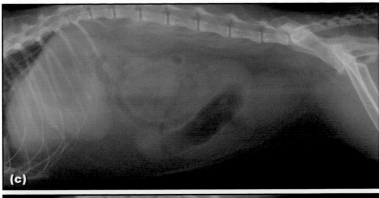

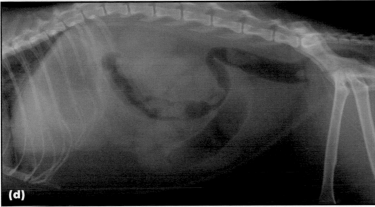

11.3 (continued) Lateral radiographs obtained **(c)** before and **(d)** after pneumocolonography. This technique was helpful for differentiating the large from the small intestine in a cat with a small intestinal obstruction. In (c) there is a severely dilated segment of intestine visible in the caudoventral abdomen. (d) The pneumocolonogram clearly demonstrated that the distended segment was not large intestine and that a mechanical small intestinal ileus was present.

bacteria and barium that causes a life-threatening septic peritonitis. In these cases, diluted (20%) ionic or non-ionic iodinated contrast media should be used instead of barium.

Lateral and VD radiographs are performed after the introduction of contrast medium to assess the entire colon, including the caecum (Figure 11.4). Additional right and left lateral oblique views as well as dorsoventral (DV) views may be required to identify a lesion.

In normal dogs and cats, the barium–mucosa interface should have a smooth appearance. Peristaltic waves appear to have a corrugated appearance and should disappear on repeat views. A common complication with infusion of contrast medium into the colon is a symmetrical narrowing at the level of the catheter tip, associated with transient local spasticity. The transient nature, lack of wall thickening and normal palpation at this site should help to identify this false lesion.

Double-contrast colonogram

After draining the positive contrast medium out of the colon, an equal volume of room air can be injected. The double-contrast study allows assessment of:

- Space-occupying lesions of the colon wall
- The location of strictures and intramural lesions.

The longitudinal mucosal folds will be visible because they are coated with barium, and contrast with the luminal air.

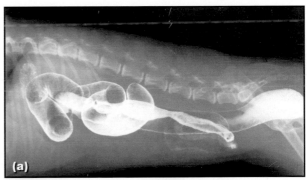

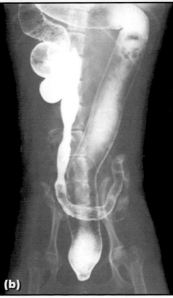

11.4 Double-contrast study of the colon in a dog in **(a)** lateral and **(b)** VD views. The barium coats the intestinal mucosa to show its smooth, thin-walled nature.

Ultrasonography

Large intestine

The colon is often observed as a bright linear hyperechoic structure that causes reverberation artefacts (Figure 11.5a). This appearance is caused by the gas and faecal content, which makes most of the colon wall difficult to observe. Only the wall closest to the transducer can be clearly identified when artefacts are present. It can be differentiated from the small intestine by its thickness and wall layering. The typical five acoustic layers are much thinner than in the small intestine and all are of approximately equal thickness (Figure 11.5b).

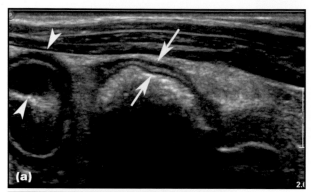

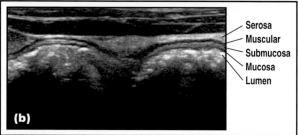

Serosa
Muscular
Submucosa
Mucosa
Lumen

(b)

11.5 Ultrasonograms of the normal colon.
(a) Transverse image. The near wall (between the white arrows) is well defined with a high-resolution transducer (17 MHz linear probe). The far wall cannot be identified because of the artefacts created by the presence of faeces and air. These appear as a diffuse hyperechoic region distal to the wall. The small intestine lying next to the colon shows the different appearance of the wall layering (between arrowheads). **(b)** Longitudinal image. Note the five layers that can be observed with a high-resolution linear transducer.

Peristalsis is rare in the large intestine. Wall thickness in typical faeces-filled segments is <1 mm, and in less full segments is approximately ≤2 mm in dogs and ≤1.7 mm in cats. The wall of the empty colon has a very irregular appearance, owing to bunching of the distensible mucosal layer, and this can be mistaken for infiltration or thickening (Figure 11.6).

The descending colon can be scanned from the pelvic inlet along the left abdominal wall, where it lies very superficially. Placing the transducer transversely at the level of the urinary bladder helps to identify the colon, which is dorsal to it and appears as a curvilinear hyperechoic structure. Continuing cranially, the colon can be observed to turn towards the right just caudal to the stomach and it then continues caudally on the right-hand side of the abdomen. The ascending colon

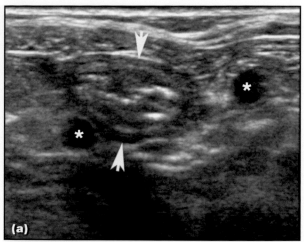

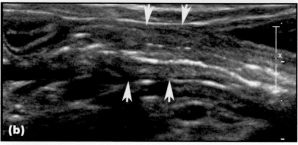

11.6 **(a)** Transverse and **(b)** longitudinal ultrasonograms of the empty and contracted descending colon (between arrows). The asterisks mark two vessels seen in cross section. When the colon is contracted, the wall layering appears irregular or stippled. This should not be confused with thickening.

and caecum can be identified medial to the descending duodenum, which serves as a good landmark. The ileum can be identified as it enters the colon at the ileocolic junction (Figure 11.7).

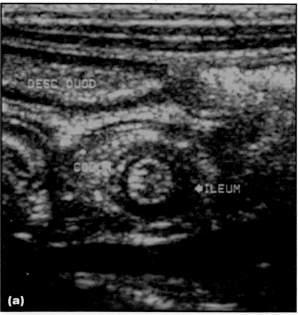

11.7 Ultrasonograms of the normal ileocolic junction in a dog and a cat. **(a)** Transverse image of the ileocolic junction in the dog. The ileum appears as a small structure with concentric rings sitting at the entrance to the colon. The duodenum (DUOD) is seen as a longitudinal small intestinal segment lateral to the ileum. (continues) ▶

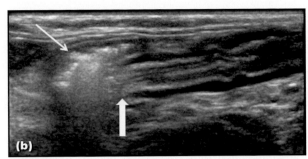

11.7 (continued) Ultrasonograms of the normal ileocolic junction in a dog and a cat. **(b)** Sagittal image of the feline ileum taken at its entrance (wide arrow) to the colon (thin arrow).

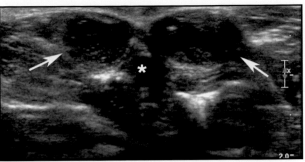

11.8 Ultrasonogram of normal anal sacs in a dog. A high-frequency linear probe was placed across the anus. The anal sacs (arrowed) appear as round to oval, thin-walled structures with content of varying echogenicity. The asterisk is placed over the anal sphincter, which appears as a poorly defined hypoechoic region.

The ileocolic junction has a distinct appearance in cats and dogs. The short ileum can be found in the right mid-abdomen where it enters the caecum. In most cats, and many dogs, the ileocolic junction can be identified. The ileum appears to end bluntly in a large intestinal segment. In cats, there is usually no gas in the caecum and reverberation artefacts are not present.

Although normal regional lymph nodes are not visible radiographically, they are visible with high-resolution transducers on ultrasonography. The right colic, medial iliac and hypogastric lymph nodes appear as small, oval to ellipsoid moderately echogenic structures with smooth borders. The right colic lymph nodes are seen at the ileocolic junction in cats. The paired medial iliac lymph nodes are located by using the aortic bifurcation as a landmark. At the first bifurcation, to the external iliac arteries, the medial iliac lymph nodes can be identified as homogenous, elliptical and smoothly bordered structures that are almost isoechoic to the surrounding tissues. Normally <1 cm in width, the medial iliac lymph nodes can range up to 3 cm in length.

Perianal region

Both curved and linear array high-frequency transducers (≥7.5 MHz) should be used to examine the perianal region because the structures of interest are fairly superficial. Indications include a swelling or mass in the perianal, rectal or anal region. Normal structures that can be identified include:

- Anus
- Anal sacs
- Rectum
- Vagina
- Urethra.

The examination can be carried out by positioning the transducer transversely across the anus so that it is located in the centre of the image; this produces a dorsal plane image. The anal sacs can be identified on either side of the anus as round, well marginated structures with a regular thin wall and hypoechoic or heterogenous content (the 'owl' appearance; Figure 11.8). Variations include gas in the anal sacs, following removal of the contents as part of the physical examination.

With ultrasonograms obtained in the dorsal plane, the anus appears as a circular and fairly well defined structure. Turning the probe through 90 degrees will show the anus and distal portion of the rectum in a sagittal section, and the rectum can be followed for a short distance to the caudal aspect of the pelvic canal. Examination beyond this point is not possible. The ultrasound transducer can also be placed lateral to the base of the tail for examination of swellings or masses in the perineal region. Intrapelvic examination of the descending colon and rectum requires alternative imaging modalities, such as CT, MRI or endoscopic ultrasonography.

Overview of additional imaging modalities

Cross-sectional imaging modalities (e.g. CT and MRI) can be used to examine the large bowel and are especially useful for diagnosing intrapelvic lesions. Owing to the lack of superimposition of the pelvis and neighbouring structures when these techniques are used, the colon, sublumbar and perianal regions can be better examined. Indications include: pre-surgical work-up before resection of lesions that may extend into the pelvic canal; examining the extent of space-occupying perianal lesions; and recognition of regional metastases.

Endoscopic ultrasonography of the pelvic canal has not been described in dogs and cats but has potential for examination of the rectum, prostate gland and regional lymph nodes. As with CT and MRI, endoscopic ultrasonography requires specialist equipment and expertise.

Large bowel diseases

Radiographic findings in the large intestine are usually non-specific. Disease processes may lead to changes in size, shape, location and opacity on survey radiographs but a multimodal approach is often required to arrive at a diagnosis. Furthermore, the finding of a radiographically normal large intestine does not rule out disease.

Congenital diseases

Short colon has been reported in dogs and cats. Radiographically, the colon appears to have a shorter course and the ascending and transverse segments are not clearly identifiable. Atresia ani (Figure 11.9), recti or coli, imperforate anus, fistulation, diverticula or duplication of the large bowel and rectum can occur, but are rare in dogs and cats. Enteric duplication is a rare congenital defect that has been described in dogs. These abnormalities generally require a barium enema to confirm the diagnosis.

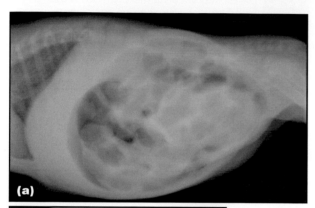

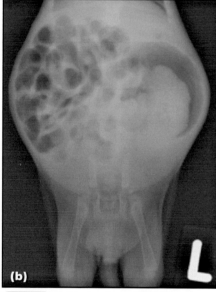

11.9 (a) Lateral and (b) VD radiographs of a 4-week-old kitten with atresia ani. The abdomen is severely distended and the entire small intestinal tract is markedly distended and filled with gas. On the VD view there is a large gas-filled structure containing a large amount of very opaque granular material, which was the descending colon.

Displacement

Displacement of the colon can create the appearance of luminal narrowing, owing to compression by the extramural lesion. However, some tumours, such as prostatic or anal sac carcinomas, may metastasize to the colon and lead to true mural thickening and stricture. Contrast radiography, colonoscopy or ultrasonography is required to rule out wall infiltration.

Perineal hernias may lead to displacement and possible entrapment of the colon and rectum, bladder and prostate gland. Radiographically, perineal hernias appear as soft tissue swellings at the tail base. Gas-filled intestinal segments may also be observed. Ultrasonography can often be used with success for determining which structures are displaced. Alternatively, positive-contrast studies (e.g. barium enema, retrograde urethrocystogram) can be used to demonstrate the herniated structures. (For further information on displacement, see Chapter 8.)

Intussusception and caecal inversion

Large intestinal intussusception occurs most commonly at the ileocolic junction. Ileocolic, caecocolic (caecal inversion), ileocaecal and colocolonic intussusceptions are all possible. Small intestinal dilatation caused by obstruction of the ileocolic region may be present. The diagnosis of a low intussusception is difficult to make on survey radiographs, owing to the variable appearance. Barium enemas, double-contrast colonogram studies and ultrasonography can be used to diagnose a lesion in the region of the ileum or caecum. A barium enema will show a colonic filling defect in the region of the ascending or transverse colon and caecum, but not necessarily an obstruction, as is seen with an intussusception. Caecal inversion occurs when the caecum inverts into the colon. The lesion appears as a soft tissue opacity in the right mid-abdomen and the normal air-filled caecum is not present.

Ultrasonography can be very helpful for diagnosing large intestinal intussusceptions and caecal inversions and is usually preferred to contrast studies. Lesions appear similar to small intestinal intussusceptions, with a multilayered appearance of the wall in the region of the ascending or transverse colon in both longitudinal and transverse views.

Ulcers and perforation

Colonic ulcers may occur in dogs receiving glucocorticoid therapy, and the risk is increased with concurrent use of non-steroidal anti-inflammatory drugs. Ulceration of the colonic mucosa is difficult to detect with either contrast radiography or ultrasonography. Positive-contrast and double-contrast procedures may show small multifocal areas of extension of barium into the mucosa. Double-contrast colonography augmented by CT is sufficiently sensitive to detect ulceration and small nodules in human patients. Ultrasonographically, ulcerated regions are difficult to detect. Colonoscopy is the modality of choice for detecting ulceration.

Colonic or rectal perforation may occur in dogs following steroid therapy, dehiscence after colonic surgery, perforating foreign body, neoplasia or trauma. Depending on the site of perforation, either peritonitis or retroperitoneal loss of detail with free air may be observed. If the anus or rectum is involved, lucent striations may be present along the wall. Communication with the retroperitoneal space is possible, with focal increased soft tissue opacities caudally. Irregular or linear lucencies may be observed. If the ascending, transverse or descending colon is affected, loss of abdominal detail and free air may be identified radiographically. The perforated colon can potentially develop a stricture or diverticulum.

Diverticula and fistulae

Colorectal diverticula are rare in dogs. They are caused by tears in the muscular layer of the colon that allow the mucosa and submucosa to protrude through the defect. They can occur secondarily to a perineal hernia or to trauma and straining. Fistula formation is often caused by trauma but may be congenital. Vaginorectal, urethrorectal and rectocutaneous fistulae have been described. Both diverticula and fistulae can be diagnosed by endoscopy or positive-contrast studies. However, a sacculation of the rectum and a diverticulum have a similar appearance following a barium enema. When a fistula between the colon and another structure is suspected, the use of iodinated contrast media is indicated. Barium is contraindicated for colonic studies for the diagnosis of perforation or fistulae. Fistulae can be diagnosed by demonstrating a connection between the colon and the vagina, urethra or skin.

Ileus

Alterations in the diameter and content of the large intestine are common abnormalities that are recognized radiographically in dogs and cats. They can be generalized or localized. A homogenous content of soft tissue opacity with a normal or increased diameter is generally associated with increased fluid volume. Homogenous soft tissue opacities can also be observed with intraluminal masses, intussusceptions or foreign bodies. Definitions of some terms associated with ileus are given below:

- Constipation: difficult, incomplete or infrequent evacuation of dry hardened faeces
- Obstipation: a severe form of constipation, defined as an inability to evacuate a mass of dry, hard faeces
- Megacolon: hypomotility and dilatation of the colon, which results in constipation and obstipation.

Common causes of megacolon include chronic constipation and nutritional, metabolic or mechanical problems. Chronic renal disease and the associated persistent subclinical dehydration are also commonly associated with megacolon. In addition, idiopathic cases of megacolon can occur, more commonly in cats. Neurological diseases associated with megacolon include spinal cord diseases such as cauda equina syndrome, sacrococcygeal agenesis in Manx cats, dysautonomia and Hirschsprung's disease. Metabolic diseases, such as hypokalaemia and hypothyroidism, have also been reported to be associated with this condition.

Radiographically it is difficult to differentiate primary constipation and obstipation from megacolon. Distension of the colon can be recognized radiographically when its diameter is greater than three times that of the small intestines or greater than the length of L7. The opacity of the contents change when long-standing obstipation and obstruction are present. The longer that faecal matter is present in the colon, the more desiccated it becomes. The faecal balls will appear to have a bony or near bony opacity (Figure 11.10).

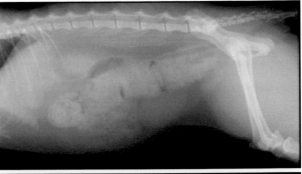
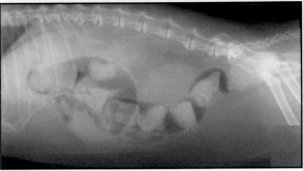

11.10 Lateral radiographs of obstipated cats demonstrating the bony opacity of the faecal content and distension of the colon. The increased opacity is caused by desiccation as the faecal balls cannot be evacuated.

The goal of the imaging examination is to rule out a mechanical cause of the obstruction. Mechanical obstruction can be caused by:

- Foreign body
- Perineal hernia
- Anorectal congenital anomaly
- Pelvic stenosis following trauma
- Prostatomegaly
- Lymphadenomegaly
- Colonic mass
- Intrapelvic mass.

Mineral opacities, representing stones and opaque metal foreign material, can be identified within the colon on survey radiographs. Pebbles and stones are not infrequent incidental findings on radiographs. Once most foreign bodies have passed through the entire small intestinal tract to reach the colon, they are usually passed through the colon without a problem.

Rectal and anal strictures can occur secondarily to trauma, chronic inflammation and neoplasia. Radiography and ultrasonography are important for helping to differentiate malignant from benign disease in the rectal region. A barium enema study can demonstrate the length of the stricture, even if the stricture is intrapelvic. This is an advantage of this technique over ultrasonography, which cannot image the complete rectum. However, ultrasonography can better demonstrate the perirectal tissues in order to rule out a mass. Demonstration of a mass with lymphadenopathy makes neoplasia a likely diagnosis. Ultrasonography can be performed from a perianal approach and guided tissue sampling can be performed.

Vascular compromise attributable to thrombo-embolism and volvulus are less common diseases that cause dilatation (Figure 11.11). Radiographic features of volvulus, which is a surgical emergency, include severe gaseous distension of the colon.

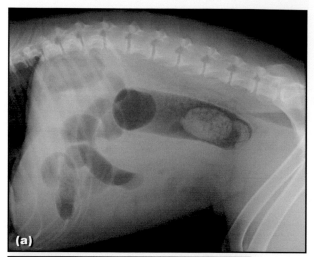

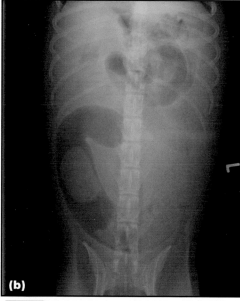

11.11 **(a)** Lateral and **(b)** VD radiographs of a dog with colonic torsion. The abdomen is distended and there is a loss of detail in the mid-abdomen. The majority of the small intestinal segments are dilated and either gas- or fluid-filled. The colon is severely dilated and is displaced.

Focal wall thickening

Colorectal neoplasms, such as polyps and carcinomas, cause focal nodules or masses. Focal masses may also be caused by pyogranulomatous colitis, such as is seen in dogs from regions endemic for histoplasmosis. Adenocarcinomas generally cause a circumferential and focal thickening of the colon with stricture. Lymphosarcoma can also affect the large intestine and may appear focal or diffuse. Both carcinomas and lymphosarcomas occur in dogs and cats. Adenocarcinoma is the most common colonic neoplasm in cats, followed by lymphosarcoma. Leiomyosarcoma can also be found in the large intestine and has been described in the caecum.

Depending on their size, masses may be difficult to identify on survey radiographs. However, often there is air surrounding the lesion that protrudes into the lumen, making the mass readily visible. Pneumo-colonography can be used to demonstrate soft tissue masses and strictures. If the mass is creating a stric-ture, the colon is often dilated cranial to it. With either negative- or positive-contrast studies, the wall of the colon is usually irregular, and positive contrast medium may extend into the lesion when neoplasia is present. Strictures caused by non-neoplastic diseases or extra-mural compression generally maintain a smooth mucosal surface against the barium contrast medium.

Ultrasonography is currently the method of choice for diagnosing large intestinal neoplasms. Survey and contrast radiographs are frequently non-specific, whereas ultrasound examination can show the exact location and extent of the mass. Limitations of ultrasonography include the inability to completely evaluate or even detect intrapelvic lesions. Neoplastic masses generally cause disruption of the normal wall layering and the lumen can appear asymmetrical and irregular. Mineralization may also be present and appear as multifocal hyperechoic structures with acoustic shadowing. Lymphoma generally has a very hypoechoic appearance and thickened wall. However, mast cell infiltration and leiomyosarcomas can have a similar appearance.

Both fungal and neoplastic disease can lead to focal mass lesions and the ultrasonographic appear-ance is too non-specific to distinguish between the two. Histological examination of biopsy or cytology specimens is always required for a definitive diagnosis. The sublumbar lymph nodes are often enlarged and can be rounded and hypoechoic when colonic neoplasia is present. However, fungal infection can also lead to lymphadenopathy. Ultrasound-guided fine-needle aspiration with a 22- or 25-gauge needle can be performed to obtain a cytological diagnosis of intestinal masses.

Diffuse thickening

Neoplastic, inflammatory and infectious diseases can cause diffuse thickening of the colonic wall. Inflam-matory bowel disease (IBD), lymphosarcoma (Figure 11.12), pythiosis and histoplasmosis can lead to simi-lar radiographic changes. However, wall thickening is typically not identified on survey radiographs. In patients with colitis, the colon may or may not be distended. The fluid-filled colon will appear with a homogenous soft tissue opacity, possibly with some gas bubbles. Other potential findings include a gener-alized gas-filled lumen. Occasionally, emphysema-tous changes of the wall can be identified in patients with gas-producing bacterial infections. Radio-graphically this appears as a lucent border at the serosal surface of the colonic wall.

Positive contrast medium examination in patients with severe colitis may show multifocal extension of the barium into the mucosa, which can also be seen with diffuse neoplasia. In ulcerative colitis, an irregular mucosa–barium interface can be observed, with extension of barium into the thickened colonic wall. Because of the non-specific nature of this finding,

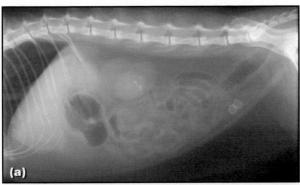

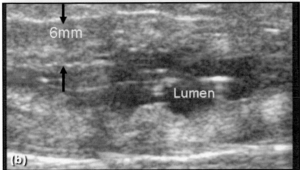

11.12 **(a)** Radiograph and **(b)** ultrasonogram of a thickened colonic wall. A pneumocolonographic study was performed and showed a rigid and thickened wall. Ultrasonography of the colon showed severe thickening with loss of wall layering. The medial iliac lymph nodes were also enlarged in this patient, but were only observed ultrasonographically. The diagnosis was confirmed as a lymphosarcoma.

histology is always required to make a definitive diagnosis. In chronic inflammatory disease, the colon may actually become shortened. The colon may also have a corrugated appearance caused by spasticity, which does not resolve on repeat radiographs. However, this appearance can occur simply owing to the administration of barium.

Ultrasonographically, the colon can be evaluated for wall thickening and loss of layering as well as regional lymphadenopathy, which gives this technique an advantage over survey radiography. Diffuse IBD with lymphocytic–plasmacytic infiltration cannot always be detected ultrasonographically. In IBD the wall layering is often preserved and normal to mild wall thickening may occur. Severe diffuse thickening of the colonic wall may occur with ulcerative colitis, fungal infections (Figure 11.13) and diffuse neoplastic processes such as lymphosarcoma. The wall can be >8 mm thick in cats with colonic adenocarcinomas.

Perianal diseases

In animals with swelling, pain or a palpable mass in the perianal region, survey radiographs should be performed. These can be used to provide an overview of the caudal abdomen, to detect bone lesions and to characterize the displacement of gas-filled bowel into the perianal region. Certain disease processes, such as neoplasia and infections, can extend into the retroperitoneal space from the anal region (Figure 11.14). Adenocarcinomas are known to metastasize

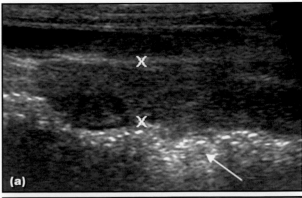

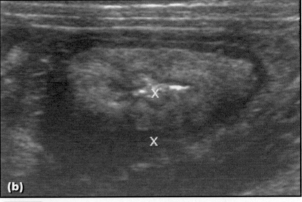

11.13 **(a)** Longitudinal and **(b)** transverse ultrasonograms of a diffusely thickened colonic wall in a dog. The colon wall (x–x) is 8 mm thick with a loss of layering. The arrow shows the air artefacts caused by the colon content distal to the near wall. The diagnosis was pythiosis. Other differential diagnoses should include neoplasia.

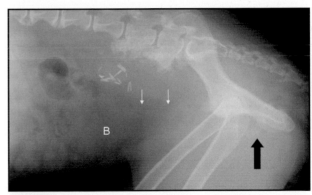

11.14 Lateral radiograph of the caudal abdomen in a dog with anal sac adenocarcinoma. There is extension of the soft tissue mass into the retroperitoneal space and severe irregular periosteal new bone formation along the ventral lumbar vertebrae. The metal clips in the caudal abdomen are attributable to previous partial resection of the infiltrating mass. The small white arrows show the ventral displacement of the colon. The space-occupying lesion was caused by a combination of extension of the tumour and sublumbar lymphadenopathy. The black arrow shows destruction of the pubic bone. B = Bladder.

locally to soft tissue and bone. The location of the bladder and prostate gland in male dogs can also be assessed. If the descending colon or rectum is suspected of being involved in the disease process, a barium enema can be performed to rule this out. If the urinary bladder cannot be visualized, then a positive-

or negative-contrast retrograde cystogram may be indicated to aid localization.

Alternatively, ultrasonography can be used to assess lesions in the perianal region. Herniated intestinal structures can be easily identified in the sac of a perineal hernia by the wall layering and reverberation artefacts that result from the gas content. The prostate gland and urinary bladder may also be displaced into a perineal hernia and are easy to recognize with ultrasonography. If extension of a perianal mass into the retroperitoneum is suspected, cross-sectional imaging with CT (Figure 11.15) or MRI is indicated. As dictated by the complexity of many intrapelvic lesions, CT imaging can be augmented with positive-contrast studies of the large intestine or urogenital tract as necessary.

Masses and nodules in the region of the anal sacs can be assessed most accurately ultrasonographically with high-resolution curved or linear array transducers. Impaction, abscessation and neoplastic disease of the anal sacs can be readily identified. Masses caused by anal sac adenocarcinomas are well described in dogs but are rare in cats. Squamous cell carcinoma is less common but is a differential diagnosis. Anal and rectal masses can be diagnosed with ultrasonography. They may appear as irregularly shaped solid structures with a heterogenous echotexture in the region of the anal sac. Neoplastic infiltration of the rectal or anal tissue can also be assessed by ultrasound examination (Figure 11.16).

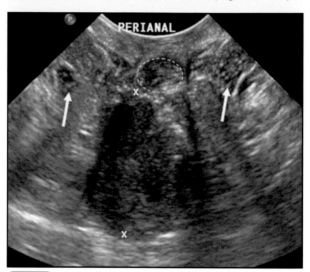

11.16 Perianal ultrasonogram of a rectal stricture caused by a lymphosarcoma. A 3 cm mass (x–x) is located next to the rectum (dotted circle). The arrows indicate the anal sacs.

If lesions are identified in the perianal region or rectum, the regional lymph nodes should be examined. The medial iliac and hypogastric nodes are common sites of metastasis of perianal neoplasms (Figure 11.17a). These sublumbar lymph nodes are located by ultrasonographically tracing the distal abdominal

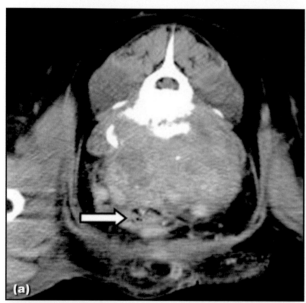

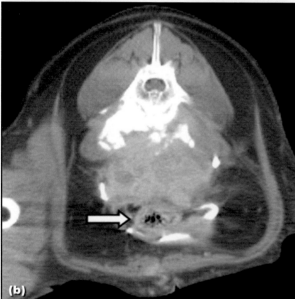

11.15 CT scan of the same dog as in Figure 11.14. **(a)** Prior to radiation therapy the image shows a large heterogenous and poorly marginated mass that fills the pelvic and retroperitoneal space with compression of the rectum (arrowed). **(b)** After radiation therapy there is a reduction in the size of the diffuse and poorly marginated mass (arrowed) with less compression of the colon.

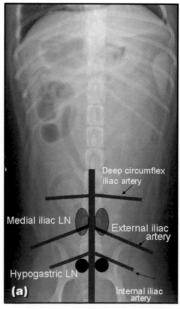

11.17

Sublumbar lymph nodes in a dog. **(a)** VD radiograph showing the location of the sublumbar lymph nodes (LN). (continues) ▶

Deep circumflex iliac artery

Medial iliac LN

External iliac artery

Hypogastric LN

Internal iliac artery

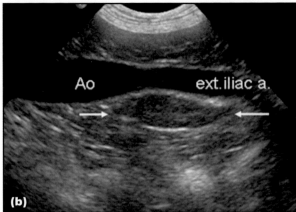

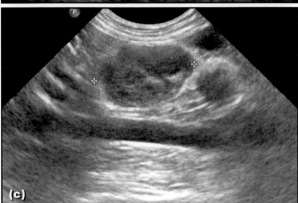

11.17 (continued) Sublumbar lymph nodes in a dog.
(b) Ultrasonogram of a normal medial iliac
lymph node (arrowed). The node is small and elliptical
with medium echogenicity. Ao = Aorta; ext. iliac a. =
External iliac artery. **(c)** Ultrasonogram of a lymph node
(x–x) containing tumour metastases. The node is
enlarged, rounded and has a heterogenous echotexture.

aorta to its bifurcation. At the first bifurcation (with the
external iliac arteries), the medial iliac lymph nodes
are observed (Figure 11.17b). Metastatic medial iliac
lymph nodes are rounded, enlarged and hypoechoic.
(Figure 11.17c).

References and further reading

Bellah JR (1983) Colonic perforation after corticosteroid and surgical treatment of intervertebral disk disease in a dog. *Journal of the American Veterinary Medical Association* **183(9)**, 1002–1003, 965

Bentley AM, O'Toole TE and Kowaleski MP (2006) Colon volvulus in dogs. *Compendium on Continuing Education for the Practicing Veterinarian* **28(2)**, 105–106

Bertoy RW (2002) Megacolon in the cat. *Veterinary Clinics of North America: Small Animal Practice* **32(4)**, 901–915

Boysen SR, Tidwell AS and Penninck DG (2003) Ultrasonographic findings in dogs and cats with gastrointestinal perforation. *Veterinary Radiology and Ultrasound* **44(5)**, 556–564

Brisson BA, Whiteside DP and Holmberg DL (2004) Metastatic anal sac adenocarcinoma in a dog presenting for acute paralysis. *Canadian Veterinary Journal* **45(8)**, 678–681

Byers CG, Leasure CS and Sanders NA (2006) Feline idiopathic megacolon. *Compendium on Continuing Education for the Practicing Veterinarian* **28(9)**, 658–664

Dennis R and Penderis J (2002) Radiology corner: anal sac gas appearing as an osteolytic pelvic lesion. *Veterinary Radiology and Ultrasound* **43(6)**, 552–553

Farrow CS, Green R and Shiveley M (1995) *Radiology of the Cat.* Mosby Inc., St Louis

Fluke MH, Hawkins EC, Elliott GS and Blevins WE (1989) Short colon in two cats and a dog. *Journal of the American Veterinary Medical Association* **195(1)**, 87–90

Goggin JM, Biller DS, Debey BM, Pickar JG and Mason D (2000) Ultrasonographic measurement of gastrointestinal wall thickness and the ultrasonographic appearance of the ileocolic region in healthy cats. *Journal of the American Animal Hospital Association* **36(3)**, 224–228

Goulden B, Bergman MM and Wyburn RS (1973) Canine urethro-rectal fistulae. *Journal of Small Animal Practice* **14(3)**, 143–150

Graham JP, Newell SM, Roberts GD and Lester NV (2000) Ultrasonographic features of canine gastrointestinal pythiosis. *Veterinary Radiology and Ultrasound* **41(3)**, 273–277

O'Brien TR (1981) *Radiographic Diagnosis of Abdominal Disorders in the Dog and Cat.* WB Saunders, Philadelphia

Sato AF and Solano M (2004) Ultrasonographic findings in abdominal mast cell disease: a retrospective study of 19 patients. *Veterinary Radiology and Ultrasound* **45(1)**, 51–57

Suess RP Jr, Martin RA, Moon ML and Dallman MJ (1992) Rectovaginal fistula with atresia ani in three kittens. *Cornell Veterinarian* **82(2)**, 141–153

Washabau RJ and Holt D (1999) Pathogenesis, diagnosis, and therapy of feline idiopathic megacolon. *Veterinary Clinics of North America: Small Animal Practice* **29(2)**, 589–603

Zoran DL (1999) Pathophysiology and management of canine colonic diseases. *Compendium on Continuing Education for the Practicing Veterinarian* **21(9)**, 824–841

12

The liver and gallbladder

Tobias Schwarz

Overview of anatomy

The canine and feline liver consists of six lobes with several processes (Figure 12.1). In dogs and cats the liver is located within the ribcage. The convex diaphragmatic surface of the liver is intimate with the concave visceral surface of the diaphragm. The visceral surface of the liver contains impressions of the adjacent organs (gallbladder, right kidney, stomach and duodenum). The strong lobation and a small film of peritoneal fluid provide high flexibility to accommodate the respiratory excursion of the diaphragm.

The gallbladder is a pear-shaped fluid-filled organ located between the quadrate and right medial liver lobes in the dog and between two parts of the right medial liver lobe in the cat. It stores and concentrates the bile that it receives from the hepatic biliary ducts. Bile is secreted into the duodenum via the cystic and common bile duct. The anatomy of the bile duct and its relationship with the pancreatic duct differs between dogs and cats (Figure 12.2). In cats, the gallbladder is frequently bilobed.

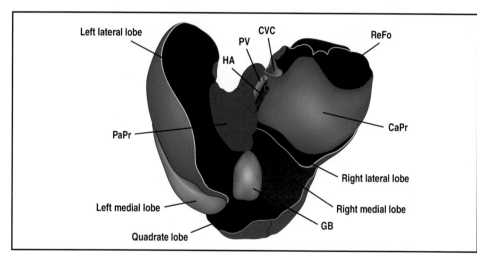

12.1 Visceral surface of the canine liver and gallbladder. The liver consists of six different lobes. The caudate lobe contains the papillary process (PaPr) centrally and the caudate process (CaPr) and renal fossa (ReFo) (for the right kidney) on the right. The porta hepatis is the central hilus of the liver, which allows passage of the hepatic artery (HA), portal vein (PV), caudal vena cava (CVC), common bile duct, nerves and lymphatics. The gallbladder (GB) is adjacent to the right medial and quadrate lobes.

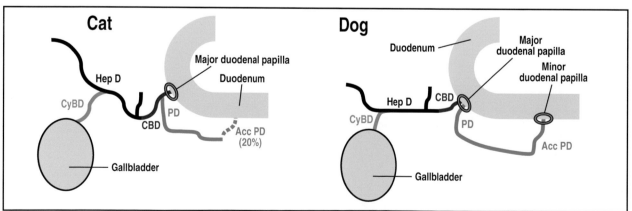

12.2 Feline and canine bile and pancreatic duct systems. The gallbladder receives bilious secretions from numerous hepatic bile ducts (Hep D) via the cystic bile duct (CyBD). Bile is excreted into the duodenum via the cystic and hepatic bile duct(s) which, after receiving the last tributary, form the common bile duct (CBD). The CBD is more tortuous in the cat. The CBD drains into the proximal descending duodenum at the major duodenal papilla. In the dog this entrance is shared with the pancreatic duct (PD), whereas in cats the PD joins the CBD before entering the sphincter. The canine pancreas has an additional larger accessory pancreatic duct (Acc PD), which drains into the minor duodenal papilla further distally into the duodenum, whereas only 20% of cats have this duct and papilla. Variations have been described in both species.

Radiographic anatomy and normal variation

The liver is the largest soft tissue organ in the body (Figure 12.3). Because of similar opacity and close proximity, the radiographic borders of the liver are normally merged with those of the gallbladder and parts of the diaphragm. This relationship is encompassed in the term 'hepatic silhouette'.

It can be difficult to delineate the border of the liver from that of the right kidney. The hepatic silhouette lies almost entirely within the costal arch. The caudoventral hepatic margin may protrude slightly beyond the costal arch and is of triangular shape. In deep-chested dogs (e.g. Dobermanns) the hepatic silhouette lies almost completely within the ribcage, whereas in barrel-chested dogs (e.g. terrier breeds) it protrudes further caudally. In young animals, the liver is

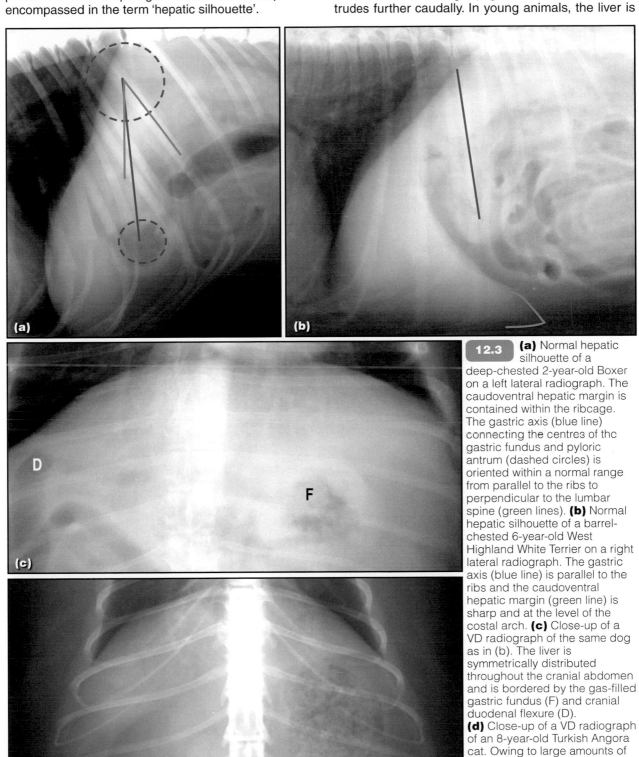

12.3 **(a)** Normal hepatic silhouette of a deep-chested 2-year-old Boxer on a left lateral radiograph. The caudoventral hepatic margin is contained within the ribcage. The gastric axis (blue line) connecting the centres of the gastric fundus and pyloric antrum (dashed circles) is oriented within a normal range from parallel to the ribs to perpendicular to the lumbar spine (green lines). **(b)** Normal hepatic silhouette of a barrel-chested 6-year-old West Highland White Terrier on a right lateral radiograph. The gastric axis (blue line) is parallel to the ribs and the caudoventral hepatic margin (green line) is sharp and at the level of the costal arch. **(c)** Close-up of a VD radiograph of the same dog as in (b). The liver is symmetrically distributed throughout the cranial abdomen and is bordered by the gas-filled gastric fundus (F) and cranial duodenal flexure (D). **(d)** Close-up of a VD radiograph of an 8-year-old Turkish Angora cat. Owing to large amounts of peritoneal fat, the liver margins are more visible than those in (c), and the right side protrudes further caudally than the left. (Courtesy of J Drees)

relatively larger than in adults. Inspiration will cause the hepatic silhouette to protrude further caudally. Falciform fat can be distinguished from the ventral hepatic margin, particularly in cats. On the right lateral view, the hepatic silhouette appears slightly larger and its caudoventral margin is more likely to be superimposed on the spleen than in the left lateral view.

On the ventrodorsal (VD) view, the hepatic silhouette is poorly marginated caudally. The caudal hepatic limits in the dog are marked by the gastric fundus on the left, the lesser curvature centrally and the pylorus and cranial duodenal flexure on the right. The caudal limits should be roughly symmetrical in dogs. In cats, an empty stomach is often more curved and the lesser curvature is not flush with the liver. The right side of the feline liver protrudes further caudally than the left.

Size of the hepatic silhouette
Using the gastric axis as a landmark on lateral films, a line can be drawn between the centre of the gastric fundus and the centre of the pyloric antrum (or the most ventral and caudal part of the stomach). This line should be angled within a range from parallel to the last ribs to perpendicular to the cranial lumbar spine (see Figure 12.3). Clockwise rotation of this axis outside the normal range indicates microhepatia. Anticlockwise rotation of this axis outside the normal range indicates hepatomegaly. There should be minimal protrusion of the caudoventral hepatic margin beyond the costal arch. Using the gastric axis as a landmark on VD films, a line can be drawn between the centre of the gastric fundus and the centre of the pyloric antrum (or the right-most part of the stomach). This line should be perpendicular to the cranial lumbar spine. Clockwise rotation of this axis outside the normal range indicates microhepatia. Anticlockwise rotation of this axis outside the normal range indicates hepatomegaly.

Position of the liver
The position of the hepatic silhouette is strongly influenced by chest conformation, diaphragmatic excursion, abdominal distension and to a lesser degree recumbency (see above). Positional variation secondary to these factors needs to be differentiated from true change in hepatic size. If there is no visible hepatic silhouette, a lack of peritoneal detail (ascites, lack of fat), abnormal thoracic opacities (diaphragmatic hernia) or microhepatia should be looked for.

Shape of the liver
The caudoventral hepatic margin should be evaluated on lateral radiographs. This margin is normally sharply pointed (see Figures 12.3b and 12.4). Rounding can be caused by a number of conditions resulting in diffuse liver enlargement, but might represent a positional artefact if the liver margin is not tangential to the X-ray beam. A change in shape may be caused by an enlarged gallbladder or disease of the liver parenchyma (Figure 12.4). Changes in shape may manifest by local displacement of adjacent organs. A localized organ displacement (e.g. caudal displacement of the right kidney) suggests a focal liver mass rather than generalized hepatopathy.

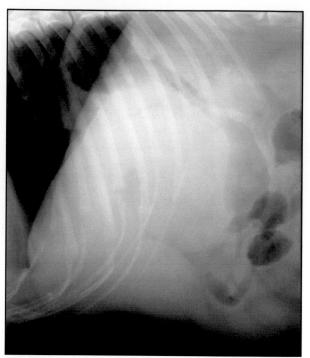

12.4   Close-up of a lateral radiograph of a 12-year-old mixed breed dog with hepatocellular carcinoma and radiographic abnormalities in liver shape. The gas-filled stomach is bent around the curved liver margin and the caudoventral hepatic margin is blunted.

Liver opacity
The liver should be a homogenous soft tissue opaque structure. Mineral or gas opacities within or superimposed on the liver (Figure 12.5) can be caused by various factors (see below).

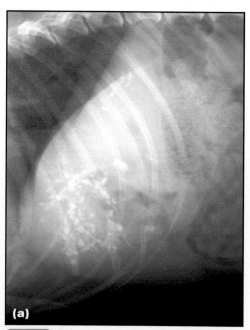

(a)

12.5   **(a)** Close-up of a lateral radiograph of a 10-year-old Cavalier King Charles Spaniel with biliary tree mineralization. Such opacities are occasionally seen incidentally in small-breed dogs but may be associated with chronic disease and bile obstruction. (continues) ▶

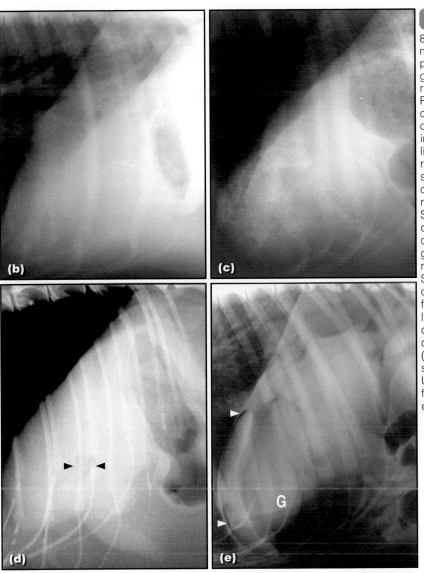

12.5 (continued) **(b)** Close-up of a lateral radiograph of an 8-year-old Old English Sheepdog with a metallic hepatic foreign body that presumably penetrated the liver via the gastric wall. **(c)** Close-up of a lateral radiograph of a 12-year-old Golden Retriever with a hepatocellular carcinoma that was treated with chemoembolization, chemotherapy and intra-arterial ethiodol. Ethiodol is a lipid-based contrast medium that remains radiographically evident for several weeks as a diffuse mineral opacity. **(d)** Close-up of a lateral radiograph of a 10-year-old Domestic Shorthaired cat with emphysematous cholecystitis. Note the irregular gas opacity (arrowheads) in the region of the gallbladder. **(e)** Close-up of a lateral radiograph of a 9-year-old German Shepherd Dog with pneumoperitoneum caused by a recent laparotomy (normal finding). The surrounding gas makes the liver and gallbladder (G) much more discernible. Separation of the diaphragmatic and hepatic silhouettes (arrowheads) is a hallmark for even small amounts of free peritoneal gas. Unless there is a benign explanation, free peritoneal gas constitutes a surgical emergency.

Significance of radiographic abnormalities

Microhepatia

A relatively small liver (Figure 12.6) is frequently seen as a normal variation. A diagnosis of cirrhosis or a portosystemic shunt is clinically relevant, but microhepatia caused by such conditions is often impossible to differentiate from normal variation on survey radiographs. Absence of liver tissue from the abdomen, caused by herniation into the thorax, may mimic microhepatia.

Generalized hepatomegaly

A large liver (Figure 12.7) is frequently seen as a normal variation. The criteria used to determine liver size often present mixed results; for example, the gastric axis may be normal but the liver may extend beyond the costal arch. Additional testing, including serology and/or ultrasonography, is usually indicated in these situations.

Pathological causes of hepatomegaly are numerous and often difficult to differentiate using any imaging modality. Passive venous congestion causes

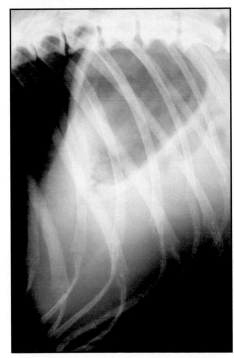

12.6 Close-up of a right lateral radiograph of a dog with microhepatia. Although the fluid-filled pylorus is difficult to discern, the gastric axis can be seen to be rotated in an anticlockwise direction beyond a line perpendicular to the lumbar spine.

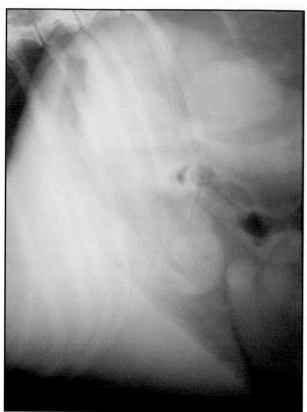

12.7 Close-up of a lateral radiograph of a 14-year-old Jack Russell Terrier with generalized hepatomegaly associated with hyperadrenocorticism. The gastric axis is rotated clockwise beyond being parallel with the rib, and the caudoventral hepatic margin is protruding into the mid-abdomen. Generalized hepatomegaly is a non-specific radiographic finding.

diffuse hepatomegaly owing to right heart failure. Concurrent signs include a distended caudal vena cava and pleural or peritoneal effusion. Causes include primary cardiac and peritoneal diseases, and an enlarged heart is usually a concurrent finding. Cardiomyopathy, tricuspid insufficiency and pericardial tamponade are major differential diagnoses. Similar findings are possible without cardiac enlargement in patients with Budd-Chiari-like syndrome and occlusion of the caudal vena cava or hepatic veins.

Many common metabolic conditions cause diffuse hepatomegaly, including hyperadrenocorticism, feline lipidosis, diabetes mellitus and hypothyroidism. Less common are liver storage diseases, such as amyloidosis. Iatrogenic vacuolar degeneration with concurrent hepatomegaly is seen in dogs, but not cats, as a result of administration of corticosteroid medications. Hepatic inflammatory conditions are common in cats and dogs. Acute and chronic hepatitis and cholangiohepatitis are common and are caused by a wide spectrum of pathogens.

Infiltrative neoplasia is also very common. Diffuse hepatomegaly is seen in dogs and cats with lymphoma. Other differential diagnoses, especially in cats, include mast cell tumours and other round cell neoplasms. Focal lesions, including those with benign and malignant aetiologies (see below), may cause the radiographic appearance of generalized hepatomegaly.

Local enlargement

Regional or local liver enlargement may be difficult to differentiate radiographically from generalized disease. Localized disease is seen more clearly when the outline of the lesion is apparent (Figure 12.8). This is the case when lesions are located on the caudal surface of the liver. Large primary neoplasms are common in cats and dogs (see Figure 12.4). Differential diagnoses for these neoplasms include hepatocellular carcinoma and bile duct carcinoma. A common lesion in cats is biliary cystadenoma. This lesion has been histologically classified as a ductal plate malformation, to indicate a benign developmental, although locally progressive, lesion. Additional neoplastic differential diagnoses include metastatic nodular infiltration.

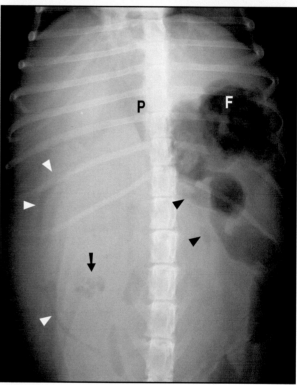

12.8 VD abdominal radiograph of a 7-year-old Cocker Spaniel with caudate liver lobe torsion. The pyloric antrum (P), duodenum and ascending colon (white/black arrowheads) are displaced towards the median plane by the enlarged lobe. The left caudal hepatic margin, outlined by the gastric fundus (F), remains normal. There are small gas bubbles within the mass attributable to central necrosis (arrowed).

Benign causes of local liver enlargement include a wide spectrum of nodular diseases. Benign nodular hyperplasia is very common, especially in older dogs. These lesions are much less common in cats. Cysts are seen in both cats and dogs, although are uncommon as a cause of radiographic hepatomegaly. Gallbladder distension may mimic localized hepatomegaly. A bulge may be seen in the mid-ventral liver contour on lateral views. Causes include anorexia, mucocele, biliary obstruction and cholecystitis (see below).

Displacement of the liver

Caudal displacement of the liver is seen as a result of increased pressure from the thoracic cavity. Simple hyperinflation is a common cause, seen very commonly in excited, hyperthyroid and asthmatic cats. Additional intrathoracic causes include marked pleural free fluid (Figure 12.9) and large pulmonary, body wall or mediastinal masses. Cranial displacement of the liver (Figure 12.10) may be caused by a diaphragmatic hernia, eventration or paralysis.

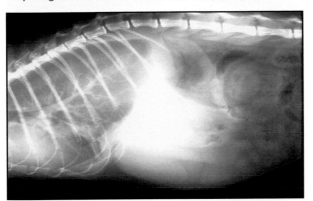

12.9 Lateral radiograph of a 2-year-old Domestic Shorthaired cat with pyothorax. The hepatic silhouette is not enlarged but the liver is displaced caudally by the space-occupying pleural effusion.

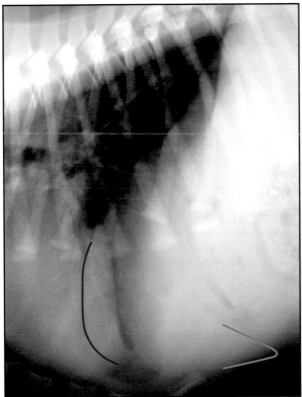

12.10 Close-up of a right lateral radiograph of a 3-month-old Boxer with right hemidiaphragmatic paralysis. Note the cranial location of the caudoventral hepatic margin (green line). This position was not caused by microhepatia but by cranial displacement of the flaccid right hemidiaphragm (red line).

Mineralization

Amorphous mineralization within the hepatic parenchyma (see Figure 12.5c) can be seen in chronic conditions with tissue necrosis attributable to abscess, torsion, neoplasia, haematoma, nodular hyperplasia or parasitic causes or as a consequence of contrast medium administration. Branching mineralization is seen occasionally in small-breed dogs without clinical signs (see Figure 12.5a). The significance of this condition is unknown.

Luminal biliary ductal and cystic calcified concretions are seen commonly in cats and occasionally in dogs. The condition is not always clinically apparent, although chronic inflammatory and obstructive causes must be considered (Figure 12.11a).

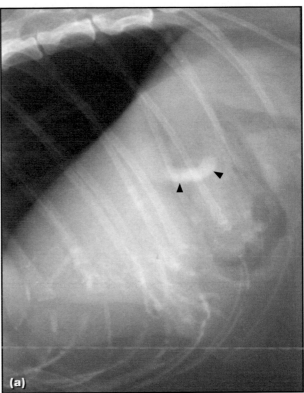

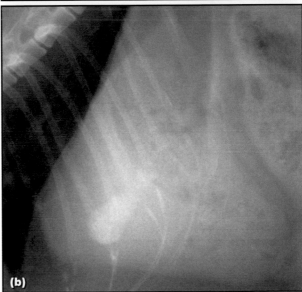

12.11 **(a)** Close-up of a lateral radiograph of a 13-year-old Domestic Shorthaired cat with mineralization of the hepatic biliary ducts and the extrahepatic common bile duct (arrowheads), leading to biliary obstruction and cholangitis. **(b)** Close-up of a lateral radiograph of a Siamese cat with gallbladder mineralization without clinical signs. The cast-like mineralization could be caused by numerous, small radiopaque choleliths or by gallbladder wall mineralization.

Mineralization of the gallbladder wall (Figure 12.11b) is rare but may occur secondary to necrosis; primary causes include abscess, neoplasia, haematoma and parasitic diseases. Branching mineralization is seen occasionally within the liver parenchyma in older terrier-breed dogs without clinical signs. The significance of this condition is unknown.

Contrast medium may accumulate in the biliary system and lead to increased opacity. Biliary excretion of water-soluble iodinated contrast medium is common in cases of anuric or oliguric renal failure; contrast medium may be seen within the gallbladder in these patients. Direct introduction of contrast media may be performed by cholecystocentesis for study of the patency of the biliary duct, or by cholecystography using iopanoic acid compounds.

Penetrating foreign bodies (e.g. needle, wire) are often incidental findings (see Figure 12.5b).

Intrahepatic gas

Abnormal gas opacities may be seen in the liver parenchyma, biliary ducts (*pneumobilia*) or branches of the portal vein (see Figures 12.5d and 12.8). Incidental reflux of gas may occur from the duodenum into the biliary ducts. This is more common in cats than in dogs. It is thought to be due to incompetence of the sphincter of Oddi with duodenal reflux. Other complicating factors may include biliary obstruction, inflammatory bowel disease or recent surgical intervention. Emphysematous cholecystitis is commonly associated with diabetes mellitus. Local necrosis is uncommon but is a clinically important differential diagnosis for local gas accumulation.

Gas in branches of the portal vein is rare in live animals. Important clinical diseases that may cause mural and luminal gas include gastric torsion, necrotizing gastroenteritis, clostridiosis, functional ileus and air embolism. It can also be seen as a normal post-mortem finding.

Ultrasonography

Technical considerations

Due to the location of the liver (Figure 12.12) within the ribcage, a curvilinear transducer is very helpful to allow full penetration of the ultrasound beam. Depending on the size of the animal and the depth of the hepatic area of interest, a transducer frequency of 7–10 MHz should be sufficient. Regardless of the position of the animal, both subxiphoid and right intracostal windows should be used for complete evaluation of the liver and gallbladder. Biopsy of the liver may require use of both windows to obtain representative samples from multiple liver lobes.

- For the subxiphoid window, the transducer is placed immediately caudal to the xiphoid process of the sternum and oriented in longitudinal and transverse directions. The entirety of the liver is scanned by rocking and fanning of the transducer to evaluate the liver and adjacent structures.
- For the subcostal window, the transducer is oriented in longitudinal and transverse planes.

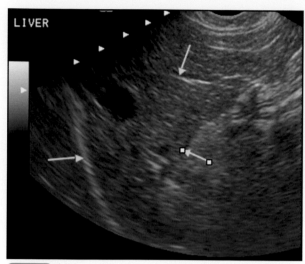

12.12 Mid-sagittal ultrasonogram of the normal liver in a cat. The liver margins are outlined with arrows.

Using this window, the right kidney and caudate liver lobe can be evaluated. Use of the transverse plane is very important for the complete evaluation of the porta hepatis, common bile duct and adjacent structures. This window is also valuable for diagnosis of portosystemic shunts.

Major ultrasonographic artefacts may affect assessment of the normal liver. The mirror artefact is commonly seen, in which an artefactual image of the liver is displayed beyond the diaphragm. This is caused by multiple echoes at the highly reflective interface with air-filled lung. Distant enhancement ('through transmission') is reliably seen in the tissues deep to a fluid-filled gallbladder, and creates an artificially hyperechoic appearance.

Hepatic size and localization of lobes

The ultrasonographic assessment of liver size can be confusing. Owing to the cross-sectional nature of this technique, the liver is never seen at once in its entirety, but just as a slice at a time. However, by using the ribcage to mark the extent of the normal caudal hepatic margin an assessment of marked microhepatia and/or hepatomegaly can be made. If finer gradations are necessary, for example assessment of the response to treatment, a lateral radiograph is recommended.

Equally, it is difficult to identify the location of the lobes ultrasonographically in the absence of peritoneal effusion because the lobar borders are barely visible on ultrasound examination. However, using anatomical or vascular landmarks (Figure 12.13) and common sense, it is usually possible to localize a hepatic lesion to a specific lobe. Clinically it may be important to place a surgical lesion to the left or right of the gallbladder. Surgical conditions in the right liver lobes are often technically more challenging than those in the left lobes.

Ultrasonography is an excellent tool for identification of liver masses and other lesions and to guide a biopsy needle to them. However, most ultrasonographic findings are non-specific and this should

Left	Centre	Right
Quadrate lobe	Gallbladder	Right medial lobe
Left lateral lobe	Oesophagus	Papillary process
Papillary process	Porta hepatis	Caudate process
Left lateral lobe	Ductus venosus	Papillary process
Right medial lobe	Caudal vena cava	Caudate process
Left medial lobe	Falciform ligament	Quadrate lobe

Cranial	Caudal
Caudate lobe	Right kidney
Left lateral lobe	Stomach
Right lateral lobe; caudate process	Duodenum

12.13 Anatomical relationships of the liver, gallbladder and adjacent organs.

be taken into account. For biliary diseases, a more specific diagnosis can often be made ultrasonographically, but ultrasound-guided biopsy samples and cholecystocentesis are also required in many cases.

Hepatic echogenicity

Great emphasis is put on hepatic echogenicity for diagnostic purposes (Figure 12.14). However, echogenicity is intrinsically related to several technical aspects of the scan that need to be standardized. Therefore, hepatic echogenicity must be assessed *only* in comparison with neighbouring organs at the same depth and preferably within the same image. If these provisions are met, normal hepatic echogenicity should be lower than that of the spleen and can range from slightly lower to slightly higher than right renal cortical echogenicity. In addition, the normally hyperechoic walls of the branches of the portal vein will be more prominent in a hypoechoic liver, and may be lost in a hyperechoic parenchyma. The use of harmonic ultrasound technology enhances the visibility of subtle differences in tissue echogenicity.

Diffusely hypoechoic liver

Generalized hypoechogenicity (see Figure 12.14c), which is usually associated with diffuse enlargement, may be difficult to verify objectively. The comparison with the spleen and right kidney can be within the normal range, but vessels appear more prominent with their hyperechoic walls in greater contrast to the surrounding hypoechoic parenchyma. Differential diagnoses for this appearance include lymphoma (and other multicentric round cell neoplasms), congestion and acute hepatitis.

Diffusely hyperechoic liver

With hyperechogenicity of the liver (see Figure 12.14d) there is indistinctness of the vessel walls (border effacement). Vacuolar diseases result in varying degrees of concurrent hyperattenuation, where the deep liver appears darker than the superficial regions. Non-vacuolar diseases, including lymphoma, usually have normally attenuating parenchyma.

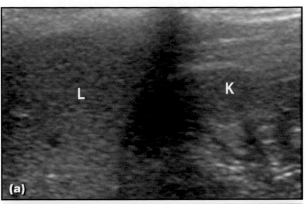

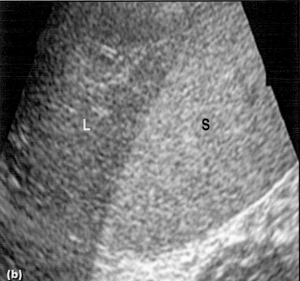

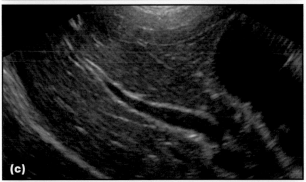

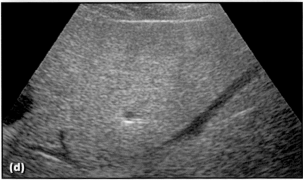

12.14 **(a)** The normal echogenicity of the canine and feline liver (L) is often higher than that of the right renal cortex (K) and **(b)** less than that of the spleen (S). **(c)** In a hypoechoic liver the margins of the portal vasculature often stand out as being particularly bright, whereas in **(d)** hyperechoic liver tissue these margins blend in with the parenchyma. (continues) ▶

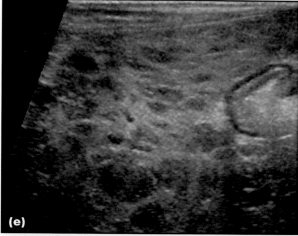

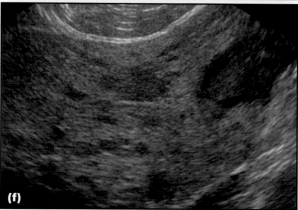

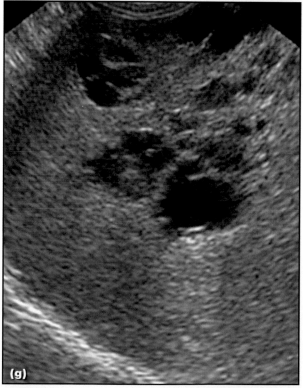

12.14 (continued) **(e)** Mixed echoic pattern with Swiss cheese-like hypoechoic nodules and hyperechoic surroundings in a dog with hepatocutaneous syndrome. **(f)** Multiple hypoechoic hepatic nodules diagnosed as benign hyperplasia on a fine-needle aspirate. **(g)** Feline biliary cystadenoma in the left lateral liver lobe with multiple anechoic cystic structures and distal enhancement.

Differential diagnoses for generalized hyper-echogenicity include vacuolar diseases, fibrosis (cirrhosis) and lymphoma. Vacuolar diseases include hyperadrenocorticism, hypothyroidism, non-specific hepatopathies and fatty infiltration. The vacuolar degeneration associated with hyperadrenocorticism is characterized by water and glycogen in the vacuoles and is caused by both exogenous and endogenous corticosteroid excess in dogs. Many dogs with mild to moderately elevated serum alkaline phosphatase have a liver biopsy specimen that shows vacuolar degeneration. This diagnosis is non-specific and the aetiology of this syndrome is currently unknown. This type of infiltration has not been documented in the cat.

Hepatic lipidosis is a clinical pathological term that describes fat vacuoles within hepatocytes. This is a consistent normal variant in obese cats without clinical signs; it is associated with a minority of hepatocytes containing fat vacuoles (usually <20%) and is termed 'mild hepatic lipidosis'. Unfortunately, the term hepatic lipidosis is also used to describe the severe form of the disease, seen in cats in hepatic failure, in which the vast majority of hepatocytes contain large distorted vacuoles (usually >80%). This can cause confusion for the unwary practitioner when reading cytological reports. Cats with mild hepatic lipidosis are not suffering from metabolic disease nor do they need specific therapy, beyond weight loss. Dogs do not deposit significant fat in the liver as a normal variant, nor do they suffer from the syndrome of hepatic lipidosis. However, fatty vacuolar degeneration is common in dogs with unregulated diabetes mellitus.

Diffusely mixed echoic liver

A mixed pattern may be caused by a single type of infiltration mixed with normal parenchyma, or by more than one form of infiltration (see Figure 12.14e). Differential diagnoses include infiltrative neoplasia, such as lymphoma or mast cell tumour, and histiocytic diseases. Patchy mixed patterns are seen with advanced fibrosis (cirrhosis), hepatocutaneous syndrome and feline amyloidosis. The classic appearance of cirrhosis is a hyperechoic parenchyma with hypoechoic regenerative nodules, free peritoneal fluid, small overall size and irregular liver margins. Hepatocutaneous syndrome is associated with mucocutaneous ulcerative lesions and liver failure. The ultrasonographic appearance is a Swiss cheese pattern with hypoechoic regenerative nodules and surrounding regions of hepatocyte collapse. Feline amyloidosis is characterized by a coarse, patchy mixed echogenicity with hyperechoic specks and hypoechoic foci.

Focal changes in echogenicity

Nodules (see Figure 12.14f) are very common in older dogs, but are not very specific. Both benign and malignant nodules can be hypoechoic, mixed or hyperechoic. It is not possible to differentiate accurately between benign and malignant hepatic nodules on routine ultrasonography. Common aetiologies include benign nodular hyperplasia, metastatic nodules, haematomas and primary liver neoplasia. A target appearance (an outer hypoechoic area surrounding a hyperechoic centre) is more commonly seen with, but is not unique to, metastatic neoplasia.

Cystic masses range in significance from primary liver neoplasia, to biliary cystadenoma, to incidental parenchymal cysts. Feline biliary cystadenomas are hyperechoic with small to large cavitated (anechoic) portions (see Figure 12.14g). They may appear uniformly hyperechoic, but they have a distinctive through transmission artefact attributable to the presence of microscopic cysts. Benign cysts are especially common in cats and are associated with polycystic kidney disease.

Liver lobe torsion may result in a local mass with a hypoechoic or mixed pattern and lack of vascular Doppler ultrasound signal.

Changes in liver contour and architecture

Interruption of the regular hepatic architecture, deviation of adjacent vascular structures and bulging of the hepatic margins are indicative of a mass lesion. Differential diagnoses include neoplasia, benign nodular hyperplasia, haematoma, abscess, granuloma, cyst and torsion. Further narrowing of the differential diagnoses requires consideration of:

- Species, breed, age, sex, history
- Echogenicity of the mass (see Figure 12.14)
- Vascularity
- Extrahepatic findings:
  - Hepatic lymphadenopathy alone is suggestive of hepatic neoplasia
  - Generalized lymphadenopathy and splenomegaly are suggestive of lymphoma
  - Peritoneal effusion and irregular margins of the liver and other organs are suggestive of carcinomatosis or cirrhosis.
- Imaging history (previous or follow-up examinations).

A common dilemma is the distinction between benign nodular hyperplasia and malignant neoplasia in the liver. Both are common, can be of similar echogenicity, size, location, vascularity and progression, are associated with organized haematoma or active haemorrhage, and each can also be present in the spleen. Therefore, no dog or cat should be euthanized based solely on the ultrasonographic diagnosis of a hepatic mass. Contrast-enhanced ultrasonography, computed tomography (CT; see Figure 12.19) and magnetic resonance imaging (MRI) have the potential to solve this issue.

Biliary abnormalities

Biliary sludge

Sludge consists of a suspension of pigment precipitates in bile and is usually seen in the gallbladder as small pieces of echogenic debris, which can be mobile or settled in a dependent location (Figure 12.15). A horizontal interface is often seen between the dependent echogenic sludge and the non-dependent anechoic bile. Positional changes cause swirling and hypostatic redistribution. The cause is

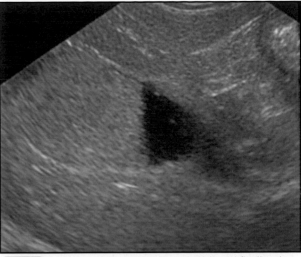

12.15 Hyperechoic sludge is an incidental finding in the canine gallbladder. Note the interface between the echoic and anechoic bile, which was parallel to the decubital plane of the dog.

not known but it is thought to be associated with cholestasis and is incidental in dogs. Biliary sludge is less common in cats. Pigment stones (non-mineralized) may obstruct the ducts.

Biliary calculi and obstruction

Mineralized stones should be gravity dependent and produce a distal shadowing artefact (Figure 12.16). Calculi may be adherent or mobile. Stones can be clinically relevant if they obstruct the cystic or common bile ducts.

Biliary obstruction is a difficult diagnosis to make in all but the most severe and chronic manifestations. The intrahepatic bile ducts are not normally visible. The common bile duct may be barely visible with a high-frequency transducer and traceable to the major duodenal papilla. Distended hepatic bile ducts can be

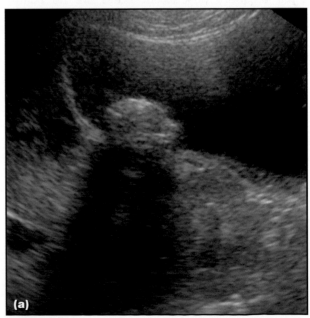

12.16 **(a)** Large mineralized gallbladder calculus with distant shadowing in a dog. This was an incidental finding. (continues) ▶

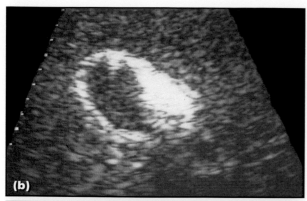

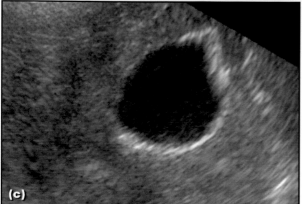

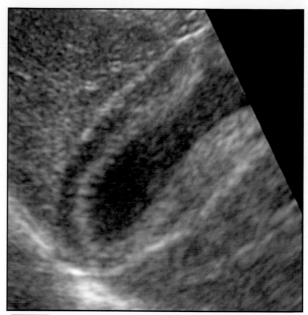

12.17 Thickened canine gallbladder wall with a layered appearance (hypoechoic central layer) indicative of mural oedema, commonly seen in cholecystitis.

12.16 (continued) **(b)** Hyperechoic partially thickened gallbladder wall associated with wall mineralization in the same cat as in 12.11b. This was an incidental finding. **(c)** Partially hyperechoic non-mineralized gallbladder wall (no distant shadowing) in a dog. This was an incidental finding.

recognized by the absence of vascular flow (negative Doppler ultrasound examination), tortuous course and intrahepatic parallelism to branches of the portal vein (*parallel channel sign*). Gallbladder and bile duct enlargement are neither very sensitive nor specific signs of biliary obstruction. There are no normal reference values for gallbladder size. The size of the gallbladder varies greatly and depends on the timing and content of the last meal. The gallbladder may not be markedly enlarged, despite obstruction. Hepatic and common bile duct distension can be the result of a current severe or a previous obstructive episode. Local discomfort has been reported in the patient with biliary obstruction when the transducer is pressed on to the cranioventral abdomen (the *Murphy sign*).

Gallbladder wall thickness and integrity

The normal gallbladder wall is <3 mm thick and is smooth and of uniform echogenicity. Moderate thickening can be mimicked by adjacent peritoneal effusion. Considerations for generalized thickening include oedema (congestion, hypoalbuminaemia), cholecystitis and cystic mucinous hyperplasia (CMH). Oedematous walls (Figure 12.17) may have a layered appearance with central hypoechoic oedema and hyperechoic inner and outer rims. CMH is a consistent finding with biliary mucocele, but not all cases of CMH have a concurrent mucocele. The wall thickening associated with CMH may be regional or diffuse, is often irregular in contour, and is associated with

varying degrees of immobile or gelatinized bile (see below). Other differential diagnoses for focal thickening include polyps and benign and malignant smooth muscle neoplasia.

Gallbladder mucocele

Mucoceles (Figure 12.18) are commonly seen in dogs but have not been reported in the cat. The underlying aetiology is unknown, but all cases have concurrent CMH. It is hypothesized that as CMH progresses, the bile becomes gelatinized. As the gelatinization progresses into the common bile duct, signs of extra-hepatic biliary obstruction are seen. Gallbladder wall necrosis, rupture and bile peritonitis are common in chronic cases. Gelatinized bile resembles a kiwi fruit in cross section and is a highly specific ultrasonographic finding.

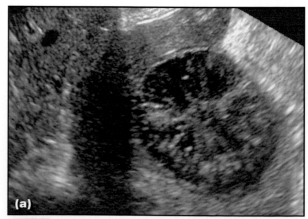

12.18 **(a)** Short axis view of the gallbladder of a 13-year-old English Springer Spaniel with a gallbladder mucocele. Note the spoke-like hyperechoic lines that resemble the cut section of a kiwi fruit (*stellate* or *kiwi pattern*). (continues) ▶

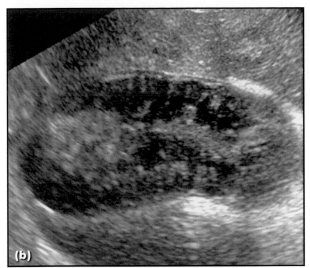

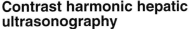
(b) Long axis view of the gallbladder of a 13-year-old English Springer Spaniel with a gallbladder mucocele.

Contrast harmonic hepatic ultrasonography

Contrast-enhanced ultrasonography is gaining more widespread use in veterinary medicine. Contrast media for ultrasonography are composed of microscopic gas bubbles that are administered intravenously. These bubbles have a non-linear oscillation when subjected to ultrasound waves and thereby enhance the echogenicity of perfused tissue. This technique has been used successfully in dogs to differentiate benign from malignant liver nodules in multiple studies. This modality has been used successfully in academic and private practice settings, and has potential for routine clinical use.

Overview of additional imaging modalities

Hepatic computed tomography

CT imaging of the liver in dogs and cats is mainly used for the identification of hepatic shunts and other vascular abnormalities (Figure 12.19). Dynamic CT studies can be used to calculate the hepatic perfusion index, which may be useful to identify occult shunting, such as that which occurs with microvascular dysplasia. CT can also be used to determine the resectability of liver and gallbladder masses and for targeted chemoembolization. Contrast-enhanced CT is used to differentiate benign from malignant nodules in human patients, although clinical studies in dogs and cats are not yet available.

Hepatic magnetic resonance imaging

MRI has been used successfully in dogs to differentiate benign from malignant liver masses, based on the intensity profile in different imaging sequences and on gadolinium-based contrast enhancement patterns.

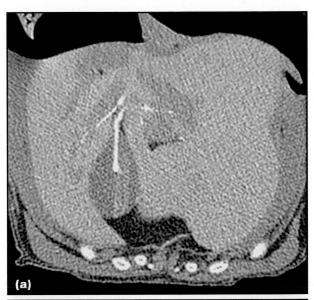

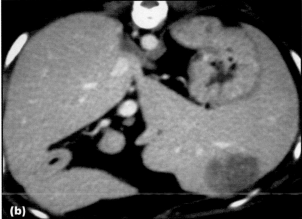

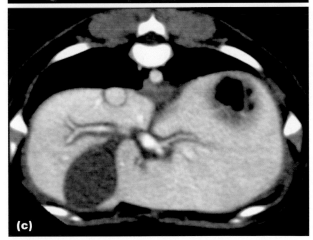

12.19 **(a)** CT image of the liver of an 11-year-old Afghan Hound that had received intravenous ionic iodinated contrast medium 1 hour earlier. Contrast-enhanced bile can be seen within the ducts and the gallbladder. This was an incidental finding. **(b)** Hypoattenuating lesion, which was diagnosed as benign hyperplasia, in the left lateral liver lobe after administration of intravenous contrast medium to a 9-year-old Jack Russell Terrier. **(c)** Image of the liver during the portal phase of CT angiography in a 6-month-old Shi Tzu without evidence of a macroscopic portosystemic shunt. There is a marked perivascular halo around the portal vein branches and the caudal vena cava, consistent with perivascular oedema, a non-specific sign of hepatopathy.

References and further reading

Beatty JA, Barrs VR, Martin PA, *et al.* (2002) Spontaneous hepatic rupture in six cats with systemic amyloidosis. *Journal of Small Animal Practice* **43**, 355–363

Brömel C, Barthez PY, Léveillé R, *et al.* (1998) Prevalence of gallbladder sludge in dogs assessed by ultrasonography. *Veterinary Radiology and Ultrasound* **39**, 206–210

Brömel C, Smeak DD and Léveillé R (1998) Porcelain gallbladder asssociated with primary biliary adenocarcinoma in a dog. *Journal of the American Veterinary Medical Association* **213**, 1137–1139

Clifford CA, Pretorius ES, Weisse C, *et al.* (2004) Magnetic resonance imaging of focal splenic and hepatic lesions in the dog. *Journal of Veterinary Internal Medicine* **18**, 330–338

Gibbs C (1981) Radiologic features of liver disorders in dogs and cats. *Veterinary Annual* **21**, 239–250

Hinkle Schwartz SG, Mitchell SL, Keating JH, *et al.* (2006) Liver lobe torsion in dogs: 13 cases. *Journal of the American Veterinary Medical Association* **228**, 242–248

Ivančić M and Mai W (2008) Qualitative and quantitative comparison of renal vs. hepatic ultrasonographic intensity in healthy dogs. *Veterinary Radiology and Ultrasound* **49**, 368–373

Lamb CR, Kleine LJ and McMillan MC (1991) Diagnosis of calcification on abdominal radiographs. *Veterinary Radiology* **32**, 211–220

Neer TM (1992) A review of disorders of the gallbladder and extrahepatic biliary tract in the dog and cat. *Journal of Veterinary Internal Medicine* **6**, 186–192

Nyland TG, Hager DA and Herring DS (1989) Sonographic evaluation of the liver, gallbladder and spleen. *Seminars in Veterinary Medicine and Surgery (Small Animal)* **4**, 13–31

O'Brien RT, Iani M, Matheson J, *et al.* (2004) Contrast harmonic ultrasound of spontaneous liver nodules in 32 dogs. *Veterinary Radiology and Ultrasound* **45**, 547–553

Rivers BJ, Walter PA, Johnston GR, *et al.* (1997) Acalculous cholecystitis in four canine cases: ultrasonographic findings and use of ultrasonographic-guided, percutaneous cholecystocentesis in diagnosis. *Journal of the American Animal Hospital Association* **33**, 207–214

Schwarz T, Störk CK, Mellor D, *et al.* (2000) Osteopenia and other radiographic signs in canine hyperadrenocorticism. *Journal of Small Animal Practice* **41**, 491–495

Vörös K, Albert M, Vetési F, *et al.* (1997) Hepatic ultrasonographic findings in experimental carbon tetrachloride intoxication of the dog. *Acta Veterinaria Hungaria* **45**, 137–150

Zwingenberger AL, Schwarz T and Saunders HM (2005) Helical CT angiography of canine portosystemic shunts. *Veterinary Radiology and Ultrasound* **46**, 27–37

13

The pancreas

Federica Morandi

Overview of anatomy

The pancreas is composed of a body and two lobes or limbs; the body separates the right and left lobes and is located just ventral to the portal vein, between the pylorus and the proximal descending duodenum. The right lobe runs in a caudal direction in the mesoduodenum, near or in contact with the body wall, just ventral to the right kidney. The left pancreatic lobe is located caudal to the greater curvature of the stomach, cranial to the transverse colon, and extends laterally to terminate close to the cranial pole of the left kidney (Figure 13.1). In the cat the left lobe may extend dorsally, caudal to the spleen.

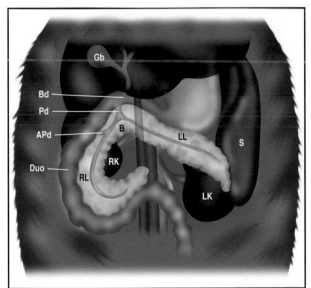

13.1 Ventral view of the pancreas and its associated anatomical landmarks. The right lobe of the pancreas (RL) runs along the medial margin of the descending duodenum (Duo). The pancreatic body (B) connects the right to the left lobe (LL), which is located caudal to the greater curvature of the stomach. The accessory pancreatic duct (APd) is the primary excretory duct in dogs and terminates at the minor duodenal papilla. The pancreatic duct (Pd) is the main excretory duct in cats and terminates at the major duodenal papilla together with the common bile duct (Bd). Gb = Gallbladder; LK = Left kidney; RK = Right kidney; S = Spleen.

The pancreas is vascularized by branches of the cranial and caudal pancreaticoduodenal arteries, and by the pancreatic branch of the splenic artery. Venous drainage of the right lobe is mostly through the caudal pancreaticoduodenal vein, the last tributary of the cranial mesenteric vein. The left lobe drains into the splenic vein. There are two excretory ducts: the accessory pancreatic duct, which terminates in the duodenum at the minor duodenal papilla; and the pancreatic duct, which terminates at the major duodenal papilla together with the common bile duct.

Normal variations

There are few major differences between dogs and cats in the anatomy of the pancreas:

- In dogs, the largest excretory duct is the accessory pancreatic duct and the pancreatic duct is often absent; in cats, the pancreatic duct is the principal excretory duct
- In cats, the left lobe and body of the pancreas are larger than the right lobe.

Radiographic detection of pancreatic disease

In the dog, the normal pancreas is not observed on plain radiographs because of its small size and silhouetting effect with the surrounding soft tissues. In some obese cats, the left pancreatic lobe can be identified on plain ventrodorsal (VD) radiographs as a focal area of soft tissue opacity located caudal to the gastric fundus, medial or caudal to the head of the spleen, and cranial to the left kidney (Figure 13.2).

Knowledge of the normal position of the pancreas is necessary in order to recognize organ displacement that may be secondary to pancreatic enlargement. Abnormalities visible in the region of the pancreas that may be associated with pancreatic disease include:

- Loss of peritoneal detail
- An irregular, ground-glass opacity in the pancreatic area
- Focal mineral opacities
- A mass effect with lateral displacement of the descending duodenum, cranial displacement of the stomach and/or caudal displacement of the colon (Figure 13.3)
- Persistent gas dilatation of regional intestinal segments, especially the descending duodenum.

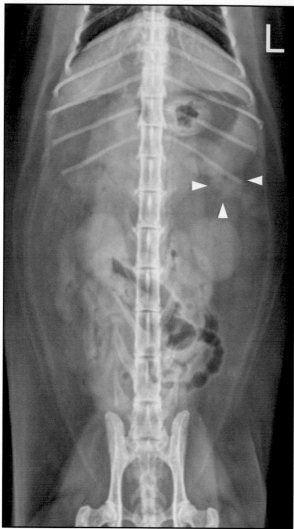

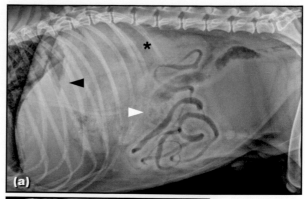

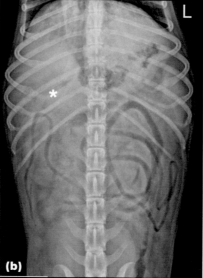

13.2 Digital VD radiograph of a 14-year-old male neutered Oriental Shorthaired cat presented for annual evaluation of chronic renal disease. The soft tissue opacity caudal to the spleen and cranial to the left kidney (arrowheads) represents the left lobe of the pancreas. Note the bilaterally small kidneys.

13.3 **(a)** Lateral and **(b)** VD digital radiographs of a 7-year-old Labrador Retriever evaluated for rapid weight loss and anorexia. There is a large mass effect in the right cranial abdominal quadrant (white asterisk) with loss of serosal detail. On the lateral view, the gastric fundus is displaced cranially (black arrowhead), the colon and small intestines are displaced caudoventrally (white arrowhead) and the kidneys are displaced caudally (black asterisk). The final diagnosis was metastatic pancreatic adenocarcinoma.

Normal plain radiographs do not rule out pancreatic disease, especially acute pancreatitis or small pancreatic masses. Barium, administered orally, can sometimes be used to assess displacement of the stomach and intestinal tract by a cranial abdominal mass, and confirm that the mass arises from the pancreatic area. Potential risks of barium studies include exacerbation of pancreatitis or aspiration. Recently, endoscopic retrograde cholangiopancreatography using an iodinated contrast medium has been reported in dogs; the procedure requires general anaesthesia and specialized skills, and its use in clinical patients has yet to be determined.

Ultrasonography

Abdominal ultrasonography is considered to be standard practice for the evaluation of the patient with suspected pancreatic disease because the pancreas is more easily identified on ultrasound examination than on plain radiographs. The low cost, widespread availability and non-invasive nature of the ultrasound examination adds to its usefulness. In addition, ultrasonography provides information on other abdominal structures that may be involved in the disease process, thereby assisting in generating differential diagnoses, and permits guided fine-needle sampling of lesions for cytological evaluation.

In the early days of ultrasonography, the pancreas was only occasionally visualized. With current ultrasonographic equipment a trained ultrasonographer should be able to identify the normal pancreas in most dogs and cats. Factors that can impair visualization of the pancreas include:

- Presence of gas or positive contrast medium in the gastrointestinal tract
- Distension of the stomach by ingesta and of the colon by faecal matter
- The presence of free abdominal air
- A large amount of intra-abdominal fat
- Deep-chested patient conformation.

Peritoneal effusion, on the other hand, does not pose a problem and can actually facilitate localization of the pancreas, especially the right lobe (Figure 13.4).

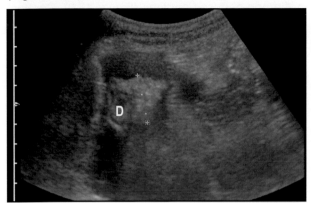

13.4 Right lobe of the pancreas (between calipers) in an 8-year-old male Labrador Retriever with ascites; the duodenum (D) is in transverse section. Note the hyperechoic appearance of the pancreas caused by distal enhancement from the surrounding fluid.

Proper patient preparation is essential for optimization of image quality. Sedation is not always necessary, but is often helpful to minimize patient discomfort and aerophagia when transducer pressure is applied. Hair clipping and liberal use of coupling gel ensure adequate transducer contact. Varying recumbency may be necessary to shift overlying gas out of the way. Dorsal recumbency is appropriate for most dogs and cats. In deep-chested dogs, lateral recumbency may provide better images, especially when an intercostal window is used. For most dogs, a 5.0–8.0 MHz transducer is adequate; small dogs and cats are best examined with an 8.0–15.0 MHz frequency. As a general rule, higher frequency provides better resolution but lower penetration and *vice versa*. The ultrasonographer should employ the highest possible frequency that provides adequate depth penetration to identify the entire pancreas.

The normal pancreas is isoechoic to slightly hypoechoic to the surrounding mesenteric fat, and can be difficult to outline in obese animals owing to the lack of a well defined capsule. The ultrasonographer must therefore rely on their knowledge of adjacent anatomical landmarks to identify this organ. In the right cranial quadrant of the abdomen, imaging the descending duodenum in the transverse plane allows identification of the right pancreatic lobe just dorsal or medial to the duodenum and ventral to the right kidney. The mid and proximal aspects of the right lobe are usually identified by the centrally located pancreaticoduodenal vein. The right lobe can then be traced caudally and cranially, until the cranial duodenal flexure is reached. Using a parasagittal image plane, the transducer can then be moved caudally and to the left, through the pylorus to the greater curvature of the stomach. The left lobe of the pancreas can be identified lying cranial to the transverse colon and can be traced laterally to the level of the spleen and cranial pole of the left kidney. The experienced ultrasonographer can also use vascular landmarks (e.g. portal vein, gastroduodenal vein) for reference.

Dogs
The normal pancreas of the dog is distinguished by the following features (Figure 13.5):

- It is isoechoic to slightly hypoechoic to the mesenteric fat; it is also less echogenic than the spleen and more echogenic than the liver
- The right lobe is triangular in shape and easily identified as it is more superficial. In addition, there is usually less overlying gas compared with the left lobe. Gastric and colonic content can often shadow over the region of the left pancreatic lobe
- The right lobe has a centrally located pancreaticoduodenal vein. The vein is large cranially and may be difficult to identify in the caudal portion of the lobe. The vascular nature can be verified with Doppler ultrasonography
- The normal pancreas is more easily identified in immature dogs, thin dogs and when abdominal effusion is present
- Reports of pancreatic size vary, but maximum thickness in Beagle-type dogs is usually considered to be about 1 cm
- Pancreatic ducts are typically not seen in dogs; the minor duodenal papilla is sometimes seen as a small nodule in the wall of the duodenum.

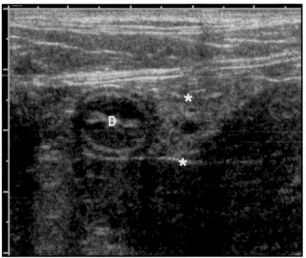

13.5 Normal right lobe of the pancreas in a 13-year-old spayed Dachshund bitch. The duodenum (D) and pancreas (between asterisks) are in transverse section. The normal duodenum appears as a target-like structure and the pancreas shows medium echogenicity. The anechoic circular structure in the centre of the pancreas is the pancreaticoduodenal vein and can be distinguished from the pancreatic duct with the use of colour Doppler ultrasonography. (Courtesy of S Hecht)

Cats
The normal pancreas of the cat is distinguished by the following features (Figure 13.6):

- It is a hypoechoic, homogenous, linear structure with well defined margins
- The body and left lobe are readily visible in most cats, whilst the right lobe is more difficult to identify

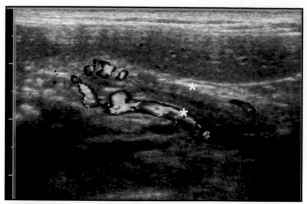

13.6 Normal body and left lobe of the pancreas in a 15-year-old male neutered Domestic Shorthaired cat. Doppler signal is visible in the splenic vein and the left pancreatic lobe is the structure of medium echogenicity seen ventral to it (between the asterisks). The normal pancreatic duct is visible in the centre of the pancreas and shows no Doppler signal. (Courtesy of S Hecht)

- The maximum thickness of the left lobe is 9.5 mm and that of the body is 8.5 mm
- The pancreatic duct is a centrally located, anechoic, tubular structure with hyperechoic walls, measuring 0.5–2.5 mm, in the left lobe
- Pancreatic size and echogenicity have been shown to remain unchanged with age, although a tendency has been found for the pancreatic duct to increase in diameter with age
- The major duodenal papilla is usually visible as a small nodule in the wall of the duodenum, and measures 2.9–5.5 mm in thickness on transverse section of the duodenum
- Pancreatic blood vessels are usually not seen without Doppler ultrasonography.

Other types of ultrasonography

Endoscopic ultrasonography allows centrally located organs, such as the pancreas, to be examined without gas interference. In humans, this technique has been reported to be more sensitive than transabdominal ultrasonography and computed tomography (CT) for the evaluation of pancreatic diseases. Endoscopic ultrasonography is not readily available in veterinary medicine; it requires specialized, expensive equipment and the use of general anaesthesia. Transducer frequency is typically 5–10 MHz. Excellent visualization of the left pancreatic lobe and body has been reported, but poor visualization of the distal right pancreatic lobe is common. The main advantage of endoscopic ultrasonography is its potential for identifying abnormalities not seen with transabdominal ultrasonography, especially in large dogs, patients with a large amount of gastrointestinal gas, or where small lesion size is suspected (insulinomas).

Contrast ultrasonography has been used to characterize the normal pancreas in cats and dogs. Normal patients have uniform enhancement of the entire gland (Figure 13.7). In dogs with pancreatitis, non-perfused areas are visible mixed with hyperperfused regions. The non-perfused regions of the pancreas in

dogs with quickly resolving clinical signs are presumed to represent oedema. Larger non-perfused regions have been associated with worsened prognosis, presumably because of haemorrhage or necrosis in the non-perfused portions (Figure 13.8). Contrast ultrasonography is easily performed as an adjunct to greyscale ultrasonography, but requires specialized ultrasound equipment and contrast media.

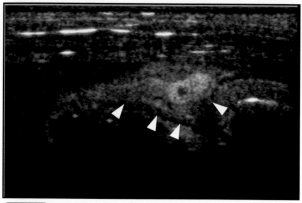

13.7 Post-contrast ultrasonogram of the pancreas (arrowheads) in a normal dog. Note the uniform hyperechoic appearance of the pancreas, indicative of uniform enhancement. (Courtesy of R O'Brien)

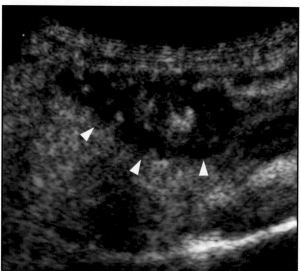

13.8 Post-contrast ultrasonogram of the pancreas (arrowheads) in a dog with severe pancreatitis. Note the heterogenous appearance of the pancreas with hypoechoic areas consistent with perfusion defects. (Courtesy of R O'Brien)

Overview of additional imaging modalities

Computed tomography

- CT is the most important tool for the diagnosis and prognostic staging of the severity of acute pancreatitis in humans.
- It is especially useful in the identification of pancreatic necrosis and its use for this purpose has been reported in veterinary medicine. Areas of necrosis do not show contrast enhancement on CT.

- Limitations of this imaging modality include the high cost and the fact that general anaesthesia is required because the patient must remain still for the entire duration of the image acquisition.
- New generation multi-slice scanners with an ultra-short acquisition time may allow scanning of small animals with the use of sedation only.
- CT may be considered in selected cases where a definitive diagnosis cannot be reached using other imaging modalities, or for pre-surgical planning (Figures 13.9 and 13.10).

Magnetic resonance imaging

- MRI has limitations similar to those of CT, with even higher costs and longer anaesthesia times.

Nuclear medicine

- Nuclear medicine (scintigraphy) with radiolabelled white blood cells (^{99m}Tc-hexamethylpropylene-amine oxime, HMPAO) has been used to diagnose pancreatitis in cats:
  - Increased uptake of the radiopharmaceutical is seen in the area of the pancreas of affected cats
  - No information on the diagnostic accuracy is available
  - Labelling leucocytes is a time-consuming procedure; furthermore, specialized equipment (gamma camera) is necessary for imaging, limiting the availability of this modality to licensed, large referral institutions.
- Somatostatin receptor scintigraphy using indium ^{111}In pentetreotide (OcreoScan®) has been used to diagnose insulinomas in dogs:
  - The radiopharmaceutical is extremely expensive
  - As for labelled leucocytes, specialized equipment is necessary for imaging, limiting the availability of this modality to licensed, large referral institutions.

Pancreatic diseases

Pancreatitis

Acute pancreatitis
Radiographic abnormalities seen with acute pancreatitis include:

- Loss of peritoneal detail in the right cranial abdomen
- Increased soft tissue opacity in the right cranial abdomen
- Widening of the gastroduodenal angle
- Mass effect at the gastroduodenal angle (Figure 13.11)
- Lateral displacement of the descending duodenum
- Gas-filled descending duodenum that does not change in appearance on subsequent radiographs (ileus) (Figure 13.12)
- The radiographs may be normal:
  - In general, the negative predictive value of radiography (i.e. the ability of normal plain radiographs to exclude the presence of acute pancreatitis) is low
  - Radiographic abnormalities consistent with acute canine pancreatitis are uncommon.

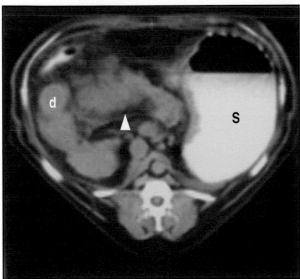

13.9 Post-contrast axial CT scan of the pancreas of an adult Golden Retriever, obtained at 10 mm slice thickness and 10 mm increments. The image is displayed in a soft tissue window (width 300 HU, level 30 HU). Diluted positive contrast medium (barium) was administered orally prior to the study and is seen in the stomach (S). Note the enlarged pancreas (arrowhead) and the surrounding striated, hyperattenuating mesentery, consistent with peritonitis. The final diagnosis was severe pancreatitis. d = Duodenum.

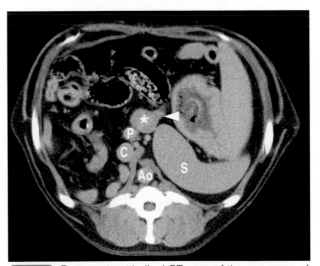

13.10 Post-contrast helical CT scan of the pancreas of a 13-year-old male neutered Weimaraner, obtained at 3 mm slice thickness, evaluated for tremor, ataxia and profound hypoglycaemia. The image is displayed in a soft tissue window (width 350 HU, level 50 HU). A focal mass (asterisk) is seen in the central abdomen; the mass has similar density and enhancement pattern to the body of the pancreas (arrowhead). At surgery, the mass was identified as a metastatic pancreatic lymph node and a small islet cell carcinoma was identified adjacent to it. Ao = Aorta; C = Caudal vena cava; P = Portal vein; S = Spleen.

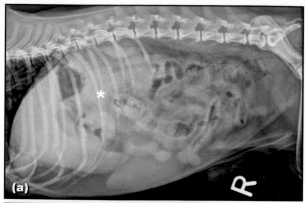

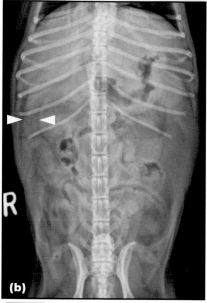

13.11 **(a)** Lateral and **(b)** VD digital radiographs of a 12-year-old male mixed breed dog evaluated for pancreatitis. Note the loss of detail in the mid-abdomen, caudal to the stomach (asterisk), and the lateral displacement of the fluid-filled duodenum (between arrowheads in b) with widening of the gastroduodenal angle.

Ultrasonographic abnormalities seen with acute pancreatitis include:

- Hypoechoic pancreatic parenchyma (Figure 13.13)
- Enlarged and irregular pancreas (>2 cm thick in longitudinal, sagittal or transverse planes) (Figure 13.14)
- Hyperechoic peripancreatic mesentery
- Peritoneal effusion (Figure 13.15)
- Solid masses or cystic lesions within the pancreas
- Dilatation of the pancreatic duct
- Duodenitis – thickened duodenum (>5 mm), with or without loss of layers and corrugated appearance (Figure 13.16)
- Extrahepatic biliary obstruction
- The ultrasonogram may be normal, especially in cats:
  - Sixty eight percent of 34 cases of acute pancreatitis in dogs showed abnormalities
  - The sensitivity of ultrasonography for the diagnosis of pancreatitis in cats ranges from 11% to 67%.

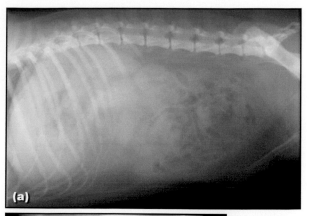

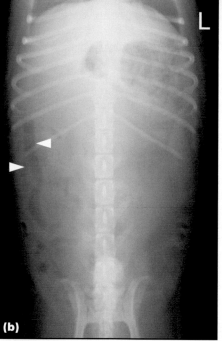

13.12 **(a)** Lateral and **(b)** VD conventional radiographs of a 5-year-old male Cocker Spaniel with severe pancreatitis. The duodenum (between arrowheads) is distended with gas and displaced laterally along the right abdominal wall. Note also the loss of serosal detail and the mass effect in the right cranial abdomen.

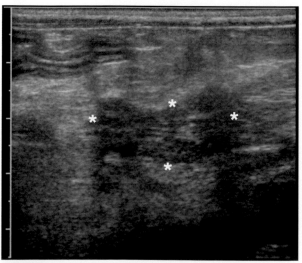

13.13 Mild pancreatitis in a 12-year-old male mixed breed dog. Note the hypoechoic right pancreatic lobe (between asterisks).

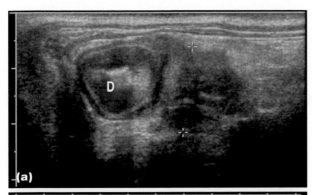

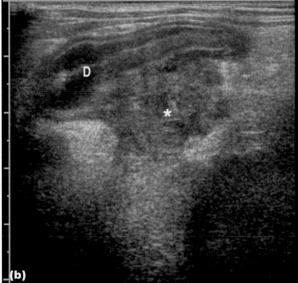

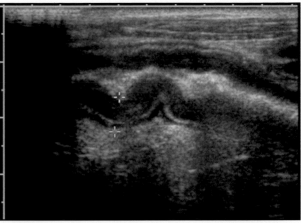

13.16 Acute pancreatitis in a 6-year-old spayed Yorkshire Terrier bitch (same dog as in Figure 13.14). The longitudinal image of the descending duodenum shows corrugation, which did not change over time, and thickening of the duodenal wall (6.2 mm between calipers). These findings are consistent with duodenitis.

Chronic pancreatitis

- The diagnosis of chronic pancreatitis is challenging.
- Radiographs are often unremarkable.
- On ultrasonography, the pancreas can be normal or decreased in size, with variable mixed echogenicity, nodular lesions, shadowing areas due to fibrosis and/or mineralization and enlargement of the pancreatic ducts.
- The accuracy of ultrasonography in the diagnosis of chronic pancreatitis is currently unknown.

Pancreatic masses

Cystic lesions

- Pseudocysts, congenital cysts and retention cysts have all been described in small animals and can be distinguished only by histopathological analysis.
    - *Pseudocysts* are a late sequel to pancreatitis; they form by accumulation of pancreatic enzymes, necrotic tissue and haemorrhage surrounded by a capsule formed by granulation and fibrous tissue. They are much more common in the left pancreatic lobe in cats, dogs and humans. Large pseudocysts can compress the stomach and cause vomiting.
    - *Congenital cysts* can vary in size and are often associated with polycystic disease of the kidneys, liver and ovaries; they are lined by epithelial cells, and, unlike pseudocysts, do not contain exudate.
    - *Retention cysts* are caused by blockage of the pancreatic ducts and accumulation of pancreatic secretions; they are often small and insignificant.
- Congenital and retention cysts are mostly anechoic structures with strong distal enhancement (through transmission) and a thin or non-visible wall.

13.14 Acute pancreatitis in a 6-year-old spayed Yorkshire Terrier bitch. **(a)** Transverse section of the left lobe of the pancreas (between calipers) and duodenum (D). Note the enlarged hypoechoic pancreas with surrounding hyperechoic mesentery. **(b)** Oblique to longitudinal plane image. The hypoechoic, irregular, enlarged left lobe of the pancreas (asterisk) is seen dorsal to the descending duodenum (D). Note the hyperechoic mesentery surrounding the pancreas.

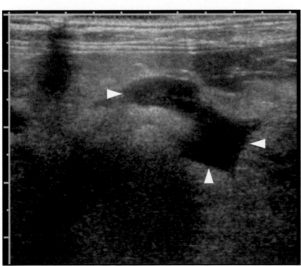

13.15 Acute pancreatitis in a 14-year-old male neutered Toy Poodle. An irregularly shaped anechoic pocket of fluid (arrowheads) is visible, together with a hyperechoic mesentery. These findings are consistent with peritonitis.

- Pseudocysts tend to have a thicker wall; they can be anechoic, but can also contain variably echogenic material, and exhibit variable distal enhancement (Figure 13.17).
- Ultrasound-guided fine-needle aspiration with a 20- or 22-gauge needle can be used to retrieve cystic fluid for cytological analysis and for therapeutic amelioration of the mass effect, especially with larger pseudocysts.

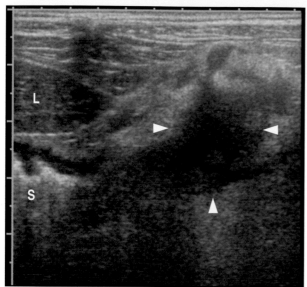

13.17   Forming pancreatic pseudocyst in a middle-aged male neutered Poodle. This image was obtained in a parasagittal plane, caudal to the stomach (S); the ventral aspect of the liver (L), which was mildly enlarged, is also visible in the near-field. The anechoic irregularly shaped area caudal to the stomach and liver (between arrowheads), with surrounding hyperechoic mesentery and mild distal acoustic enhancement, was an organizing collection of fluid and necrotic tissue that developed into a pseudocyst.

Abscesses

- Abscesses form as a complication of pancreatitis.
- The ultrasonographic appearance of abscesses varies greatly depending on the amount of suppurative content, the consistency of the material, the presence or absence of gas and the stage of maturation.
- Abscesses can have a thin or thick echogenic wall; they can contain anechoic (Figure 13.18a) or variably echogenic material as well as hyperechoic speckles (Figure 13.18b) showing reverberation artefacts (gas), or can resemble solid masses of mixed echogenicity.
- Due to the variable spectrum of the ultrasonographic appearance of abscesses, fine-needle aspiration is necessary to characterize the content, and can be used for percutaneous drainage.

Neoplasia

- Nodular lesions can represent benign nodular hyperplasia, especially in cats, and there is no conclusive way to distinguish a benign from a

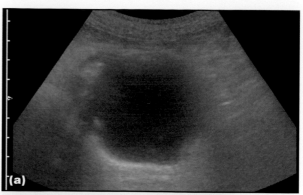

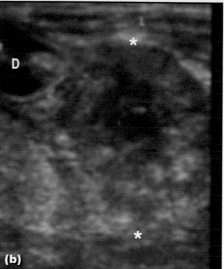

13.18   **(a)** Pancreatic abscess in a 9-year-old male neutered Labrador Retriever with a 1-month history of severe pancreatitis. The abscess is a well defined, anechoic cyst-like structure with strong distal enhancement. Ultrasound-guided drainage was performed successfully. **(b)** Pancreatic abscess of the right lobe in an 8-year-old spayed Miniature Schnauzer bitch. The duodenum (D) is in transverse section. The abscess (between asterisks) is a well defined mass of mixed echogenicity, with a thick echogenic wall and anechoic centre, containing numerous hyperechoic speckles in the distal aspect. Surgical exploration confirmed the diagnosis.

malignant nodule or mass without cytology or histopathology.
- However, large solitary masses are more likely to be neoplastic (Figure 13.19).
  - Additional abnormalities that suggest a malignancy include: regional lymphadenopathy, although mild reactive lymphadenopathy can also be seen with severe pancreatitis (Figure 13.20); the presence of hypoechoic nodular lesions in the mesentery (carcinomatosis, the dissemination of neoplasia to the peritoneal lining); and abdominal effusion (effusion of malignancy). The classic lesion in dog, cat and human patients is invasion of the duodenal wall, resulting in localized loss of duodenal layering and confluence of margins.
  - Adenocarcinoma is the most common malignancy of the pancreas.

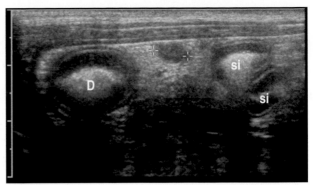

13.20 Rounded, hypoechoic mildly enlarged (7 mm between calipers) pancreatic lymph node. This patient had severe chronic pancreatitis and diabetic ketoacidosis. D = Duodenum; si = Small intestine.

- Insulinomas:
  - Can be microscopic and not visible with ultrasonography
  - Metastatic adenopathy may be difficult to differentiate from the primary lesion.

Other conditions

- Exocrine pancreatic insufficiency is caused by a loss of pancreatic acinar cells, resulting in inadequate production of digestive enzymes with subsequent malabsorption; it can be due to spontaneous atrophy (dogs) or chronic pancreatitis (cats):
  - In cats, heterogenous pancreatic parenchyma with nodular lesions is seen.
- Pancreatolithiasis has been reported in cats:
  - Pancreatic calculi are hyperechoic structures with strong distal acoustic shadowing. These may be incidental or cause obstruction.
- Pancreatic oedema can be seen with any cause of systemic vasculitis, hypoalbuminaemia or portal hypertension:
  - Accumulation of fluid in the pancreas results in thickening with multiple linear anechoic striations
  - This can usually be differentiated from pancreatitis by the lack of concurrent findings, such as peripancreatic hyperechoic fat, duodenal corrugation or local pain.

References and further reading

Caceres AV, Zwingenberger AL, Hardam E, *et al.* (2006) Helical computed tomographic angiography of the normal canine pancreas. *Veterinary Radiology and Ultrasound* **47**, 270–278

Edwards DF, Bauer MF, Walker MA, *et al.* (1990) Pancreatic masses in seven dogs following acute pancreatitis. *Journal of the American Animal Hospital Association* **26**,189–198

Etue SM, Pennick DG, Labato MA, *et al.* (2001) Ultrasonography of the normal feline pancreas and associated anatomic landmarks: a prospective study of 20 cats. *Veterinary Radiology and Ultrasound* **42**, 330–336

Gaschen L, Kircher P and Wolfram K (2007) Endoscopic ultrasound of the canine abdomen. *Veterinary Radiology and Ultrasound* **48**, 338–349

Head LH, Daniel GD, Becker TJ, *et al.* (2006) Use of computed tomography and radiolabeled leukocytes in a cat with pancreatitis. *Veterinary Radiology and Ultrasound* **46**, 263–266

Hecht S and Henry G (2007) Sonographic evaluation of the normal and abnormal pancreas. *Clinical Techniques in Small Animal Practice* **22**, 115–121

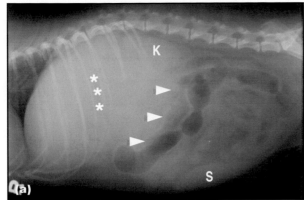

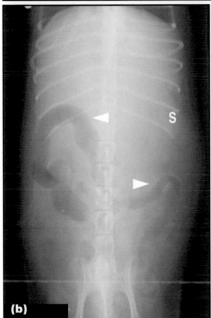

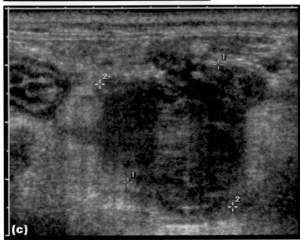

13.19 **(a)** Lateral and **(b)** VD conventional radiographs of a 7-year-old male Yorkshire Terrier with weight loss, inappetence and abdominal distension. There is a very large craniodorsal abdominal mass, originating from the left cranial quadrant. There is displacement of the colon and small intestines caudally, ventrally and towards the right (arrowheads). The spleen (S) and kidneys (K) are visible. The stomach (asterisks) is visible on the lateral view. The final diagnosis was carcinoma. **(c)** The same dog as in Figure 13.3. A large (3.2 cm x 2.7 cm) mass with irregular margins and mixed echogenicity is seen arising from the body of the pancreas. The final diagnosis was metastatic pancreatic adenocarcinoma.

Hecht S, Penninck DG and Keating JH (2007) Imaging findings in pancreatic neoplasia and nodular hyperplasia in 19 cats. *Veterinary Radiology and Ultrasound* **48,** 45–50

Hess RS, Saunders HM, VanWinkle TJ, *et al.* (1998) Clinical, clinicopathological, radiographic and ultrasonographic abnormalities in dogs with fatal acute pancreatitis: 70 cases (1968–1995). *Journal of the American Veterinary Medical Association* **213,** 665–670

Iseri T, Yamada K, Chijiwa K, *et al.* (2007) Dynamic computed tomography of the pancreas in normal dogs and in a dog with pancreatic insulinoma. *Veterinary Radiology and Ultrasound* **48,** 328–331

Jaeger JQ, Mattoon JS, Bateman SW, *et al.* (2003) Combined use of ultrasonography and contrast-enhanced computed tomography to evaluate acute necrotizing pancreatitis in 2 dogs. *Veterinary Radiology and Ultrasound* **44,** 72–79

Lester NV, Newell SM, Hill RC, *et al.* (1999) Scintigraphic diagnosis of insulinoma in a dog. *Veterinary Radiology and Ultrasound* **40,** 174–178

Moon-Larson M, Panciera DL, Ward DL, *et al.* (2005) Age-related changes in the ultrasound appearance of the normal feline pancreas. *Veterinary Radiology and Ultrasound* **46,** 238–242

Morita Y, Takiguchi M, Yasuda J, *et al.* (1998) Endoscopic ultrasonography of the pancreas in dogs. *Veterinary Radiology and Ultrasound* **39,** 552–556

Newell SM, Graham JP, Roberts GD, *et al.* (2000) Quantitative Magnetic Resonance Imaging of the Normal Feline Cranial Abdomen. *Veterinary Radiology and Ultrasound* **41,** 27–34

Ohlerth S and O'Brien RT (2007) Contrast Ultrasound: general principles and veterinary clinical applications. *The Veterinary Journal* **174,** 501–512

Probst A and Kneissl S (2001) Computed tomographic anatomy of the canine pancreas. *Veterinary Radiology and Ultrasound* **42,** 226–230

Ruaux CG (2003) Diagnostic approaches to acute pancreatitis. *Clinical Techniques in Small Animal Practice* **18,** 245–249

Spillmann T, Happonen I, Kahkonen T, *et al.* (2005) Endoscopic retrograde cholangio-pancreatography in healthy Beagles. *Veterinary Radiology and Ultrasound* **46,** 97–104

VanEnkevort BA, O'Brien RT, Young KM (1999) Pancreatic pseudocysts in 4 dogs and 2 cats: ultrasonographic and clinicopathological findings. *Journal of Veterinary Internal Medicine* **13,** 309–313

14

The spleen

Laura Armbrust

Normal radiographic anatomy

The normal spleen in dogs is an elongated flattened organ, which is triangular in cross section. In cats it is more ovoid in cross section. The spleen is located in the left hypogastric region and has dorsal ('head') and ventral ('tail') extremities. The head of the spleen is located in the dorsal cranial left abdomen, attached to the fundus of the stomach by the gastrosplenic ligament, through which the left gastroepiploic and short gastric arteries and veins course. The body and tail of the spleen exhibit greater mobility, are usually very superficial, and variably located in the mid- to ventral abdomen.

On ventrodorsal (VD) radiographs, the head of the spleen is seen as a triangular soft tissue opacity along the left body wall, caudal and lateral to the fundus of the stomach and cranial to the left kidney, in both the dog and the cat (Figure 14.1). The cranial–caudal position may change depending on body position, degree of distension of the stomach and splenic size. On the VD view, the body and tail of the spleen may be oriented parallel to the long axis of the body, adjacent to the left lateral body wall, or to the right, perpendicular to the long axis of the body. Often the body and tail regions are poorly visualized due to superimposition with other structures.

On the lateral view in the cat, the head of the spleen is seen as a triangular soft tissue opacity in the dorsal abdomen between the fundus of the stomach and the kidneys. This is less common in the dog. In addition, as the spleen is proportionately shorter in the cat than in the dog, the tail and body of the spleen are generally not visible on the lateral view in cats. The body and tail of the spleen may be visible on the lateral view in dogs (Figure 14.2) as a triangular soft tissue opacity located anywhere between the caudal ventral margin of the liver and the apex of the urinary bladder. The tail and body of the spleen are more commonly seen along the mid-ventral body wall on a right lateral recumbent view than on a left lateral recumbent view.

Normal variations

Dogs that are young and athletic generally have larger spleens than geriatric or sedentary dogs. German Shepherd Dogs (and closely related breeds) have larger spleens than other similar sized dogs. Some normal cats have larger spleens that reach the ventral abdominal wall on the lateral view. Occasionally,

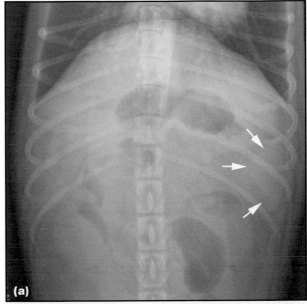

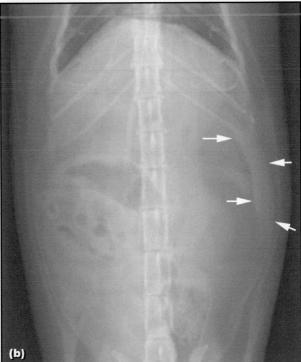

14.1 The normal spleen (arrowed) can be seen on the VD radiograph in both **(a)** the dog and **(b)** the cat. The head and body of the spleen are seen in the dog on this view, whilst the entirety of the spleen is seen along the left lateral body wall in the cat.

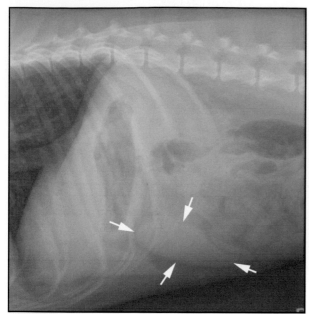

14.2 Lateral radiograph of a dog showing the normal body and tail of the spleen (arrowed) caudal to the stomach and liver.

bends or folds are noted in otherwise normal spleens of both species.

Determination of splenic size

Splenomegaly

Radiographic and ultrasonographic assessment of spleen size in dogs and cats is exclusively subjective. In the dog, an assessment can be made of the thickness of the spleen and the degree of rounding or blunting of the margins (Figure 14.3a). On the lateral view, enlargement of the body or tail of the spleen results in dorsal and caudal displacement of the intestines. Enlargement of the head of the spleen results in rightward and caudal displacement of the intestines and caudal displacement of the left kidney. Splenic size in the cat is much less variable; an enlarged spleen is presumed if the body and tail are seen on the lateral view (Figure 14.3b).

Microsplenia

Reduction in the size of the spleen is uncommonly reported. The most common cause of a diffusely small spleen is contraction following an acute bleeding episode. Developmental or degenerative changes are additional aetiologies. Splenic contraction is a well documented component of the dive reflex in many species, although the importance in dogs and cats is not known.

Detection of shape changes

The splenic surfaces should be smooth and the margins at each border should be sharp. Irregularity of the surface contours is considered abnormal and can be diffuse or focal in nature (Figure 14.4). Indented regions are noted with fibrosis, possibly secondary to trauma or infarction.

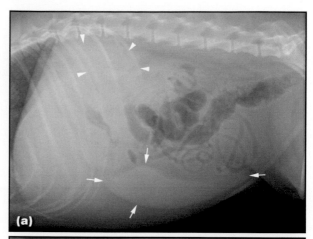

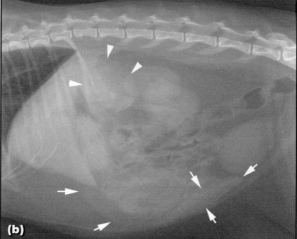

14.3 **(a)** Lateral radiograph showing diffuse splenomegaly in a dog. The body and tail of the spleen (arrowed) are increased in thickness and show rounding of the margins. The enlarged head of the spleen (arrowheads) results in increased opacity in the dorsocranial abdomen. The intestines are displaced in a dorsal and caudal direction. **(b)** Lateral radiograph showing diffuse splenomegaly in a cat. Normally, the body and tail of the spleen (arrowed) are not visible in the cat. The enlargement of the head of the spleen (arrowheads) is identified by the increased soft tissue opacity in the dorsocranial abdomen.

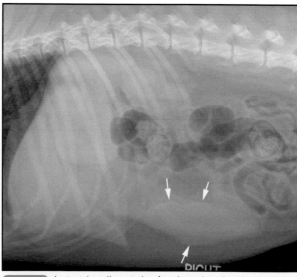

14.4 Lateral radiograph of a dog showing irregularity of the splenic margins (arrowed).

Ultrasonography

The head of the spleen is often located within the ribcage in the cranial left dorsal abdomen in dogs; therefore, a left intercostal approach may be necessary to fully evaluate the spleen. The entire spleen in the cat is caudal to the ribcage and can be fully evaluated from a ventral approach.

The spleen should be uniform in echogenicity. In the cat, the spleen may be hypoechoic or similar in echogenicity to the renal cortex. In the dog, the normal spleen (Figure 14.5a) is hyperechoic to the liver and renal cortices. The spleen is uniform in echotexture and has a smoothly marginated, hyperechoic capsule. The echogenicity of the capsule is best appreciated when the interrogating ultrasound beam is perpendicular to the capsule surface (Figure 14.5b). The splenic veins are visualized at the splenic hilus and for a short distance within the parenchyma. The splenic veins can be evaluated with colour Doppler ultrasonography for assessment of blood flow. Doppler ultrasonography interrogation of splenic vein blood flow (Figure 14.6) is important for evaluation of splenic torsion, thrombosis and certain mass lesions. Compared to the high accuracy in the liver of dog and human patients, contrast ultrasonography seems less accurate for differentiation between benign and malignant focal disease in the spleen. No difference was noted between the perfusion pattern of haematomas and haemangiosarcomas in the spleen of dogs.

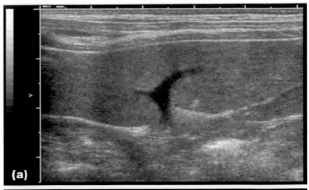
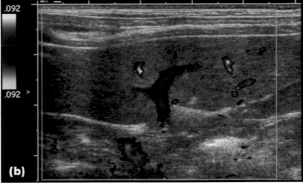

14.6 Ultrasonograms of the spleen in a normal dog showing a splenic vein **(a)** without and **(b)** with colour Doppler examination.

Overview of additional imaging modalities

Computed tomography (CT) and magnetic resonance imaging (MRI) can also be used to evaluate splenic disease. CT and MRI are not widely used due to the need for general anaesthesia and the ease of complete splenic evaluation using ultrasonography. On CT, the spleen is homogenous and similar in density to the musculature, and is hyperattenuating compared with the kidney (Figure 14.7). Contrast

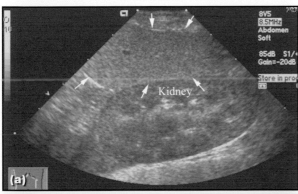
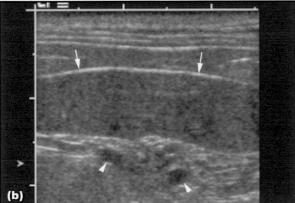

14.5 **(a)** Ultrasonogram of the spleen in a normal dog. The splenic parenchyma (arrowed) is uniform in echotexture and hyperechoic relative to the kidney cortex. **(b)** Ultrasonogram of the normal spleen in a cat. The splenic capsule is easily visible in the near-field (arrowed) and the splenic veins can be seen close to the hilus (arrowheads).

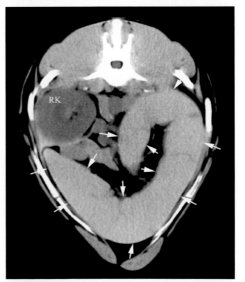

14.7 CT image of the cranial abdomen of a dog that was anaesthetized with thiopental. The spleen (arrowed) is enlarged and hyperattenuating compared with the right kidney (RK). (Window width = 300 HU, window level = 50 HU)

enhanced CT has been used to compare malignant and non-malignant splenic masses. A significant difference was seen in pre- and post-contrast imaging between malignant and benign masses. CT has also been used to confirm diagnosis of splenic torsion in a dog when abdominal radiography and ultrasonography were inconclusive. Findings included an enlarged, non-enhanced spleen and a soft tissue mass effect, representing the rotated pedicle. Use of MRI for evaluation of splenic disease is not commonly performed due to cost and anaesthesia concerns. MRI may be more accurate than CT for characterization of focal splenic lesions.

Splenic diseases

The differential diagnoses for abnormalities of the spleen are given in Figure 14.8.

	Diffuse splenomegaly: smooth margins	Diffuse splenomegaly: irregular margins	Focal or multifocal masses
Anaesthetics/ tranquillizers (phenothiazine, barbiturates)	X		
Infection: splenitis	X	X	
Infection: abscess(es)		X	X
Immune-mediated disease	X		
Nodular hyperplasia		X	X
Neoplasia: haemangiosarcoma			X
Neoplasia: lymphoma; mast cell tumour; histiocytosis	X	X	X
Venous congestion (right heart failure, portal hypertension)	X		
Infarct(s)		X	
Torsion (note also abnormal location)	X	X	
Extramedullary haemopoiesis	X	X	X
Haematoma(s)			X

14.8 Differential diagnoses for abnormalities of the spleen. The expected radiographic appearance of the splenic disease processes are represented with an X.

Vascular conditions

Splenic congestion

Passive congestion of the spleen can result from anaesthetics or tranquillizers, haemolytic anaemia, toxaemic conditions or portal hypertension. Radiographic findings with splenic congestion include diffuse enlargement of the spleen. The margins

remain smooth, but the thickness of the spleen increases and the borders are rounded. The intestines are displaced in a dorsal and caudal direction on the lateral view and medially on the VD view (Figure 14.9). Ultrasonographic changes noted in dogs after tranquillization with acepromazine and thiopental included an increase in splenic size and increased attenuation. No changes were seen with propofol administration. Chronic congestion may result in increased echogenicity.

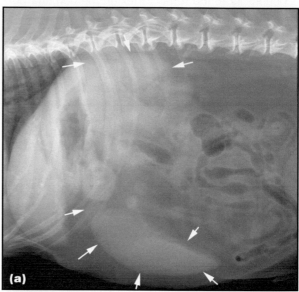

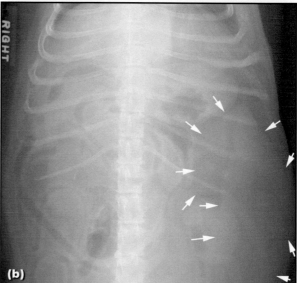

14.9 An 11-year-old mixed breed dog sedated with acepromazine prior to abdominal radiography. The spleen (arrowed) is diffusely enlarged noted by increased thickness and rounding of the margins. This has resulted in **(a)** dorsal and caudal displacement of the intestines on the lateral view and **(b)** medial displacement of the small intestines on the VD view.

Splenic torsion

Splenic torsion most often occurs in large-breed, deep-chested dogs and can be an isolated finding or in association with gastric dilatation and volvulus. Great Dane and German Shepherd Dogs are over-represented breeds. Radiographic findings of splenic torsion are severe enlargement with increased thickness and rounding of the splenic margins. A hallmark of the disease is an abnormal position of the spleen; this may manifest as a lack of ability to visualize the head of the spleen in its normal left cranial location on a VD view or as a large C-shaped soft tissue opacity in the central abdomen on both views (Figure 14.10). Often there is poor serosal

detail due to the presence of peritoneal fluid. The fundus of the stomach may be displaced caudally and medially. In addition, if necrosis of the spleen is present, regions of gas may be present within the parenchyma (Figure 14.11).

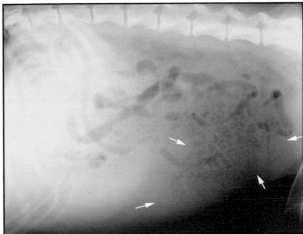

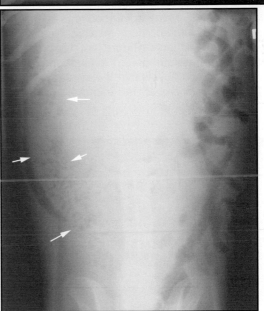

14.11 Radiographs of an 8-year-old German Shepherd Dog showing multifocal small gas pockets within the right mid- to caudal abdomen. There is diffuse loss of serosal detail and the intestines are displaced away from the abnormal gas-filled structure (arrowed). Splenic torsion with necrosis was diagnosed.

Ultrasonographic findings with splenic torsion include severe enlargement with a lacy hypoechoic appearance. The key findings in 15 dogs were immobile intraluminal echoes with an absent Doppler ultrasonography signal in the splenic veins (Figure 14.12). However, these findings may also be seen in cases of diffuse lymphoma with malignant thrombosis. A hilar hyperechoic perivenous triangle has also been seen associated with splenic torsion.

Thromboembolic disease

Splenic infarction is commonly associated with autoimmune haemolytic anaemia and thrombocytopenia and concurrent high-dose corticosteroid administration. It has also been reported secondary to

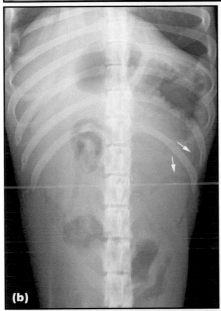

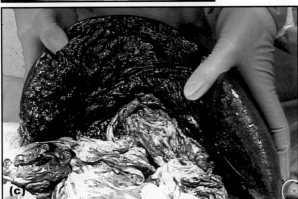

14.10 Abdominal radiographs of a 4-year-old Belgian Tervuren presented with a 4-day history of lethargy, depression and anorexia. Serosal detail is poor throughout the abdomen. **(a)** There is a reverse C-shaped soft tissue opacity in the mid-abdomen (arrowed) on the lateral view. **(b)** On the VD view there are loops of small intestine (arrowed) occupying the region normally occupied by the head of the spleen. **(c)** Splenic torsion was confirmed during abdominal exploratory surgery.

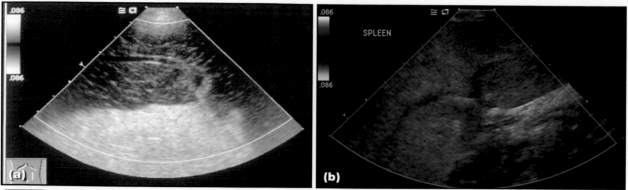

14.12 Colour Doppler ultrasonograms from two dogs with splenic torsion. **(a)** Typical hypoechoic, lacy parenchymal appearance of the spleen. **(b)** The spleen has a more uniform echogenicity, but no flow was identified in the splenic vessels.

inflammatory diseases (e.g. pancreatitis, septicaemia), hypercoagulable conditions, renal disease, hyper-adrenocorticism, neoplasia and cardiovascular disease. Thromboembolic disease is not recognized on radiographs. On ultrasound examination, acute infarction may be occult. More advanced cases have a characteristic well demarcated, swollen hypoechoic region in the periphery (Figure 14.13a). Colour Doppler and contrast ultrasound evaluation demonstrate a lack of blood flow within these areas (Figure 14.13b). Chronic or complicated infarcts may have a more variable appearance.

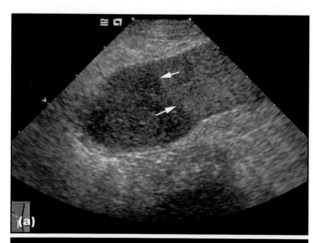

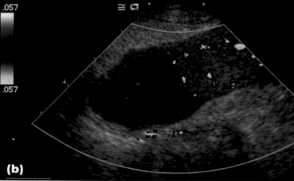

14.13 Ultrasonograms of a dog with a splenic infarct. **(a)** There is a sharp line of demarcation (arrowed) between the normal hyperechoic splenic parenchyma and the hypoechoic infarcted region. **(b)** With colour Doppler evaluation, lack of blood flow is noted in the infarcted area.

Splenic masses

Splenic masses can be divided into general categories of neoplastic and non-neoplastic disease. Differential diagnoses for masses or nodules include:

* Neoplasia
* Haematoma
* Abscess
* Granuloma
* Cyst
* Nodular hyperplasia
* Extramedullary haemopoiesis.

Neoplasia, extramedullary haemopoiesis and haematomas are most commonly recognized in the dog.

Radiographic findings of splenic masses depend on location. If the mass is in the head of the spleen, there is rightward and caudal displacement of the small intestine and descending colon (Figure 14.14). The left kidney may also be displaced caudally. A

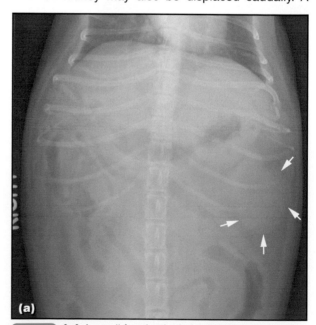

14.14 **(a)** A small focal splenic head mass (arrowed) was only visible on the VD view in this dog. Due to the small size of the mass there was minimal displacement of the colon and small intestines. (continues) ▶

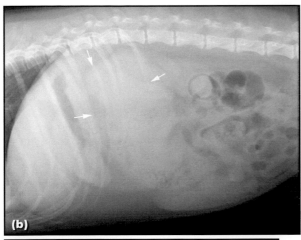

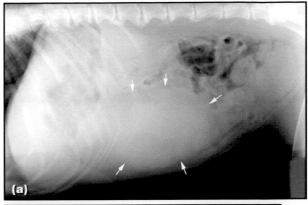

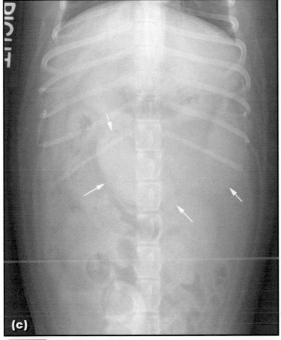

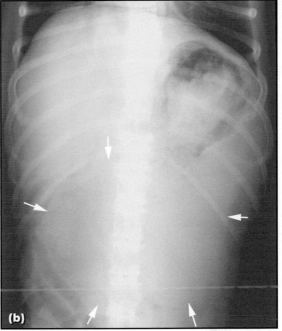

14.14 (continued) **(b,c)** A large mass involving the head and body of the spleen, resulting in caudal and rightward displacement of the small and large intestines.

14.15 Splenic haemangiosarcoma involving the body and tail of the spleen is seen as **(a)** a ventral mass (arrowed) on the lateral view, resulting in caudal and dorsal displacement of the intestines. **(b)** On the VD view, the mass (arrowed) is central and to the left of midline, resulting in rightward and caudal displacement of the small intestines.

mass affecting the body and tail of the spleen (Figure 14.15) results in a cranial ventral mass or mass effect on the lateral view. This, in turn, results in caudal and dorsal displacement of the small and large intestines. On the VD view, a mass in the body and/or tail of the spleen is more variable and may be left-sided, central or right-sided. The aetiology of splenic masses and nodular lesions can not be definitively determined based on ultrasonography alone as there is overlap in the appearance of benign and neoplastic disease. For example, target-like lesions (hypoechoic rim with a hyperechoic centre) are most commonly neoplastic, although less frequently they can be caused by nodular hyperplasia.

Benign masses

Most benign diseases, such as haematoma, abscess and nodular hyperplasia, can not be distinguished from neoplastic disease based on radiography and

ultrasonography. One exception is noted with myelolipoma, which has a unique hyperechoic and very atypical hyperattenuating appearance on ultrasonography.

Splenic haematoma: Splenic haematomas can be of variable size. They may not be apparent on radiographs or may present as large, well circumscribed splenic masses (Figure 14.16). Haematomas vary greatly in appearance on ultrasound examination, depending on age, and are indistinguishable from haemangiosarcomas. Haematomas can be parenchymal or subcapsular in location and are variably echoic. Free abdominal fluid is not usually present.

Splenic abscess: Splenic abscesses are uncommon but may occur as a solitary mass, multifocal masses or be associated with splenic torsion. Associated with torsion, the radiographic findings

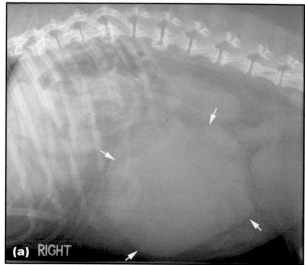

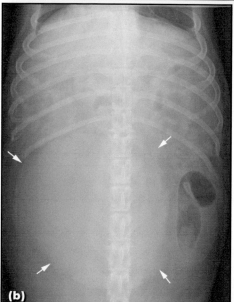

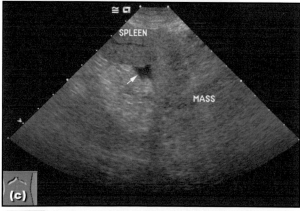

14.16 **(a,b)** A well circumscribed splenic haematoma present in the ventral mid-abdomen (arrowed). **(c)** The normal spleen can be seen (SPLEEN) and is confluent with the haematoma (MASS). A small amount of anechoic abdominal fluid (arrowed) is also visible.

include an enlarged, abnormally located spleen with multifocal gas bubbles. Abscesses can be hypoechoic to hyperechoic on ultrasound examination. Intraparenchymal gas will be very hyperechoic with a ring down or dirty shadow artefact.

Nodular hyperplasia: Hyperplasia is often not detected on radiographs. Nodular hyperplasia may cause focal masses or diffuse splenomegaly with irregular margins. Hyperplastic nodules in the spleen are variable in appearance on ultrasonography. They may be hypoechoic, hyperechoic or of mixed echogenicity.

Neoplasia

Sarcomas are the most common histological type of focal splenic neoplasm in dogs. Metastatic carcinoma is less common. A focal mass or mass effect (see above) is the most common radiographic finding with neoplasia (Figure 14.17). Lack of serosal margin detail due to haemoperitoneum is often seen with haemangiosarcoma (Figure 14.18).

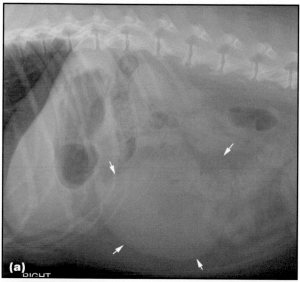

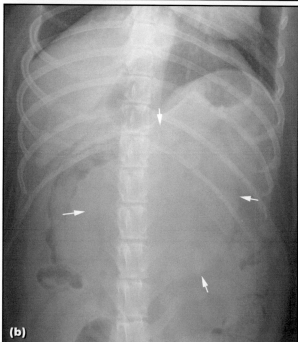

14.17 A 10-year-old Labrador Retriever diagnosed with splenic haemangiosarcoma. A well circumscribed mass (arrowed) is present in the ventral mid-abdomen on **(a)** lateral and **(b)** VD radiographs. (continues) ▶

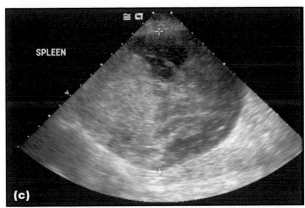

14.17 (continued) A 10-year-old Labrador Retriever diagnosed with splenic haemangiosarcoma. **(c)** The mass was of mixed echogenicity with hyperechoic, hypoechoic and anechoic regions being identified on ultrasound examination. Note the similarity in appearance of the radiographs in this dog with neoplastic disease compared with a dog with benign disease (see Figure 14.16).

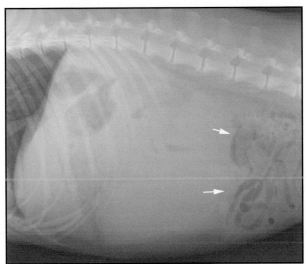

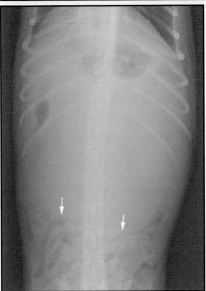

14.18 Radiographs from a dog with splenic haemangiosarcoma and haemoabdomen. The splenic margins are not well defined due to the loss of abdominal serosal detail. A mass effect is present due to the caudal displacement of the small intestines (arrowed).

On ultrasound examination, haemangiosarcomas are generally poorly defined and usually of complex echogenicity; both hyperechoic and hypoechoic portions with anechoic regions. However, other lesions, including haematomas, other sarcomas and atypical benign nodules, may also have this appearance. The larger the mass, without concurrent free fluid, nodules in other organs or other signs of metastases, the more likely it is that the mass is benign. Contrast ultrasonography is unable to differentiate between hemangiosarcomas and haematomas based on perfusion pattern.

In cats, lymphosarcoma and mast cell neoplasia are the most common neoplastic diseases to affect the spleen. Although diffuse enlargement is commonly present, multifocal nodules and a solitary mass can be seen on radiographs. On ultrasound examination, neoplasia is most commonly hypoechoic, but can be hyperechoic or of mixed echogenicity. There are no pathognomonic changes to distinguish neoplastic from non-neoplastic disease in dogs or cats.

Other splenic diseases

Splenitis
Bacterial and fungal diseases may result in secondary splenomegaly. Diffuse splenitis may appear similar to a splenic torsion, with a hypoechoic, lacy parenchymal pattern. Generally, blood flow can still be identified within the splenic vessels, which helps distinguish the two diseases. Chronic inflammation can result in more variable patterns of decreased to increased echogenicity.

Extramedullary haemopoiesis
Extramedullary haemopoiesis can cause mild to moderate splenomegaly. As a focal lesion, extramedullary haemopoiesis is often seen ultrasonographically as hyperechoic or hypoechoic nodules.

Diffuse neoplastic disease
Lymphocytic (Figure 14.19), histiocytic, mastocytic, myelomatous and leukaemic infiltrates may result in diffuse splenomegaly. In the cat, generalized splenomegaly is most common with a lymphoma

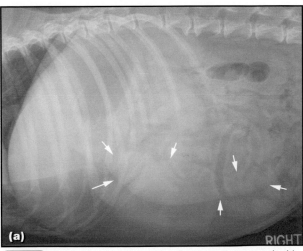

14.19 **(a)** Lateral radiograph of a dog diagnosed with multicentric lymphoma. (continues) ▶

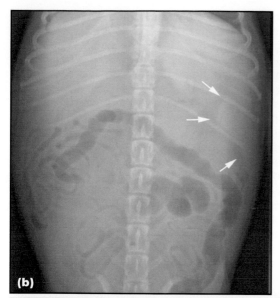

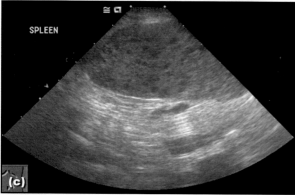

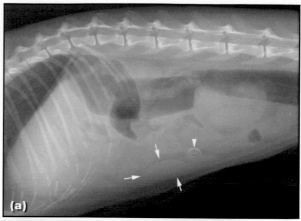

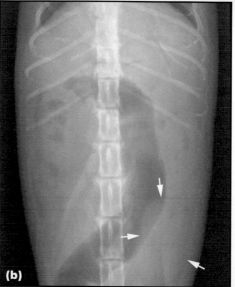

14.19 (continued) **(b)** VD radiograph of a dog diagnosed with multicentric lymphoma. The spleen is diffusely enlarged (arrowed). **(c)** Small hypoechoic nodules are noted throughout the splenic parenchyma on ultrasonography.

(Figure 14.20) or mast cell tumour. Although these diseases are generally hypoechoic on ultrasonography, they can be mottled or normal in echogenicity.

References and further reading

Balcar I, Seltzer SE, Davis S, *et al.* (1984) CT patterns of splenic infarction: a clinical and experimental study. *Radiology* **151**, 723–729

Clifford CA, Pretorius ES, Weisse C, *et al.* (2004) Magnetic resonance imaging of focal splenic and hepatic lesions in the dog. *Journal of Veterinary Internal Medicine* **18**, 330–338

Cuccovillo A and Lamb CR (2002) Cellular features of sonographic target lesions of the liver and spleen in 21 dogs and a cat. *Veterinary Radiology and Ultrasound* **43**, 275–278

Fife WD, Samii VF, Drost WT, *et al.* (2004) Comparison between malignant and nonmalignant splenic masses in dogs using contrast-enhanced computed tomography. *Veterinary Radiology and Ultrasound* **45**, 289–297

Hanson JA, Papageorges M, Girard E, *et al.* (2001) Ultrasonographic appearance of splenic disease in 101 cats. *Veterinary Radiology and Ultrasound* **42**, 441–445

Mai W (2006) The hilar perivenous hyperechoic triangle as a sign of acute splenic torsion in dogs. *Veterinary Radiology and Ultrasound* **47**, 487–491

Neath PJ, Brockman DJ and Saunders HM (1997) Retrospective analysis of 19 cases of isolated torsion of the splenic pedicle in dogs. *Journal of Small Animal Practice* **38**, 387–392

Newell SM, Graham JP, Roberts GD, *et al.* (2000) Quantitative magnetic resonance imaging of the normal feline cranial abdomen. *Veterinary Radiology and Ultrasound* **41**, 27–34

O'Brien RT, Waller KR and Osgood TL (2004) Sonographic features of drug-induced splenic congestion. *Veterinary Radiology and Ultrasound*

14.20 A 13-year-old Domestic Shorthaired cat with lymphoma of the spleen and intestines. **(a)** The spleen (arrowed) is visible on the lateral view, which denotes splenomegaly in the cat. Mineralization of the peritoneal fat (arrowhead) is also seen near the spleen. **(b)** On the VD view, the margins of the spleen are difficult to visualize, but the left kidney (arrowed) is caudally displaced by the enlarged spleen. **(c)** Ultrasonogram showing the spleen is diffusely hypoechoic and mottled in echogenicity.

45, 225–227

Patsikas MN, Rallis T, Kladakis SE, *et al.* (2001) Computed tomography diagnosis of isolated splenic torsion in a dog. *Veterinary Radiology and Ultrasound* **42**, 235–237

Saunders HM, Neath PJ and Brockman DJ (1998) B-mode and Doppler ultrasound imaging of the spleen with canine splenic torsion: a retrospective evaluation. *Veterinary Radiology and Ultrasound* **39**, 349–353

15

The adrenal glands

Paul Mahoney

Introduction

Adrenal gland imaging is performed as part of the assessment of a patient when there is suspicion of abnormal adrenal gland function. Information that is of interest to a veterinary surgeon includes the size, shape and location of both glands, the internal structure, the presence of any local invasion into adjacent vessels or organs, and whether there is any evidence of distant metastases. Adrenal gland imaging alone cannot be used as an indicator of adrenal gland function, and findings should be interpreted in the light of the clinical presentation and results of other diagnostic tests.

Overview of anatomy

The adrenal glands are paired retroperitoneal structures usually located ventral to the second and third lumbar vertebrae. They are composed of two functionally different tissues: the outer cortex and the inner medulla. The adrenal gland cortex produces steroid hormones (aldosterone, cortisol and adrenal androgens) whilst the medulla produces adrenaline and noradrenaline.

In dogs, the right adrenal gland (Figure 15.1a) is more cranially positioned than the left. It lies cranial to the right renal artery, medial to the cranial pole of the right kidney and in the region of the origin of the coeliac artery or the cranial mesenteric artery. It is in close apposition to the dorsal surface of the caudal vena cava. In some dogs the capsule of the right adrenal gland is continuous with the tunica externa of this vessel. The left adrenal gland (Figure 15.1b) is located cranial to the left renal artery (close to the origin of the cranial mesenteric artery), ventral to the aorta, and has a variable relationship with the cranial pole of the left kidney, depending on the position of the kidney. Normal adrenal glands typically measure between 15 mm and 30 mm in length, and between 4 mm and 10 mm in diameter at the widest point. The left adrenal gland often has a bilobed (peanut-shaped) appearance whilst the right adrenal gland may be thickest towards its centre or caudal pole and resembles an arrowhead pointing cranially.

In cats, the adrenal glands have a similar location to those of dogs, relative to the major vessels. However, the relationship between the left adrenal

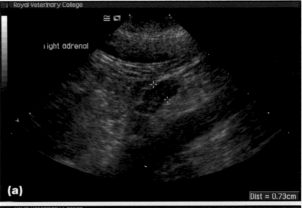

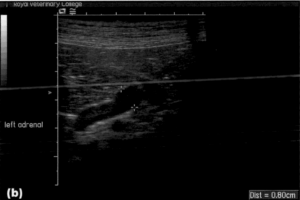

15.1 Ultrasonograms of the normal canine adrenal glands. **(a)** Right adrenal gland. **(b)** Left adrenal gland.

gland and the cranial pole of the left kidney is more variable owing to the greater mobility of the feline kidney. The adrenal glands are usually oval-shaped structures (Figure 15.2) and typically measure between 5 mm and 13 mm in length, and between 3 mm and 4.6 mm in width.

Both adrenal glands receive their blood supply from several major vessels, including the phrenicoabdominal artery, the abdominal aorta, the lumbar arteries and the renal arteries. Each adrenal gland vein drains into the corresponding phrenicoabdominal vein, and then into the caudal vena cava, although the left phrenicoabdominal vein may also drain into the left renal vein as a normal variation. The adrenal gland lymphatics drain into the lumbar aortic lymph nodes and then into the lumbar lymphatic trunk and/or the cisterna chyli.

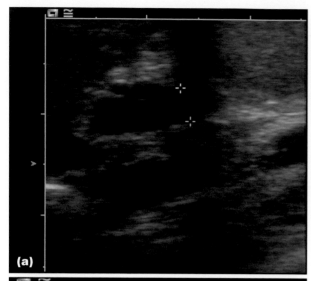

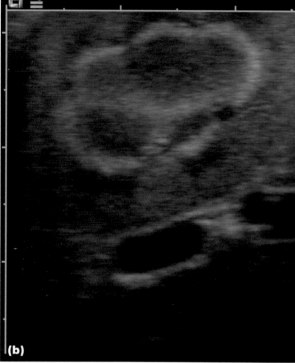

15.2 Ultrasonograms of the normal feline adrenal glands. **(a)** Right adrenal gland. **(b)** Left adrenal gland.

Normal variations

Although the relationship to each other remains relatively constant, normal adrenal glands can vary in association with surrounding anatomical structures. They should always be located cranial to the ipsilateral renal artery, and they are usually adjacent to the origins of the coeliac and cranial mesenteric arteries. Although most normal adrenal glands are located ventral to the second and third lumbar vertebrae, occasionally they may be located as far cranially as the line of the T12–T13 intervertebral space in dogs.

The measurements of the adrenal glands given above should not be considered a reference cut-off for disease, because functionally normal adrenal glands may be beyond this range and abnormal adrenal glands may be within this range. Normal adrenal glands may also occasionally show variation in shape. Canine adrenal glands may have a more uniform diameter along their length; feline adrenal glands may occasionally have a bilobed appearance.

Approximately one-third of healthy aged cats may develop microscopic evidence of adrenal gland mineralization. This does not often develop to such an extent as to be detectable with conventional imaging, but when it is seen it should not be considered a significant finding (Figure 15.3).

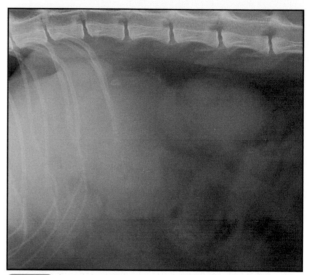

15.3 Lateral radiograph showing mineralization of the adrenal glands in an aged cat. This is considered an insignificant finding.

Radiography

The routine radiographic assessment of a dog or cat with clinical suspicion of adrenal gland disease should include lateral and ventrodorsal (VD) abdominal radiographs, as well as dorsoventral (DV), left lateral and right lateral thoracic radiographs. A lack of any radiographic findings does not rule out the possibility of adrenal gland disease.

Contrast radiography

Non-selective angiography can be performed to help identify a tumour thrombus invading the caudal vena cava. The left or right saphenous vein is catheterized and a bolus of water-soluble iodinated contrast medium is injected. Lateral and VD radiographs centred on the retroperitoneal area ventral to T12–L3 are taken towards the end of the injection. The person injecting the contrast medium should take care with regard to radiation safety by wearing appropriate protective clothing and standing as far away from the primary beam as possible. A tumour thrombus can be identified as a filling defect in the vessel lumen (Figure 15.4), extending cranially from the region of the renal veins. The length of the tumour thrombus can be quite variable, and in some dogs it may even extend beyond the line of the diaphragm.

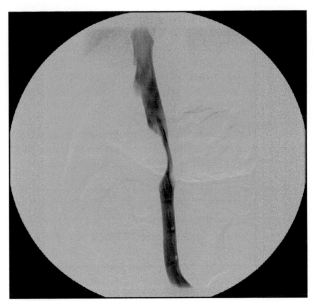

15.4 Subtraction fluoroscopic image of a tumour thrombus creating a filling defect in the caudal vena cava.

Ultrasonography

Consistent visualization of both adrenal glands requires experience, patience, equipment of sufficient quality and a cooperative patient. These small structures are located in a region that is difficult to assess, and imaging may be hampered by edge shadowing artefacts from adjacent organs and vessels. The inability to visualize one or both adrenal glands should never be used as an indicator of disease.

The landmarks for locating the left adrenal gland are the aorta, the left renal artery, the left kidney and the paired coeliac and cranial mesenteric arteries. Using a longitudinal plane, the probe is placed just ventral to the lumbar musculature on the left side. The aorta is identified as the closer of the two large vessels that run in a craniocaudal direction. As it is followed cranially from the iliac region, the left renal artery can be seen as a large branch projecting laterally, which then arcs cranially or cranioventrally. It is often seen to pulsate. The left kidney can then be identified by following this vessel, and is typically lateral or ventrolateral to the aorta. The region ventral to the aorta and cranial to the left renal artery should then be interrogated in both longitudinal and transverse imaging planes to locate the adrenal gland.

The landmarks for locating the right adrenal gland are the caudal vena cava and the right kidney. Using a longitudinal plane, the probe is placed just caudal to the 13th rib and ventral to the lumbar musculature. The caudal vena cava is identified as the nearer of the two large vessels, and it diverges away from the aorta as it approaches the diaphragm. Vena caval diameter can vary considerably depending on the pressure applied to the abdomen by the probe. At the 13th rib, the probe may need to be angled cranially and dorsally to allow visualization of the right renal hilus. Maintaining the longitudinal plane along the vessel, the caudal vena cava is imaged in the region of the renal hilus. By then slightly tilting the probe dorsally, the right

adrenal gland may be seen as an elongated hypoechoic structure adjacent to the dorsal or dorsolateral surface of the caudal vena cava. Because of their close proximity in many dogs, the caudal vena cava and the right adrenal gland may be difficult to differentiate owing to volume averaging.

Both adrenal glands are usually uniformly hypoechoic compared with the surrounding tissue. Occasionally, one or both glands may be seen to have a slight variation in echogenicity, where the cortex is hypoechoic and the medulla is hyperechoic (Figure 15.5).

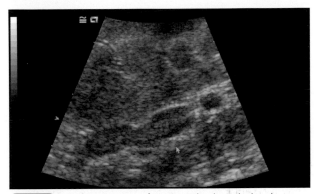

15.5 Ultrasonogram of a normal adrenal gland showing the cortex and medulla.

Overview of additional imaging modalities

Computed tomography

Spiral computed tomography (CT) allows rapid cross-sectional X-ray imaging of the retroperitoneal space. Unlike conventional abdominal radiography, CT allows the adrenal glands to be visualized without any overlying structures obscuring the glands. This technique is more sensitive for the detection of adrenal gland masses than radiography and, when CT angiography is performed, is more reliable for detecting invasion of a neoplasm into the surrounding vessels than non-selective angiography or ultrasonography (Figure 15.6). Thoracic CT is more sensitive and specific than thoracic radiography for detecting pulmonary metastases and can be used to image the pituitary gland in animals with pituitary-dependent hyperadrenocorticism.

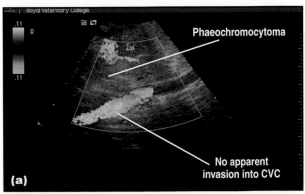

Phaeochromocytoma

No apparent invasion into CVC

(a)

15.6 **(a)** Ultrasonogram of a phaeochromocytoma showing no invasion into the adjacent caudal vena cava (CVC). (continues) ▶

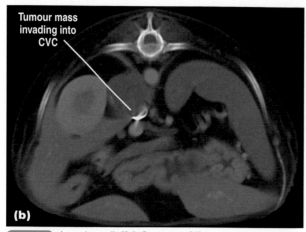

15.6   (continued) **(b)** Contrast CT image of the same dog as in Figure 15.4, showing tumour invasion into the caudal vena cava (CVC).

The limitations of CT are its expense, limited availability and the need for deep sedation or general anaesthesia. A high level of expertise is required to interpret these images. In the coming years, it is likely that affordable machines will become increasingly available to the veterinary market. The need for a high level of expertise to interpret the images will remain.

Magnetic resonance imaging

The use of magnetic resonance imaging (MRI) gives superior soft tissue contrast compared with conventional CT and allows imaging in multiple planes without the need to reformat images. It can be used to image the adrenal glands (Figure 15.7) and

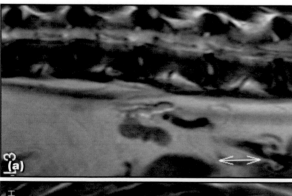

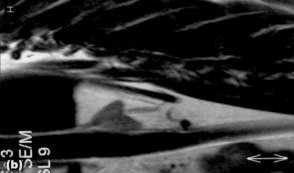

15.7   Magnetic resonance images of **(a)** the normal canine left adrenal gland and **(b)** the normal canine right adrenal gland.

adjacent vessels without the need for iodinated contrast medium, as well as imaging the pituitary gland in animals with pituitary-dependent disease. The quality of the images is dependent on the strength of the magnet and the coils being used, and meaningful interpretation of the images requires a high level of expertise.

The current limitations of MRI are its expense, limited availability, the requirement for general anaesthesia, prolonged scanning times and the need for a high level of expertise to interpret the images.

Nuclear medicine

There is very limited veterinary experience in the use of radioactive substances to evaluate the adrenal glands in dogs. [123]Iodine-metaiodobenzylguanidine has been used to image phaeochromocytomas and [131]Iodine-19-iodocholesterol has been used to image the adrenal gland cortex. The requirement for radioactive substances, health and safety issues, the limited availability of gamma cameras, and the increasing access to ultrasonography, MRI and CT has meant that scintigraphic evaluation of the adrenal glands remains a rare procedure.

Adrenal gland diseases

Radiography and ultrasonography remain the primary imaging modalities for assessing dogs and cats when there is suspicion of adrenal gland disease. Ultrasonography is preferred when assessing the size, shape and internal structure of the glands, and for determining the presence of local invasion or intra-abdominal metastases. Radiography gives a better overview of the patient and provides information on the pulmonary and cardiovascular systems, the presence of non-adrenal gland organomegaly and dystrophic mineralization at distant sites.

Changes in the appearance of the adrenal gland

Adrenal gland mineralization

On abdominal radiographs, adrenal gland mineralization appears as a focal area of opacity, craniomedial to the left and/or right kidney.

- Although this may occasionally be seen in hyperplastic adrenal glands, in the dog it is more suggestive of neoplasia.
- Mineralization cannot be used to differentiate tumour type: it is found in approximately 50% of adrenal gland adenomas; 50% of adrenal gland carcinomas; and 10% of phaeochromocytomas.
- In the cat, mineralization is an uncommon age-related finding and not usually of clinical significance.
- Mineralization appears as a hyperechoic surface with deeper acoustic shadowing when viewed with ultrasonography (Figure 15.8). This shadowing may impede the ability to evaluate local vessels.

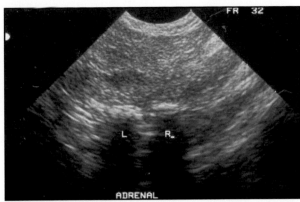

15.8 Ultrasonogram showing mineralization of the left (L) and right (R) adrenal glands of an aged cat. Note the distal shadowing impeding the view of the deeper structures.

Unilateral adrenal gland mass

Radiographic evidence of an adrenal gland mass is an uncommon finding. Fewer than 20% of dogs with naturally occurring hyperadrenocorticism have an adrenal gland neoplasm and these are not usually radiographically apparent unless they are larger than 2 cm in diameter and/or mineralized. Invasion into adjacent structures by a neoplasm will not be detected on plain abdominal radiographs.

In experienced hands, ultrasonography will detect much smaller adrenal gland masses than those seen by radiography.

- Although most adrenal gland masses are primary adrenal gland neoplasms (Figure 15.9), differential diagnoses include metastatic disease, myelolipoma, haemorrhage and granuloma.
- Cytology of such masses will not reliably differentiate adenomas from adenocarcinomas.
- Invasion of local vessels or other organs is a marker for malignancy, giving primary differential diagnoses of carcinoma and phaeochromocytoma.
- Occasionally dogs with pituitary-dependent hyperadrenocorticism show asymmetrical adrenal gland enlargement, which must not be misinterpreted as adrenal gland-dependent disease.

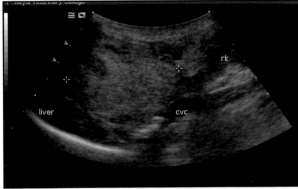

15.9 Ultrasonogram of a right adrenal gland carcinoma; thoracic radiographs demonstrated nodular pulmonary metastatic disease. CVC = Caudal vena cava; rk = Right kidney.

- Occasionally a unilateral adrenal gland mass may be benign and an incidental finding. The history and clinical findings should always be reviewed to ensure that pointers to hyperadrenocorticism or phaeochromocytoma were not missed during the initial consultation.

Bilateral adrenomegaly

A diameter of 7.4 mm has been proposed as an upper limit of normal adrenal gland size when measured ultrasonographically. However, it must be noted that although many patients with pituitary-dependent hyperadrenocorticism have adrenal glands beyond this measurement, a considerable number do not. Equally important, patients with no adrenal gland disease may have adrenal glands larger than this cut-off. The sensitivity and specificity of adrenal gland ultrasonography is not high enough to use it reliably as a screening test for hyperadrenocorticism.

- Bilateral adrenal gland neoplasms have been reported infrequently in the veterinary literature. These may be separate neoplasms of differing origin, bilateral adrenocortical tumours (benign or malignant), bilateral phaeochromocytomas or bilateral myelolipomas.
- Dogs and cats with diabetes mellitus may develop mild bilateral adrenomegaly (Figure 15.10).

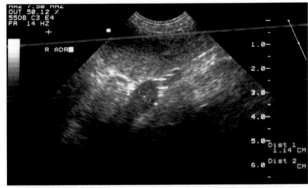

15.10 Ultrasonogram of a dog with diabetes mellitus showing mild bilateral adrenomegaly.

- Trilostane is a 3β-hydroxysteroid dehydrogenase inhibitor that is authorized for use in the treatment of canine pituitary-dependent hyperadrenocorticism. Most treated dogs show significant adrenal gland enlargement within 6 months; the difference between the cortical and medullary echogenicities may become quite pronounced, and occasionally one or both glands may become misshapen (Figure 15.11). Trilostane should not be used unless the clinician is confident in the diagnosis of hyperadrenocorticism and pre-treatment imaging studies are complete. Once treatment has begun, imaging may prove confusing and unhelpful in differentiating pituitary-dependent from adrenal gland-dependent disease.

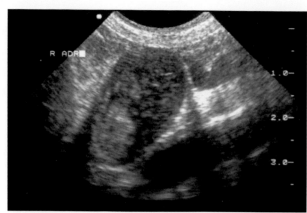

15.11 Ultrasonogram of an adrenal gland 6 weeks after beginning treatment with trilostane. The adrenal gland is enlarged and shows marked variation in its internal echogenicity.

Reduced adrenal gland size

- Dogs with hypoadrenocorticism typically have adrenal glands that are thinner (often <3 mm wide) (Figure 15.12) than those animals with normal adrenal gland function. However, this finding should be used with caution; the normal adrenal gland is difficult to image and if not imaged completely, the less experienced operator may assume that the adrenal glands are small. If the clinical presentation is suggestive of hypoadrenocorticism, adrenal gland function should be tested with an adrenocorticotrophic hormone stimulation test.
- Animals receiving corticosteroid supplementation can have adrenal glands that are difficult to visualize. One or both may be reduced in size and they may show an increase in echogenicity with a loss of corticomedullary differentiation.

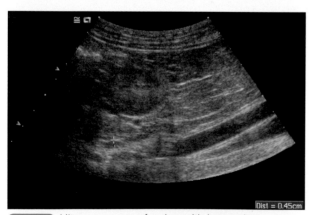

15.12 Ultrasonogram of a dog with hypoadreno-corticism; both adrenal glands were thin.

Other changes associated with adrenal gland disease

Canine hyperadrenocorticism
Most of the radiographic changes that are commonly seen are non-specific.

- Between 75% and 90% of affected animals will have radiographic evidence of mild, moderate or severe hepatomegaly; hepatic size is not an

indicator of duration or severity of the disease. Hepatomegaly is a contributor to the 'pot-bellied' appearance seen in >50% of affected dogs.
- The urinary bladder is often distended (even after the patient has urinated) (Figure 15.13) because relative bladder atony may develop, leaving the patient unable to empty their bladder completely.

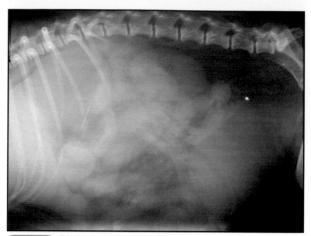

15.13 Right lateral abdominal radiograph of a dog with pituitary-dependent hyperadrenocorticism, showing mild hepatomegaly, a 'pot-bellied' appearance and moderate distension of the bladder.

- A very small number of cases will have radiopaque calcium phosphate or calcium oxalate calculi in the bladder.
- Pulmonary metastases are rarely seen at presentation, but this finding has important consequences in the further assessment and treatment of the case.
- Dystrophic calcification of soft tissues is infrequently seen. When identified, it is usually in the cutis and subcutis (calcinosis cutis; Figure 15.14), but may also occur in the renal pelves, gastric mucosa and/or the wall of the abdominal aorta and its branches. Generalized pulmonary interstitial mineralization may occasionally be visible and contributes to the generalized reticular interstitial pattern sometimes seen in affected dogs. Tracheal and mainstem bronchial wall calcification is a normal age-related finding and should not be used as an indicator of hyperadrenocorticism.

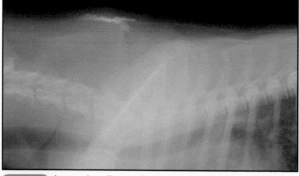

15.14 Lateral radiograph showing calcinosis cutis in the soft tissue structures dorsal to the cervicothoracic region of the spine.

- The hypercoagulable state that exists in dogs with hyperadrenocorticism predisposes them to the formation of pulmonary thromboemboli. This is a rare complication but one that should be considered if dyspnoea develops. Thoracic radiographs may be unremarkable or there may be blunting of the pulmonary arteries, areas of hyperlucent lung (Figure 15.15), localized alveolar infiltrates and/or pleural fluid.
- Although generalized osteopenia develops in dogs with hyperadrenocorticism, it is usually mild, may not be radiographically apparent and is of no clinical significance. Radiography of the skull to screen for a pituitary neoplasm is of no value at all.
- Non-traumatic rupture of an adrenal gland neoplasm may result in haemoretroperitoneum (Figure 15.16) or haemoabdomen, seen radiographically as a loss of serosal detail caused by fluid accumulation in the abdomen or retroperitoneum.

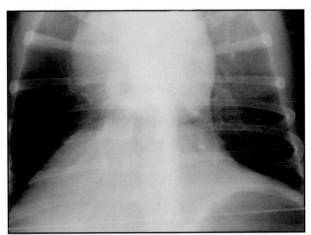

15.15 DV radiograph of the caudal thorax showing hyperlucent right caudal lung fields caused by pulmonary thromboembolism.

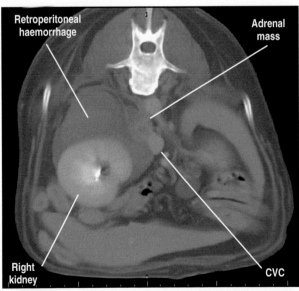

15.16 Contrast CT image showing haemorrhage within the retroperitoneal space dorsal to the right kidney. A 2 cm diameter adrenal gland carcinoma can be seen opposed to the right dorsal surface of the opacified caudal vena cava (CVC).

Feline hyperadrenocorticism

Feline hyperadrenocorticism is a rarely reported condition.

- As with dogs, cats may develop a 'pot-bellied' appearance as well as hepatomegaly.
- Unlike dogs, cats do not suffer from steroid hepatopathy and liver enlargement is usually caused by concurrent diabetes mellitus.

Hypoadrenocorticism

- Dogs with hypoadrenocorticism that present with clinical signs of hypovolaemia may show radiographic evidence of microcardia and pulmonary hypovascularity (Figure 15.17). On a lateral thoracic radiograph, the heart may appear short and narrow, and may show slight indentation over its cranioventral margin.
- The normal elongated cardiac silhouette in some deep-chested breeds should not be mistaken for microcardia.
- Concurrent reversible megaoesophagus is a rare finding in this condition.
- Abdominal radiographs are expected to be unremarkable.

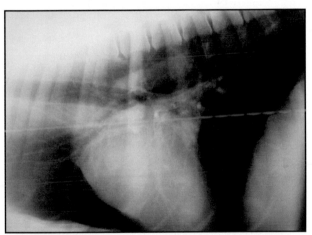

15.17 Lateral thoracic radiograph demonstrating microcardia and hypovascular lung fields, which may be evident in dogs with hypoadrenocorticism.

Phaeochromocytoma

Phaeochromocytoma is a malignant neoplasm of the adrenal gland medulla. Animals may present with clinical signs referable to a functional neoplasm, they may have signs associated with a large space-occupying mass and/or metastatic disease, or the neoplasm may be an incidental finding. A relatively large number of dogs with this type of neoplasm present with clinical signs referable to other diseases, including unrelated neoplasms elsewhere, diabetes mellitus, hyperadrenocorticism, hepatic disease and renal disease.

Abdominal radiographic findings can be quite variable.

- In 25–56% of cases the neoplasm is large enough to be visualized and approximately 10% show mineralization of the mass.

- Other findings may include hepatomegaly, ascites and renal displacement.
- Thoracic radiography detects pulmonary metastases in approximately 10% of cases.
- Mild left-sided cardiac enlargement caused by systemic hypertension may be seen.
- Non-traumatic rupture of a phaeochromocytoma results in haemorrhage within the retroperitoneum or peritoneum.

Feline primary hyperaldosteronism

Feline primary hyperaldosteronism (Conn's syndrome) is a condition caused by unilateral or bilateral adrenal gland neoplasia. Affected cats may present with hypokalaemia and clinical signs of polymyopathy. There are no specific radiographic findings that confirm this condition; however, in the appropriate clinical scenario, this condition should be considered as a differential diagnosis if an abdominal radiograph identifies a soft tissue mass in the cranial retroperitoneal space. Diagnosis is much more likely to be made ultrasonographically (Figure 15.18).

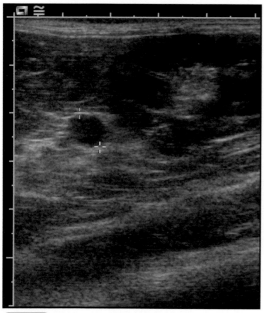

15.18 Ultrasonogram of an adrenal gland mass in a cat with primary hyperaldosteronism.

References and further reading

Ash RA, Harvey AM and Tasker S (2005) Primary hyperaldosteronism in the cat: a series of 13 cases. *Journal of Feline Medicine and Surgery* **7**, 173–182

Barthez PY, Marks SL, Woo J, *et al.* (1997) Pheochromocytoma in dogs: 61 cases (1984–1995). *Journal of Veterinary Internal Medicine* **11**, 272–278

Barthez PY, Nyland TG and Feldman EC (1998) Ultrasonography of the adrenal glands in the dog, cat, and ferret. *Veterinary Clinics of North America: Small Animal Practice* **28**, 869–885

Berry CR, Hawkins EC, Hurley KJ, *et al.* (2000) Frequency of pulmonary mineralization and hypoxemia in 21 dogs with pituitary-dependent hyperadrenocorticism. *Journal of Veterinary Internal Medicine* **14**, 151–156

Feldman EC and Nelson RW (2004) Canine Hyperadrenocorticism. In: *Canine and Feline Endocrinology and Reproduction, 3rd edn,* ed. EC Feldman and RW Nelson, pp. 283–288. Saunders, Missouri

Feldman EC and Nelson RW (2004) Canine Hypoadrenocorticism. In: *Canine and Feline Endocrinology and Reproduction, 3rd edn,* ed. EC Feldman and RW Nelson, pp. 320–325. Saunders, Missouri

Feldman EC and Nelson RW (2004) Hyperadrenocorticism in Cats. In: *Canine and Feline Endocrinology and Reproduction, 3rd edn,* ed. EC Feldman and RW Nelson, pp. 379–381. Saunders, Missouri

Feldman EC and Nelson RW (2004) Hypoadrenocorticism in cats. In: *Canine and Feline Endocrinology and Reproduction, 3rd edn,* ed. EC Feldman and RW Nelson, p. 416. Saunders, Missouri

Feldman EC and Nelson RW (2004) Pheochromocytoma and Multiple Endocrine Neoplasia. In: *Canine and Feline Endocrinology and Reproduction, 3rd edn,* ed. EC Feldman and RW Nelson, pp. 447–450. Saunders, Missouri

Huntley K, Frazer J, Gibbs C, *et al.* (1982) The radiological features of canine Cushing's syndrome: a review of forty-eight cases. *Journal of Small Animal Practice* **23**, 369–380

Llabrés-Díaz FJ and Dennis R (2003) Magnetic resonance imaging of the presumed normal canine adrenal glands. *Veterinary Radiology and Ultrasound* **44**, 5–19

Locke-Bohannon LG and Mauldin GE (2001) Canine pheochromocytoma: diagnosis and management. *Compendium on Continuing Education for the Practicing Veterinarian* **23**, 807–814

Mantis P, Lamb CR, Witt AL, *et al.* (2003) Changes in ultrasonographic appearance of adrenal glands in dogs with pituitary-dependent hyperadrenocorticism treated with Trilostane. *Veterinary Radiology and Ultrasound* **44**, 682–685

Zimmer C, Horauf A and Reusch C (2000) Ultrasonographic examination of the adrenal gland and evaluation of the hypophyseal-adrenal axis in 20 cats. *Journal of Small Animal Practice* **41**, 156–160

16

The kidneys and ureters

Martha Moon Larson

Introduction

Plain radiographic evaluation of the feline and canine kidneys is limited, but renal size, shape and opacity may be adequately assessed. Surrounding retroperitoneal fat is necessary for visualization because the more radiolucent fat contrasts with the renal soft tissue silhouette and separates it from adjacent viscera. Visualization of the kidneys in a thin patient, or in patients with retroperitoneal fluid, is nearly impossible because of lack of contrast. In many patients, superimposition of intestinal gas or faecal material prevents complete evaluation of the kidneys.

Normal radiographic anatomy

In the dog, the kidneys are bean-shaped or elongated ovals (Figure 16.1). The right kidney is located more cranially, usually at the level of T12 to L1. The 13th rib typically crosses the cranial pole. Visualization of the right kidney is often poor owing to silhouetting with the caudate liver lobe, as well as superimposed gastric and intestinal gas and colonic faecal material. The left kidney is located more caudally, typically at the level of L1–L3, and is more consistently visualized.

On lateral views, the kidneys are located dorsally within the retroperitoneal space. Typically, the cranial pole of the right kidney is superimposed on the gastric fundus and the proximal extremity of the spleen. The caudal pole of the right kidney usually overlaps the cranial pole of the left kidney, and the right lateral abdominal radiograph shows greater longitudinal separation of the kidneys. Large amounts of retroperitoneal fat sometimes lead to a more vertical orientation of the kidney on lateral views.

Radiographic visualization of the kidneys in the cat is more consistent than in the dog. The kidneys are typically located between L1 and L4, and have a more rounded, ovoid shape (Figure 16.2). The right kidney may be more cranial or at the same level as the left kidney.

Ventrodorsal (VD) radiographs are best used to assess renal size in dogs and cats, because lateral views can result in renal superimposition, rotation and some disproportionate magnification of the kidneys. The cranial–caudal dimension (length) of the kidney is compared with the cranial–caudal dimension of the second lumbar vertebral body. Renal length in the dog ranges from 2.5–3.5 times the length of L2 (Figure

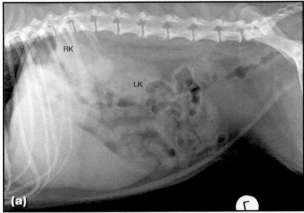

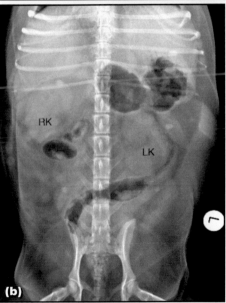

16.1 **(a)** Left lateral view of the canine abdomen. The right kidney (RK) is located slightly cranial to the left kidney (LK) in the retroperitoneal space. The caudal pole of the right kidney is superimposed on the cranial pole of the left kidney. Hepatomegaly is present. **(b)** VD view of the canine abdomen. The 13th rib crosses the cranial pole of the right kidney. The left kidney is located slightly more caudally, adjacent to L2–L4. Superimposed small opacities represent nipple shadows.

16.3). Early reports of feline renal measurements suggested that the normal kidney length was 2.4–3 times the length of L2. However, later reports state that smaller kidneys (1.9–2.6 times the length of L2) may be present in older cats without signs of renal disease. This continues to be the subject of mild

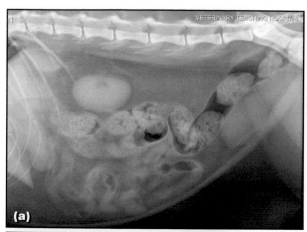

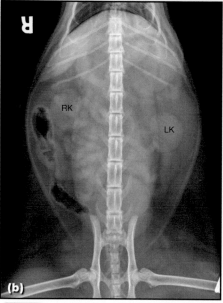

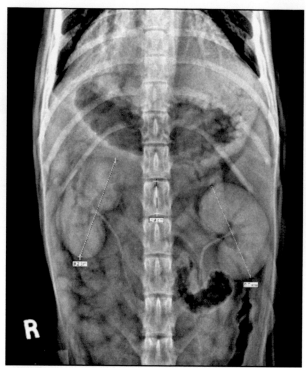

16.3   The cranial–caudal dimension of the left kidney is compared with the cranial–caudal length of L2. This kidney measures approximately 3.5 times the length of L2.

16.2   **(a)** Left lateral view of the feline abdomen. The kidneys are superimposed and surrounded by retroperitoneal fat. A focal area of fat opacity is present at the superimposed renal hilus. **(b)** VD view of the feline abdomen. The left kidney (LK) is adjacent to L3 and L4, and is well visualized. The right kidney (RK) is slightly cranial to the left kidney and is less well visualized owing to superimposed small bowel loops.

controversy, because 'without clinical signs' is not necessarily the same as 'without histological evidence of disease'. Utilization of 2.4 times the length of L2 as the lower limit of normal may result in greater sensitivity for the detection of chronic renal changes, or a decrease in specificity. Intact cats tend to have larger kidneys than neutered cats: for neutered cats the range is 1.9–2.6 times the length of L2; and for intact cats the range is 2.1–3.2 times the length of L2.

The kidneys should be of homogenous soft tissue opacity, although the feline renal pelvic area can appear as a focal, slightly more radiolucent space because of fat deposition (see Figure 16.2). Mineral opacity within the renal parenchyma is not normal, although it may be incidental. Gas in the kidney is most commonly iatrogenic, attributable to retrograde extension of air into the ureters and renal collecting system during double-contrast studies or pneumocystography. Rarely, gas may be produced by bacteria *in situ* or may reflux from the ureter.

The ureters are not normally visualized on plain abdominal radiographs owing to their small size. On rare occasions, the ureters may be seen as thin, linear soft tissue opacities running caudally through the retroperitoneal space in dogs and cats with large amounts of retroperitoneal fat. It is important not to mistake the end-on deep circumflex iliac artery, as seen in the dorsocaudal abdomen on the lateral view, for a ureteral calculus.

Incomplete visualization of the kidneys on plain abdominal radiographs is not uncommon, but does necessitate additional imaging procedures. Contrast studies or alternative imaging techniques such as ultrasonography, computed tomography (CT), magnetic resonance imaging (MRI) or nuclear scintigraphy will add information regarding renal size, shape, internal architecture or function.

Contrast radiography

Excretory urography

The most commonly performed radiographic contrast procedure for renal evaluation is the excretory urogram. Iodinated contrast medium is administered intravenously at a typical dose of 600–700 mg iodine/kg, and is then followed as it is taken up, and excreted, by the kidneys. An excretory urogram study enhances the evaluation of renal size and shape, and allows visualization of the contrast medium-filled renal pelvis, diverticula (pelvic recesses), ureters and bladder. In addition, the excretory urogram provides a crude assessment of renal function, although only 5% of renal function is necessary for excretion of iodinated contrast media. Excretory urography is unable to provide differentiation between solid and cystic renal masses.

Indications for an excretory urogram include:

- Haematuria
- Urinary incontinence (suspected ectopic ureter)
- Uroabdomen (suspected ruptured kidney, ureter or bladder)
- Retroperitoneal fluid
- Dorsal abdominal mass
- Evaluation of renal size, shape or location.

Contraindications for an excretory urogram are:

- Anuria
- Dehydration
- Known hypersensitivity to iodinated contrast media.

Intravenous administration of ionic iodinated contrast agents (meglumine diatrizoate, meglumine/ sodium diatrizoate, meglumine iothalamate) is safe in the vast majority of patients, but both mild and potentially severe reactions can occur, primarily because of the hypertonicity of the contrast agent. Reactions are usually mild and self-limiting (nausea, hives, vomiting), although rarely pulmonary oedema and cardiac arrest can occur. Contrast medium-induced nephrotoxicity has been well studied in human patients, and renal insufficiency has been identified as a major risk factor, although the incidence and severity have recently become somewhat controversial. Contrast medium reactions are much less frequent when using a non-ionic agent (such as iohexol or iopamidol) compared with an ionic contrast agent, owing to the lower osmolality. Non-ionic contrast agents, although considerably more expensive, should be considered in patients with pre-existing renal disease.

The three contraindications for an excretory urogram are dehydration, anuria and known iodine contrast medium sensitivity. Dehydration is the most common contraindication to the administration of intravenous contrast agents, and the patient should be stabilized and well hydrated prior to any studies. Anuria, associated with severe nephritis, toxicity or trauma, is an absolute contraindication. Determination of anuria may be difficult unless urine output is closely monitored over a period of hours. Contrast medium-induced renal failure should be considered when a good initial nephrogram is followed by increasing or persistent renal opacity and a delayed pyelogram.

Technique
Food should be withheld from the patient for at least 12 hours prior to an elective excretory urogram, although water should be available at all times. Again, dehydration is a contraindication for intravenous contrast medium administration. Cleansing enemas should be performed at least 2 hours prior to the procedure, thus allowing time for the colon to be free of both faeces and gas. Lateral and VD plain abdominal radiographs must be taken prior to contrast medium administration to check for remaining faecal material and to assess the urogenital system. Small calculi that are visible on plain abdominal radiographs may be obscured by the contrast medium. Urinalysis and culture should be performed prior to contrast medium administration as the agent may affect the measurement of specific gravity and may inhibit the growth of some bacteria. Urinalysis results are not accurate for at least 24 hours after contrast medium administration.

For an elective excretory urogram, general anaesthesia may be used to minimize restraint of the patient and to decrease the number of repeat films resulting from poor patient compliance. However, hypotension secondary to sedation/anaesthesia may predispose the patient to the negative effects of the contrast agent.

The contrast agent is administered intravenously as a bolus, at a dose of 600–700 mg iodine/kg bodyweight. The intravenous catheter should be left in place for the duration of the study in case adverse reactions occur. The patient should remain in dorsal recumbency throughout the early phase of the excretory urogram, until the ureterogram phase is reached or a lesion needs to be evaluated with lateral views. VD views are taken immediately post-injection (at 5 seconds) and then at 1, 5, 20 and 40 minutes post-injection. Lateral and oblique VD views may be taken 5–10 minutes post-injection for visualization of the individual ureters. The timing and views are fairly flexible, although the renal silhouette is most consistently visualized during the nephrogram phase, from 5 seconds to 5 minutes post-injection, the renal pelvis at 10 and 20 minutes post-injection, the ureters at 5, 10 and 20 minutes post-injection, and the bladder at 40 minutes post-injection.

The excretory urogram may be inadequate for a true positive-contrast cystogram, as the contrast medium will become diluted with residual urine and the bladder may not be well distended with contrast medium. However, it may be used as a substitute if direct bladder catheterization is not possible.

Radiological findings
The nephrogram is the initial phase of the excretory urogram, and occurs when contrast medium is present in the terminal glomerular renal vessels (vascular nephrogram) and the renal tubules (tubular nephrogram). During this phase (peak opacity: 10–30 seconds) the kidneys have a homogenous increased opacity. In some normal animals, there may be a more pronounced opacity in the renal cortex relative to the medulla (Figure 16.4). The intensity and duration of the opacity of the kidneys in the nephrogram phase depends on the dose of intravenous contrast agent, renal perfusion, glomerular filtration of the contrast medium, tubular resorption of water and the patency of the renal outflow tract. The nephrogram phase usually lasts for approximately 2 minutes; it then starts to fade as the pyelogram phase becomes apparent. During this second phase, opacification of the renal pelvis, diverticula and ureter occurs following concentration and excretion of the contrast medium by the renal tubules and collecting ducts. The pyelogram phase may last for 2 or more hours after contrast medium injection.

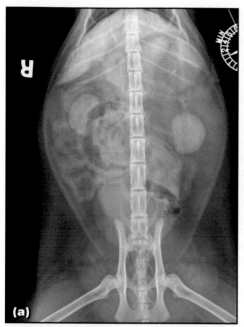

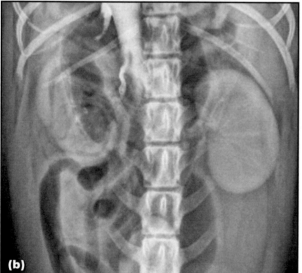

16.4 **(a)** VD view of a normal feline abdomen taken 1 minute following intravenous contrast medium injection. A uniform nephrogram is present bilaterally. **(b)** VD view of a normal canine abdomen taken immediately after intravenous contrast medium injection. There is a more pronounced opacity in the renal cortex relative to the medulla during this nephrogram phase.

The normal contrast medium-filled renal pelvis is a well defined, narrow curvilinear structure at the renal hilus, measuring ≤2 mm in width (Figure 16.5). Diverticula appear as paired linear 'spikes' extending towards the periphery and measure ≤1 mm in width. In some normal dogs, the diverticula are not well defined after contrast medium injection. This is considered a normal variation as long as the renal pelvis and proximal ureter are normal in size and shape. Abdominal compression may be used to obstruct the distal ureters partially, resulting in better diverticular filling and visualization, although this technique is not used by the author. The diverticula are often more prominent in the cat, although normal measurements for the feline diverticula and pelvis have not been reported.

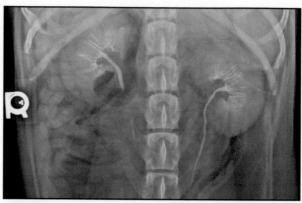

16.5 VD view of a normal canine abdomen taken 10 minutes after intravenous contrast medium injection. A normal contrast medium-filled renal pelvis and diverticula are present bilaterally. Both ureters are also visualized. Gaps in the contrast medium-filled ureters are caused by ureteral peristalsis.

Contrast medium-filled ureters are visualized descending caudally towards the bladder trigone (Figure 16.6). Ureteral diameter is inconsistent owing to intermittent ureteral peristalsis. Normal proximal

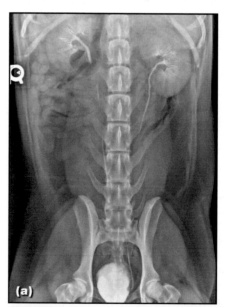

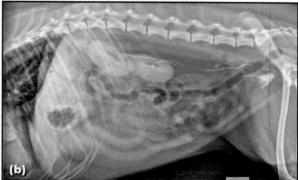

16.6 **(a)** VD view of a normal canine abdomen taken 10 minutes after intravenous contrast medium administration. The ureters are visualized extending caudally and entering the caudodorsal aspect of the bladder. **(b)** Lateral view of a normal canine abdomen taken 3 minutes after intravenous contrast medium administration. The ureters are visible coursing caudally to the minimally distended bladder.

ureteral width is 2–3 mm. The terminal portions of the ureters make a short cranial diversion before entering the bladder at the cranial border of the trigone.

The pattern and extent of changes in opacity in the nephrogram and pyelogram phases of the excretory urogram must be followed carefully, as several factors can affect the appearance. Normally, the nephrogram should have a phase of intense uniform opacity, followed by a gradual decrease in opacity during the next 1–3 minutes as the pyelogram phase takes over.

- A nephrogram that is poor initially and then fades immediately usually indicates an insufficient dose of contrast medium or primary polyuric renal failure.
- A poor initial nephrogram followed by persistent opacity may indicate severe generalized renal disease.
- If the initially poor nephrogram is followed by increasing opacity, prior systemic hypotension, acute extrarenal obstruction or renal ischaemia may be the cause.
- A good initial nephrogram followed by persistent or increasing opacity may indicate hypotension or renal failure induced by the contrast medium itself (Figure 16.7), acute renal tubular necrosis or acute renal obstruction.
- The opacity of the pyelogram phase may be decreased in the face of renal failure, as a result of increased urine volume and decreased concentrating ability.

The overall appearance of the contrast medium-filled renal pelvis, diverticula and ureters should be examined closely because changes in the normal structure can aid in the diagnosis of several renal diseases.

Percutaneous antegrade positive-contrast pyelography

Percutaneous positive-contrast pyelography introduces the contrast agent directly into the renal pelvis, thus avoiding the adverse reactions that may occur if the contrast medium is administered systemically. Positive-contrast pyelography is not limited by poor renal function and allows consistent visualization of the contrast medium-filled renal pelvis and ureter. Pelvic and ureteral size, shape, diameter and patency can be evaluated (Figure 16.8). This procedure is very useful to test the patency of a ureter, especially in cases of concurrent unilateral hydronephrosis and hydroureter, and to determine the degree and location of any ureteral obstruction.

A 25-gauge spinal needle is inserted through a thin portion of the renal cortex into the dilated pelvis under ultrasound guidance. The view and exact angle used will vary, depending on patient factors. The large hilar and interlobar vessels should be avoided. A volume of urine is removed, the amount that can be removed safely depending on the degree of hydronephrosis, and the equivalent of one half of the removed volume of ionic or non-ionic iodinated contrast agent is slowly introduced. Pelvic and ureteral

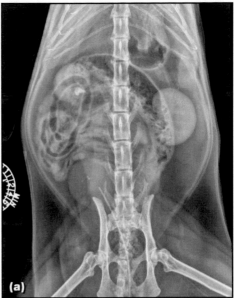

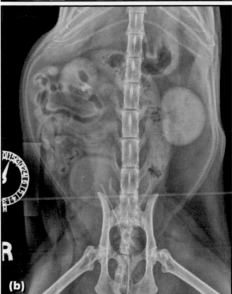

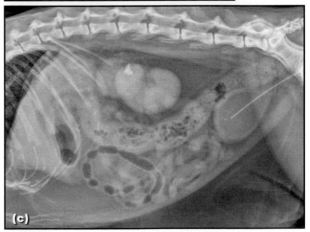

16.7 **(a)** VD view of a feline abdomen taken 1 minute after intravenous contrast medium administration. A normal nephrogram is present. A radiopaque calculus is present in the right renal pelvis. **(b)** VD and **(c)** lateral views taken 15 minutes later. A persistent nephrogram is present and no contrast medium is visible in the renal pelvis, ureters or bladder lumen (contrast medium is visible enhancing the bladder wall). Contrast medium-induced renal failure was diagnosed.

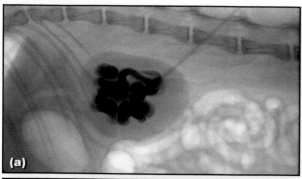

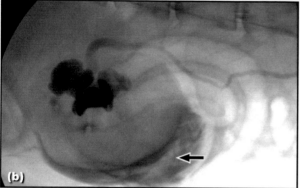

16.8 **(a)** Fluoroscopic image of the left kidney taken immediately after ultrasound-guided contrast medium injection directly into the dilated renal pelvis. The renal pelvis and dilated diverticula are visible. **(b)** Fluoroscopic image of the left kidney taken 1 minute after injection of contrast medium into the renal pelvis. Some positive contrast medium has leaked into the perirenal area (arrowed).

filling is demonstrated by fluoroscopy, as available, followed by VD and lateral abdominal radiographs. The most common complications are leakage of contrast medium from the renal pelvis secondary to inadvertent needle puncture, and capsular leakage at the site of needle insertion. Subcapsular haemorrhage and haemorrhage into the renal pelvis can be serious complications.

Retrograde urethrography and vaginourethrography are additional contrast procedures that can be used to evaluate the termination sites of ureters suspected of being ectopic (see Chapter 17).

Ultrasonography

Ultrasonography of the kidneys provides excellent visualization of renal size, shape and internal architecture, especially when conditions prevent adequate radiographic evaluation. Whilst ultrasound examination using Doppler techniques can provide information regarding renal perfusion, renal function cannot be assessed.

Technique

The kidneys may be imaged from either a lateral or ventral (with the patient in dorsal recumbency) abdominal window. The right kidney is often more difficult to view in the dog as it lies partially under the ribcage and may be obscured by bowel gas. It is especially difficult to image in deep-chested or large breeds of dog. Right lateral intercostal approaches from the 11th and 12th intercostal spaces are often needed for complete visualization of the right kidney in these dogs. The left kidney is easier to image consistently because of its more caudal location. The spleen often lies ventral to the left kidney and may be used as an acoustic window for the ventral approach. The kidneys are more caudally located in cats and are easier to image consistently. Longitudinal and transverse scans of the entire kidney should be performed. In cats and small dogs, a ≥7.5 MHz transducer works well for both kidneys. In larger dogs, a 5.0 MHz probe may be needed for the right kidney. The ≥7.5 MHz probe may be adequate for the left kidney even in large dogs because of the more superficial location.

Additional ultrasonography modalities can also be used with specific diseases. Doppler ultrasonography can be used to verify vascular structures and may help to differentiate a hydroureter from the surrounding normal vasculature. Acute infarction results in a lack of Doppler signal in the affected interlobar or interlobular vessels. More chronic-appearing infarcts (wedge-shaped hyperechoic regions) may be reperfused.

Contrast ultrasonography has been used to provide a more global assessment of renal perfusion. Normal dogs and cats have uniform cortical enhancement followed by less intense medullary enhancement. Many lesions that are occult on greyscale ultrasonography, including infarction and metastatic neoplasia, are easily demonstrated as poorly perfused lesions using contrast enhancement (Figure 16.9).

Normal ultrasonographic anatomy

The renal capsule is a thin, linear hyperechoic structure, but is usually not seen around the entire kidney (Figure 16.10). The renal cortex is uniformly echoic, usually slightly hypo- or isoechoic compared with the liver. The right kidney is easily compared with the caudate liver lobe in dogs. However, in some normal obese cats, the renal cortex may be hyperechoic to the liver. This is likely to be due to fat vacuoles in the cortical–tubular epithelium. The renal cortex should be hypoechoic to the spleen, using the left kidney for comparison.

There should be a clear demarcation between the cortex and medulla. The renal medulla is very hypoechoic and is separated into compartments by linear hyperechoic interlobar vessels and diverticula, which radiate from the renal sinus. The renal sinus is hyperechoic owing to peripelvic fat and dense fibrous connective tissue, and is centrally located at the renal hilus. The renal pelvis is a potential space and not usually visualized. However, with high-frequency transducers, a narrow anechoic fissure, 1–2 mm wide, may be seen at the renal hilus (Figure 16.11). The pelvis may also be slightly dilated in some normal patients secondary to physiological (diuresis) or

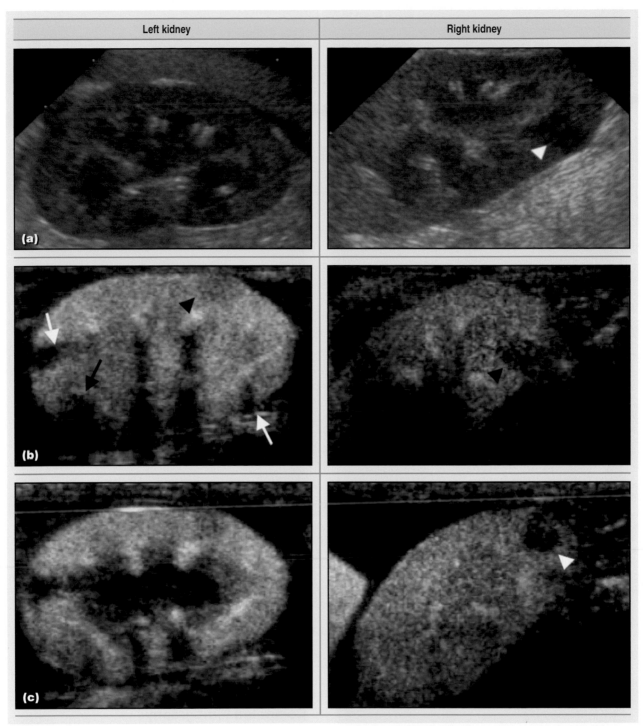

Left kidney	Right kidney

16.9 **(a)** Greyscale and **(b,c)** contrast ultrasonograms of the left and right kidneys with metastatic histiocytic sarcoma. (a) On the greyscale image the left kidney appeared normal but a hypoechoic nodule was seen in the caudal pole of the right kidney (arrowhead). (b) Fifteen seconds after administration of intravenous contrast medium, additional poorly perfused wedge-shaped lesions were seen in the left kidney (white arrows) and discrete nodule-shaped lesions were seen in the right (black arrowhead) and left (black arrowhead and black arrow) kidneys. The lesion in the right kidney corresponded to the lesion seen on the greyscale image. (c) Thirty seconds after contrast administration the same lesions were still seen in the left kidney and an additional lesion was seen in the right kidney (arrowhead).

pathological polyuria. High-intensity echoes can be seen at the renal periphery, the corticomedullary interface and in the renal sinus, and are produced by reflective fibrous or fat interfaces.

Kidney measurements in cats have been reported to range from 3.0–4.3 cm, with the cortex measuring 2–5 mm in thickness. In dogs, because of breed variation, renal measurements range from 3–10 cm, with cortical thickness measuring 3–8 mm. The ureters are not normally visualized.

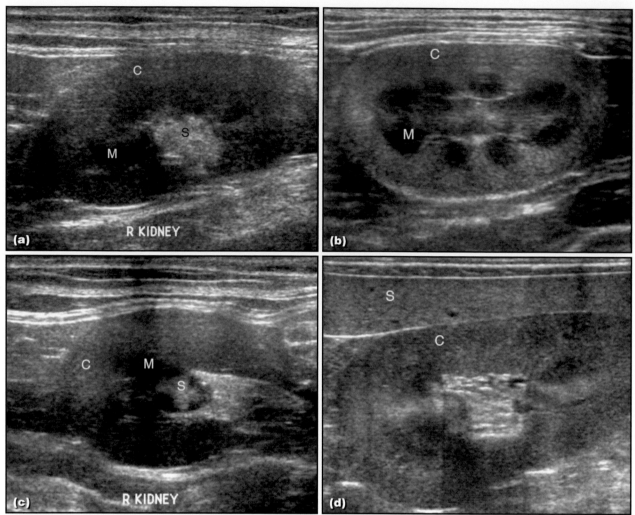

16.10 **(a)** Longitudinal ultrasonogram of the right kidney taken at the renal hilus. The renal sinus is a bright, echogenic structure at the centre of the kidney. Cranial is to the left and ventral is at the top of the image. **(b)** Longitudinal ultrasonogram of the right kidney taken lateral to the renal hilus. The hypoechoic medullary portions of the kidney are more prominent and are separated by echogenic diverticula and interlobar vessels. Cranial is to the left and ventral is at the top of the image. **(c)** Transverse ultrasonogram of the right kidney taken at the level of the renal hilus. Ventral is at the top of the image and right is on the left side. **(d)** Longitudinal ultrasonogram of the spleen and left kidney. The spleen is hyperechoic compared with the renal cortex. C = Cortex; M = Medulla; S = Renal sinus.

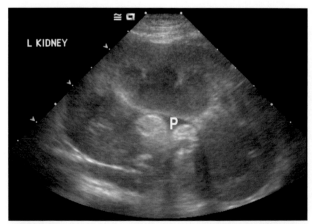

16.11 Longitudinal ultrasonogram of the left kidney. The renal pelvis (P) is visualized as a thin anechoic slit at the renal hilus. Cranial is to the left and ventral is at the top of the image.

Additional imaging modalities

Computed tomography

Computed tomography (CT) offers some advantages in renal and ureteral imaging. The entire urinary tract can be evaluated accurately owing to lack of superimposition of the adjacent viscera and skeletal structures, and the ability to perform multiplanar and 3D reconstructions facilitates diagnosis. The normal kidneys appear as homogenous soft tissue structures surrounded by retroperitoneal fat. Intravenous contrast medium provides parenchymal enhancement of the kidney and hyperattenuating contrast agent within the renal pelvis, diverticula, ureters and bladder (Figure 16.12).

CT appears to be able to detect lower concentrations of contrast medium in the renal collecting system than conventional radiography,

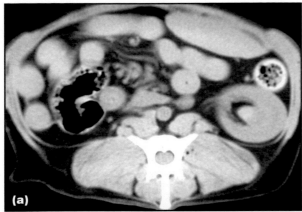

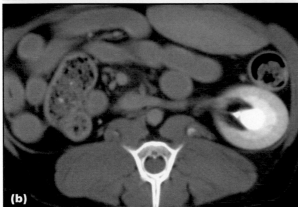

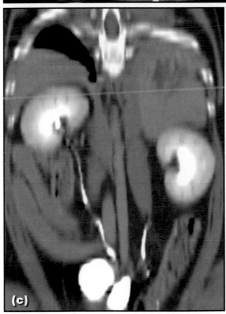

Magnetic resonance imaging

Magnetic resonance imaging (MRI) is useful in the diagnosis of renal disorders and can be used as a complementary imaging modality, in addition to CT and ultrasonography. The appearance of the kidneys following administration of intravenous contrast medium (gadolinium) is similar to the phases of an excretory urogram. Disadvantages of MRI include the expense of the equipment, the need for anaesthesia and the artefacts caused by respiratory and peristaltic motion.

Renal scintigraphy

Renal scintigraphy provides rapid, non-invasive assessment of renal function and morphology. The percentage of an injected dose of [99m]Technetium (Tc)-DTPA (diethylene triamine penta-acetic acid) excreted by the kidneys over a short time period is a good estimate of glomerular filtration rate, and provides information about both global and individual kidney function. This procedure is used commonly to evaluate contralateral renal function prior to nephrectomy, and can be used serially to evaluate the progression of disease and response to therapy.

Renal diseases

Abnormal renal size

Normal size does not rule out renal disease. Many parenchymal diseases, such as toxicity, amyloidosis, glomerulonephritis, acute nephritis and pyelonephritis, may be present without a marked change in renal size.

Increase in size

Enlarged kidneys (>3.5 times the length of the L2 vertebral body in dogs; >3.0 times the length of the L2 vertebral body in cats) may be diagnosed on plain abdominal radiographs. When severe, unilateral or bilateral renomegaly results in ventral, caudal and lateral displacement of the abdominal viscera (Figure 16.13). Enlarged kidneys may be associated with primary parenchymal disorders, pericapsular disease or collecting system dilatation. Typically, additional imaging studies, such as intravenous contrast or ultrasound examinations, are necessary to determine the aetiology of the renomegaly.

Differential diagnoses for smoothly enlarged kidneys include:

* Amyloidosis (usually mild enlargement)
* Compensatory hypertrophy
* Renal hypertrophy secondary to portosystemic shunts (usually mild; more often seen in dogs than in cats)
* Lymphosarcoma
* Hydronephrosis
* Perinephric pseudocyst
* Acromegaly
* Acute nephritis
* Toxicity
* Acute renal failure (usually mild enlargement).

16.12 **(a)** Pre-contrast and **(b)** post-contrast transverse CT scans of a normal dog showing the left renal pelvis. **(c)** Post-contrast dorsal planar reconstruction CT image of a normal dog showing the left and right kidneys and ureters.

which may be helpful in patients with renal disease and poor concentrating ability. CT has been used in the diagnosis of ectopic ureters very effectively and may be the imaging modality of choice for this disease. Percutaneous positive-contrast pyelography can also be augmented with CT.

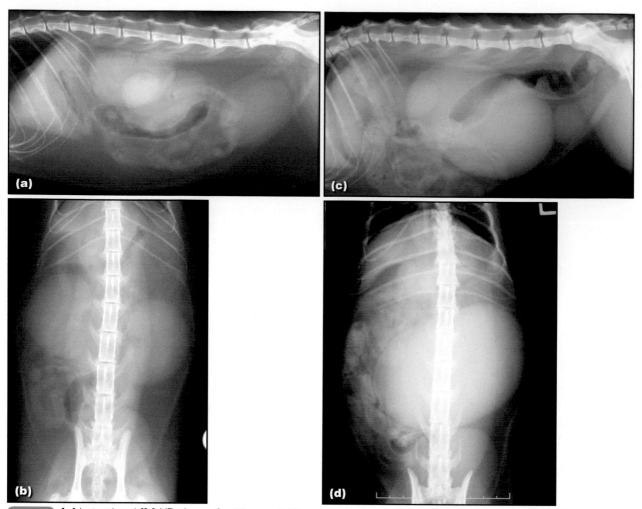

16.13 **(a)** Lateral and **(b)** VD views of a 10-year-old Domestic Shorthaired cat with renal lymphosarcoma. Both kidneys are symmetrically enlarged. There is ventral displacement of the abdominal viscera by the enlarged kidneys on the lateral view. **(c)** Lateral and **(d)** VD views of a 3-year-old Domestic Shorthaired cat with left-sided hydronephrosis. The left kidney is markedly enlarged, resulting in right-sided and ventral visceral displacement.

Differential diagnoses for enlarged, irregularly marginated kidneys include:

- Neoplasia, both primary and metastatic
- Focal renal cyst
- Polycystic kidney disease
- Feline infectious peritonitis
- Abscess/haematoma
- Renal cystadenoma.

Diffuse and focal parenchymal diseases cause variable changes in the nephrogram and pyelogram phases of the excretory urogram. The contrast study may be normal if renal function is sufficient and there is minimal architectural change. If renal function is poor, non-opacification of the nephrogram and/or pyelogram phase may occur (Figure 16.14). Differential diagnoses for enlarged, non-opacified kidneys include hydronephrosis, neoplasia, inflammation, severe cystic disease, renal trauma and renal vein thrombosis. Neoplastic masses, cysts, abscesses, infarcts and haematomas may result in focal or multifocal non-opacified disruptions of the normally uniform and homogenous nephrogram (Figure 16.15). With excretory urography alone, it is

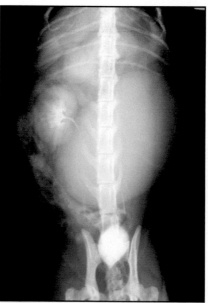

16.14 VD view of the cat in Figure 16.13cd taken 10 minutes after intravenous contrast medium administration. The hydronephrotic left kidney is non-functional and no pyelogram is present. No nephrogram was seen earlier in the study.

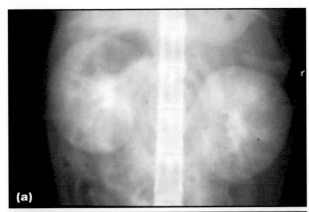

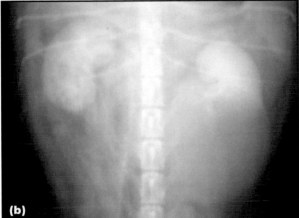

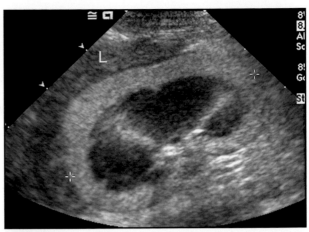

16.16 Longitudinal ultrasonogram of the right kidney in a dog with glomerulonephritis. The renal cortex is hyperechoic to the liver (L) and there is marked corticomedullary distinction. Cranial is to the left and ventral is at the top of the image.

16.15 **(a)** VD view of a 7-year-old Persian cat with polycystic kidney disease, taken 5 minutes after intravenous contrast medium administration. There are multiple poorly defined radiolucent filling defects within the renal silhouette where the renal cysts are located. **(b)** VD view of an 8-year-old mixed breed dog taken 2 minutes after intravenous contrast medium administration. A large non-opacified defect is present in the caudal pole of the left kidney. A large renal cortical cyst was diagnosed on ultrasound examination.

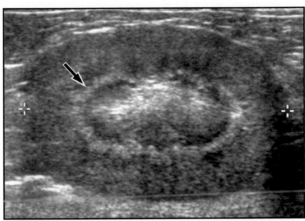

16.17 Longitudinal ultrasonogram of the left kidney in a normal dog. A hyperechoic rim (medullary rim sign) is present at the corticomedullary junction (arrowed).

not possible to determine whether a non-opacified kidney or kidney mass is solid or cystic. If mass lesions are adjacent to, or involve, the renal pelvis or diverticula, distortion or compression may be seen during the pyelogram phase.

The ultrasonographic appearance of diffuse parenchymal renal disease may be normal, but in many cases the cortex becomes hyperechoic with enhanced corticomedullary differentiation (Figure 16.16). This is a non-specific change but can occur with glomerulonephritis, interstitial nephritis, acute tubular necrosis, end-stage renal disease, lymphosarcoma, feline infectious peritonitis, hypercalcaemic nephropathy, pyelonephritis, congenital renal dysplasia and nephrocalcinosis. In progressive disease, the medullary areas may also increase in opacity, resulting in overall poor definition of the renal architecture. A medullary rim sign is a thin hyperechoic band in the outer medulla (Figure 16.17), which can be seen in both normal and diseased canine and feline kidneys on ultrasound examination, making its significance questionable. Due to the non-specific nature of increased cortical echogenicity, a biopsy is necessary for a more definitive diagnosis.

Acute renal failure secondary to ethylene glycol toxicity typically results in severely hyperechoic cortices. The medulla may also be affected. Renal hypertrophy secondary to loss of contralateral renal function or portosystemic shunts should appear normal in echogenicity and architecture. More severe generalized renomegaly can occur with diffuse neoplasia (lymphosarcoma) or feline infectious peritonitis. Renal margins may be smooth or irregular in outline with hyperechoic cortices. There is often a striking difference between the cortex and medulla. Lymphosarcoma occasionally results in hypoechoic cortices, or hypoechoic nodules or masses. A subcapsular hypoechoic rim or crescent surrounding the renal cortex has been reported to be an indication of renal lymphosarcoma, although it has also been seen with renal carcinoma and feline infectious peritonitis (Figure 16.18).

Enlarged, irregular kidneys may result from renal cysts, abscesses, haematomas or neoplastic disease. Polycystic kidney disease is a genetic disorder in which there is progressive displacement of normal renal tissue by multiple enlarging cysts; it is typically seen in Persian cats or Persian cross-breeds.

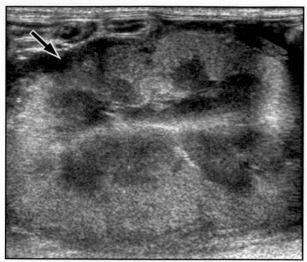

16.18 Longitudinal ultrasonogram of the left kidney in a 6-year-old Domestic Shorthaired cat with renal lymphosarcoma. The kidney is enlarged, irregular and has a hyperechoic cortex. A hypoechoic rim is present surrounding the renal cortex (arrowed). Cranial is to the left and ventral is at the top of the image.

Anechoic, variably sized thin-walled cysts, most with acoustic enhancement, are noted in the cortex and corticomedullary junction on ultrasound examination (Figure 16.19). Multiple tiny cysts may appear as a focal area of hyperechoic tissue. In dogs, focal or multifocal renal cortical cysts are considered to represent a benign change and, whilst they can be quite large, they are usually an incidental finding. However, polycystic kidney disease has been reported in Cairn and Bull Terriers. Cystadenocarcinomas in German Shepherd Dogs may appear as cystic, complex masses on ultrasound examination and are associated with dermatofibrosis.

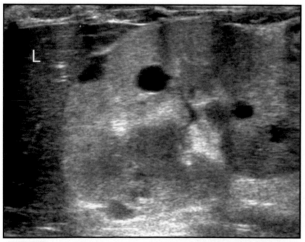

16.19 Longitudinal ultrasonogram of the right kidney in a 5-year-old Persian cat with polycystic kidney disease. Multiple anechoic cysts are present. Cranial is to the left and ventral is at the top of the image. L = Liver.

Renal abscesses and haematomas are rare, but can result in focal renal disease. Abscesses may occur secondary to adjacent infections or haematogenous spread of bacteria, and result in irregular renal enlargement. The ultrasonographic appearance of renal abscesses is variable, but a cavitated mass, often with thick, irregular walls, is common (Figure 16.20). Hyperechoic shadowing may be seen if gas is present within the abscess. Haematomas may be secondary to trauma, coagulopathy or renal biopsy, and can be located within the parenchyma (focal hyperechoic or hypoechoic areas) or in the subcapsular area. Haematomas may also occur within the renal pelvis, resulting in obstructive hydronephrosis. Abscesses and haematomas may both have an identical appearance to focal renal neoplasia.

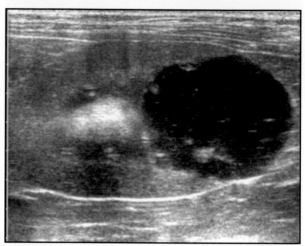

16.20 Longitudinal ultrasonogram of the left kidney in an 8-year-old Shetland Sheepdog. There is an irregular cystic mass in the caudal pole, containing some echogenic debris. A fine-needle aspirate of the mass revealed an abscess. Cranial is to the left and ventral is at the top of the image.

Whilst neoplasia (e.g. lymphosarcoma) may cause diffuse renomegaly, it can also cause focal or multifocal enlargement. Neoplasms of epithelial origin, such as carcinomas, are the most common primary renal neoplasm in the dog and typically result in a mass at either the cranial or caudal pole. Although these are usually unilateral, both kidneys can be affected. The neoplasm results in non-uniform opacification of the kidney in the area of the mass, and may distort or deviate the pelvis and diverticula (Figure 16.21). On ultrasound examination, a renal carcinoma may be hypoechoic, hyperechoic or complex, completely obliterating the normal renal architecture. Metastatic masses in the kidneys will also result in focal masses, either hyperechoic, hypoechoic (Figure 16.22) or isoechoic (see Figure 16.9). Haemangiosarcoma, osteosarcoma, melanoma, mast cell tumour and carcinoma of the lung, mammary gland and gastrointestinal tract have all been reported to metastasize to the kidneys. Transitional cell carcinoma may occur in the renal pelvis, resulting in disruption of the collecting system that is seen on ultrasound examination.

Renomegaly associated with subcapsular or perirenal disease typically results in smooth, generalized enlargement. However, subcapsular haematomas or abscesses can cause irregular borders. Perinephric (perirenal) pseudocysts have been reported most often in cats and result in focal fluid accumulation around one or both kidneys. These are not true cysts because they are characterized by a non-secretory

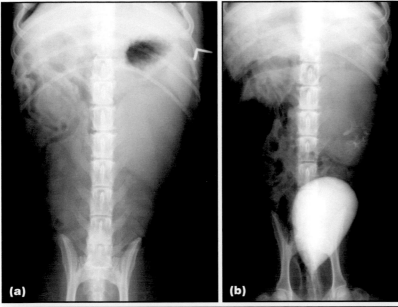

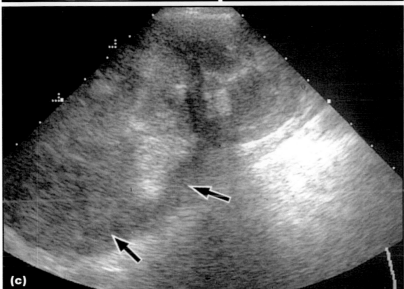

16.21 VD views of the abdomen in a 12-year-old Golden Retriever taken **(a)** before and **(b)** 20 minutes after intravenous contrast medium administration. The survey film shows an irregular, enlarged left kidney with a mass effect on the cranial pole. The pyelogram demonstrates distortion of the renal pelvis and the cranial pole mass. **(c)** Longitudinal ultrasonogram of the left kidney. A non-homogenous echogenic mass is present in the cranial pole (arrowed). The caudal pole is normal. Cranial is to the left and ventral is at the top of the image.

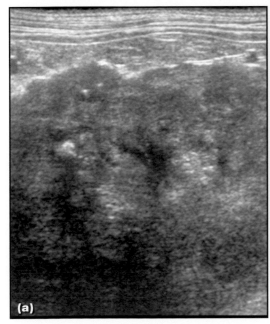

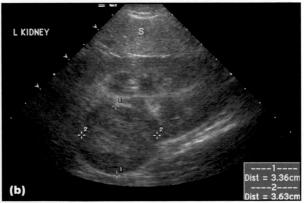

16.22 **(a)** Longitudinal ultrasonogram of the left kidney in a 12-year-old Schnauzer with renal carcinoma. The renal architecture is unrecognizable owing to replacement by neoplastic tissue. Cranial is to the left and ventral is at the top of the image. **(b)** Longitudinal ultrasonogram of the left kidney in a 10-year-old mixed breed dog with primary pulmonary carcinoma. A focal hypoechoic mass (between calipers) is present in the cranial pole. Metastatic carcinoma was diagnosed on fine-needle aspiration. Cranial is to the left and ventral is at the top of the image. S = Spleen.

epithelial lining. The fluid is most often a low protein transudate and the reason for its development is unknown. Intravenous contrast medium administration will demonstrate a small or normal sized kidney surrounded by a fluid opacity with smooth external borders. The opacity of the kidney depends on renal function and there is often concurrent renal disease. On ultrasound examination, the kidney is visible surrounded by anechoic fluid. Renal hyperechogenicity may be artefactual, resulting from the surrounding fluid (acoustic enhancement), or secondary to diffuse renal disease.

Decrease in size

Differential diagnoses for small, smoothly marginated kidneys include:

- Renal hypoplasia
- Amyloidosis
- End-stage renal disease; although the kidneys are usually irregular.

Differential diagnoses for small, irregularly marginated kidneys include:

- Chronic renal disease of numerous aetiologies (end-stage renal disease).

Small kidneys may be caused by congenital renal disease (which is present at birth), familial renal disease (which may result in chronic renal failure at a young age) or chronic renal disease of any acquired aetiology (Figure 16.23). Small kidneys secondary to chronic renal disease may be irregular in outline owing to cortical infarction. The appearance on an excretory urogram depends on renal function. Ultrasound examination of the affected kidneys typically shows small, irregular, hyperechoic kidneys with decreased corticomedullary distinction. Chronic infarction appears as a hyperechoic wedge-shaped lesion in the cortex, with the point of the infarct towards the renal hilus.

Diseases of the collecting system

Abnormalities of the collecting system (renal pelvis and diverticula) can occur secondary to inflammation (pyelonephritis) or obstruction (hydronephrosis). The abnormalities are best visualized with intravenous contrast medium studies or ultrasonography.

Pyelonephritis

Pyelonephritis (Figure 16.24) can result in mild pelvic dilatation (pyelectasia) along with blunted, poorly defined diverticula. The proximal ureter is often mildly dilated. Poor opacification may also be present, depending on renal function. Renal size may be normal or slightly enlarged with acute disease, whilst chronic pyelonephritis may result in decreased renal size. A normal excretory urogram does not rule out pyelonephritis.

Ultrasonographic changes associated with pyelonephritis, if present, reflect the changes in the collecting system seen on an excretory urogram. The pelvis is typically slightly dilated (dilatation to >3 mm is considered abnormal), as is the proximal ureter.

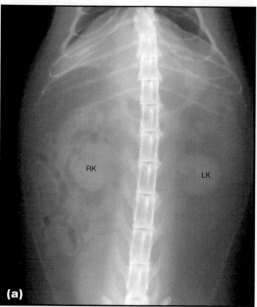

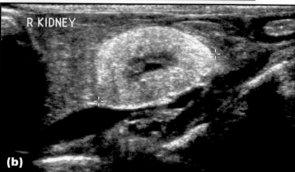

16.23 **(a)** VD view of a 10-year-old Domestic Shorthaired cat with chronic renal failure. The kidneys are small, measuring approximately the same as the length of the vertebral body of L2. LK = Left kidney; RK = Right kidney. **(b)** Longitudinal ultrasonogram of the right kidney of a 9-month-old Golden Retriever with congenital renal dysplasia. The kidney is small (approximately 2.5 cm) and hyperechoic, with poor renal architecture. Cranial is to the left and ventral is at the top of the image.

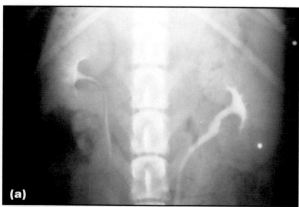

16.24 **(a)** VD view of a dog taken 20 minutes following intravenous contrast medium administration. The left renal pelvis is slightly dilated, the diverticula are poorly defined and blunted, and the proximal ureter is dilated. These findings are all consistent with pyelonephritis. The right kidney is normal. (continues) ▶

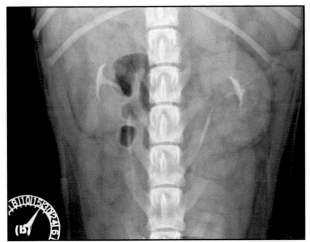

16.24 (continued) **(b)** VD view of a dog taken 20 minutes following intravenous contrast medium administration. Both renal pelves are slightly dilated with indistinct diverticula. These changes are consistent with bilateral pyelonephritis.

Hyperechoic renal cortices can occur with both acute and chronic pyelonephritis (Figure 16.25). Other reported changes attributable to pyelonephritis include: a hyperechoic line paralleling the renal sinus fat within the pelvis, proximal ureter or both; focal/multifocal hyperechoic or hypoechoic cortical echogenicities; focal/multifocal hyperechoic medullary echogenicities; and a poorly defined corticomedullary junction.

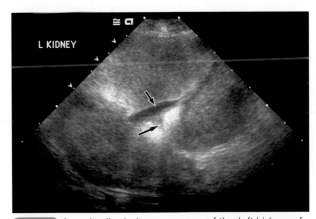

16.25 Longitudinal ultrasonogram of the left kidney of an 8-year-old Dobermann. The renal pelvis and proximal ureter are slightly dilated (arrowed), consistent with pyelonephritis. Cranial is to the left and ventral is at the top of the image.

Hydronephrosis

Hydronephrosis (Figure 16.26) results in smoothly enlarged kidneys (either unilateral or bilateral) on plain abdominal radiographs. Intravenous contrast medium administration demonstrates a contrast medium-filled dilated renal pelvis and diverticula, depending on renal function. In severe hydronephrosis, there may be only a small rim of cortical tissue surrounding the markedly dilated pelvis (see Figures 16.13 and 16.14). Ultrasonography provides excellent visualization of hydronephrosis. Anechoic fluid separates and replaces the centrally located echogenic renal sinus. Dilated diverticula may also be seen, unless the pelvis is severely dilated (Figure 16.26c). If

the ureter is also dilated, it should be followed caudally to determine the cause of obstruction. Common causes of obstructive hydronephrosis include: bladder trigone neoplasia; ureteral calculi; ureteral stricture secondary to trauma or chronic ureteritis; renal calculi; blood clots following renal biopsy; or combinations of these factors.

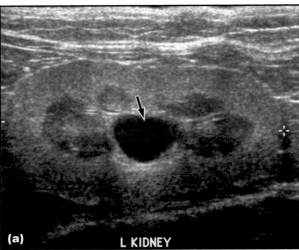

(a) L KIDNEY

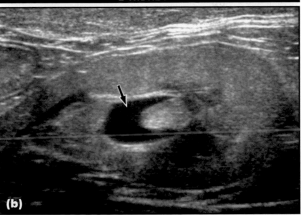

(b)

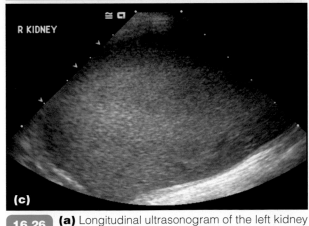

(c) R KIDNEY

16.26 **(a)** Longitudinal ultrasonogram of the left kidney in a cat with moderate hydronephrosis. The renal pelvis is dilated and anechoic (arrowed). Cranial is to the left and ventral is at the top of the image.
(b) Transverse ultrasonogram of the left kidney in the cat in (a). The renal pelvis (arrowed) is dilated and anechoic. Right is to the left and ventral is at the top of the image.
(c) Longitudinal ultrasonogram of the right kidney in a dog with severe hydronephrosis. The renal pelvis is completely dilated with echogenic fluid, with minimal renal parenchyma remaining. Cranial is to the left and ventral is at the top of the image.

Renal mineralization

The most common causes of mineralization include nephrocalcinosis and nephrolithiasis. Calculi may be located within the diverticula or pelvis, and may extend into the proximal ureter (Figure 16.27). Only radiopaque calculi (i.e. phosphates or oxalates) are visible on plain abdominal radiographs. Ultrasonography is able to detect both radiolucent and radiopaque calculi; a focal, very echogenic interface is noted, with distal shadowing (Figure 16.28). If the calculus is causing an obstruction, anechoic fluid will be visible dilating the affected portion.

Nephrocalcinosis is characterized by dystrophic parenchymal mineralization and may be difficult to differentiate from nephrolithiasis on either radiography or ultrasonography. Both conditions cause mineral opacities on radiographs and bright interfaces with shadowing on ultrasound examination. Faint linear mineralizations are often seen in the renal parenchyma, adjacent to the diverticula and renal crest; these are very common in older patients and of questionable significance. Unless there is urine dilatation of the affected segment, differentiation between renal crest peripelvic nephrocalcinosis and small pelvic nephrolithiasis may not be possible. Other sites of dystrophic mineralization include haematomas, cysts, abscesses, granulomas and neoplasms.

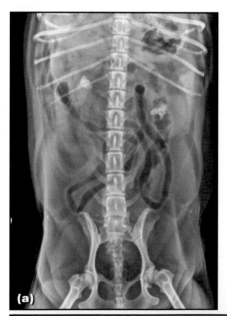

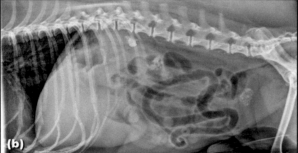

16.27 **(a)** VD and **(b)** lateral abdominal radiographs of a 7-year-old Schnauzer. Radiopaque calculi are visible in both renal pelves, extending into the proximal ureters. Multiple small radiopaque calculi are also present in the urinary bladder.

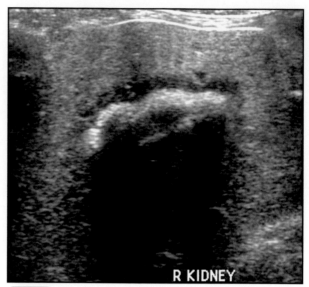

16.28 Longitudinal ultrasonogram of the left kidney in a dog with renal calculi. A curvilinear echogenic interface with distal shadowing is present.

Renal failure

Acute renal failure may result in free fluid in the retroperitoneal space, adjacent to the kidneys. This is often occult or subtle on radiography. Ultrasonographically, the volume of fluid may be only mild to moderate. The fluid may accumulate adjacent to a failing kidney with unilateral ureteral obstruction, or in a patient without systemic signs of renal failure (azotaemia). The amount of fluid does not correlate with the severity of the renal failure. Often the fluid extends into the peritoneal space. The pathogenesis may involve excess hydrostatic pressure or vasculitis of capsular vessels in the affected kidney.

Renal secondary hyperparathyroidism is a common complication of chronic kidney disease in both dogs and cats, and can manifest in the skeletal system with visible radiographic changes. The skull and mandible show the earliest and most dramatic changes, with marked demineralization (Figure 16.29). The teeth may appear much more opaque than the other

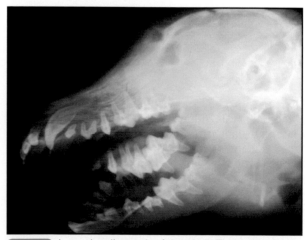

16.29 Lateral radiograph of the skull. The bone density in the skull is poor, with only the teeth showing any bone opacity. This dog had renal secondary hyperparathyroidism, which was secondary to congenital renal dysplasia.

structures of the skull because of severe mineral loss in the lamina dura. The changes are most marked and occur most rapidly in the immature patient. Metastatic calcification is an additional sequel of chronic renal disease and occurs when there is an elevated calcium:phosphate ratio. Mineralization is most prominent in the stomach (uraemic gastritis), arteries, joints and kidneys, although mineral opacities can also be seen in the myocardium, lungs and liver.

Ureteral diseases

Ureteral calculi

Ureteral calculi can often be visualized on plain abdominal radiographs (Figure 16.30), if the compo-

sition provides for sufficient radiopacity. Calcium oxalate calculi are the most common type of ureteral calculus in cats, with both calcium oxalate and struvite occurring in dogs. Both of these types are routinely radiopaque and well visualized. However, focal mineralized opacities in the area of the ureters should be followed with additional studies to determine whether they are true ureteral calculi. Mineralized opacities in the colon superimposed on the kidneys or ureters, as well as the end-on deep circumflex iliac artery, can be mistaken for calculi (Figure 16.31). Radiopaque ureteral calculi are most easily visualized as a discrete round or ovoid mineral retroperitoneal opacity on lateral abdominal radiographs. However, side of the body and symmetry cannot be easily determined on lateral views. Superimposition

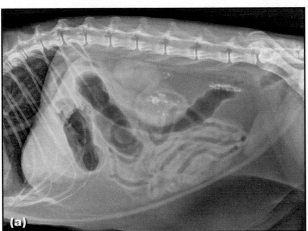

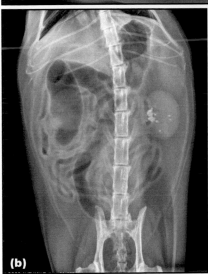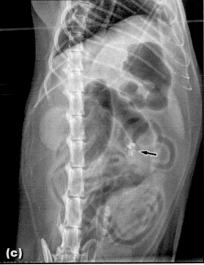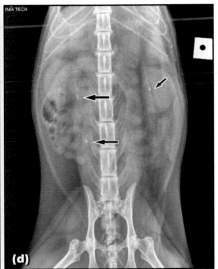

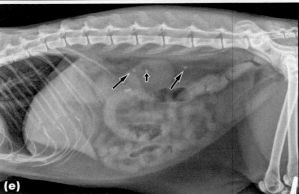

16.30 (a) Lateral, (b) VD and (c) VD oblique views of a cat with renal pelvic and ureteral calculi. Multiple radiopaque calculi are visible in the left renal pelvis, as well as the more peripheral diverticula. Multiple left-sided ureteral calculi are seen best on the VD oblique view (arrowed). (d) VD and (e) lateral views of a cat with ureteral and renal pelvic calculi. A left renal pelvic calculus (small arrow) and two right ureteral calculi are visible (large arrows). A more ventral radiopacity on the lateral view is likely to represent mineralized material in the colon.

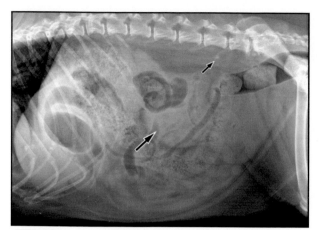

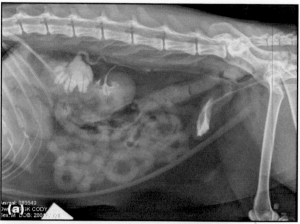

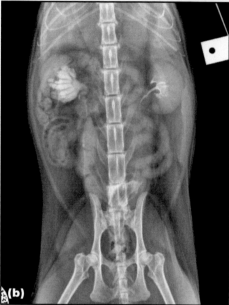

16.31 Lateral abdominal radiograph of a dog with an enlarged, irregular left kidney secondary to a large renal cyst (large arrow). The deep circumflex iliac artery is visible as a radiopaque end-on vessel immediately ventral to L6 (small arrow). This should not be mistaken for a ureteral calculus.

of gas and faecal material on the VD view may mask the appearance and location of calculi.

Additional imaging studies are often necessary to confirm the presence and stage of ureteral calculi, especially radiolucent stones. On excretory urography, calculi should cause a filling defect within the contrast medium-filled ureteral lumen and proximal dilatation of the ureter. In addition, it may be possible to visualize the renal pelvis (assuming adequate renal function). It is important not to mistake transient ureteral peristalsis for a true filling defect, and serial radiographs should be examined to help differentiate between the two conditions.

Ureteral dilatation

Ureteral dilatation usually occurs secondary to obstruction, although atony and ureteral inflammation should also be considered. Ureteral obstruction can occur at any level. A mass in the bladder trigone often causes dilatation of both ureters. Other causes include strictures, ureteral calculi (Figure 16.32), ureteral rupture, ectopic ureters and luminal or extraluminal masses. Inadvertent ligation of a ureter during abdominal surgery is also a consideration. Calculi, strictures and mural mass lesions should cause a filling defect within the affected segment with proximal dilatation. Smooth filling defects are consistent with calculi, strictures and extrinsic masses. Irregular filling defects may indicate neoplasia, inflammation or fibrosis. Ureteral atony can occur secondary to ureteritis or to surrounding tissue inflammation. Pyelonephritis (see Figure 16.25) commonly results in proximal ureteral dilatation, although the dilatation is usually mild compared with cases of obstructive hydroureter.

Ectopic ureters

Ectopic ureter is a congenital disorder of one or both ureters that causes termination in a location distal to the bladder trigone. Excretory urography can be very helpful in the diagnosis, although additional imaging studies may be necessary. The most common termination sites for ectopic ureters are the bladder neck

16.32 **(a)** Lateral and **(b)** VD abdominal radiographs of the cat in Figure 16.30de, taken 20 minutes after intravenous contrast medium administration. The right renal pelvis and diverticula are dilated secondary to partial obstruction by ureteral calculi.

and urethra, although vaginal termination also occurs. The affected ureter is often tortuous and dilated on excretory urography, although it may appear normal. Obstruction of urine flow at stenotic ureteral orifices or infection and ureteral atony result in dilatation. The ureters are best visualized at 5, 10 and 20 minutes following contrast medium injection, and oblique VD views taken at this time are helpful in visualizing the ureteral termination site without superimposition of the spine. Moderate distension of the urinary bladder with negative contrast medium prior to administration of positive contrast medium is helpful in visualizing ureteral termination (Figure 16.33).

Even with these procedures, location of ureteral termination may not be possible owing to superimposition of the pelvic structures. Ureters with abnormal termination sites close to the bladder trigone are particularly difficult to diagnose, especially if the ureter is not dilated. Intramural ectopic ureters appear externally to enter the bladder at the normal location, but tunnel below the mucosa and open at an abnormal caudal site. If ureteral

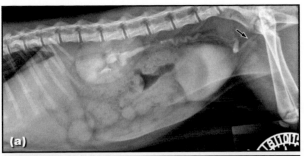

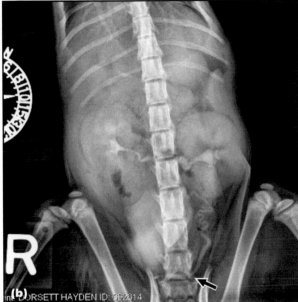

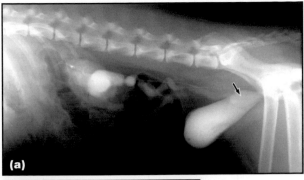

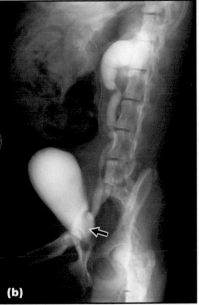

16.33 **(a)** Lateral and **(b)** VD abdominal radiographs of a 5-month-old bitch taken 10 minutes after intravenous contrast medium administration. The left ureter is dilated and tortuous and extends beyond the bladder trigone, entering in the area of the urethra (arrowed).

16.34 **(a)** Lateral and **(b)** VD oblique abdominal radiographs of a 6-month-old bitch with incontinence. These radiographs were taken 10 minutes following intravenous contrast medium injection. The right renal pelvis is dilated and the right ureter is dilated and tortuous. It appears to terminate in a contrast medium-filled sac located at the bladder neck (arrowed). A ureterocele was diagnosed at surgery.

evaluation is incomplete on excretory urography, positive-contrast vaginography and urethrography can be performed (see Chapter 17). Spiral CT has recently been reported to have good success in the diagnosis of ectopic ureters and may be the imaging modality of choice for this condition.

Ureterocele

Ureteroceles are cystic dilatations of the distal ureter near the termination site, and may accompany ectopic ureters. After excretory urography, the contrast medium-filled dilatation is visible within the bladder (especially if pre-filled with negative contrast medium) or urethra (Figure 16.34). On ultrasound examination, a round, thin-walled, fluid-filled cystic structure is visible, usually within the bladder lumen.

Ureteral rupture

Ureteral rupture typically results in fluid accumulation in the retroperitoneal space with loss of radiographic detail. This is most often seen after abdominal trauma. This diagnosis is made best with contrast radiography. After contrast medium administration, the affected ureter becomes visible as a dilated and somewhat tortuous structure proximally, with contrast medium leakage at the rupture site (Figure 16.35). A ruptured ureter may be difficult to identify with ultrasonography.

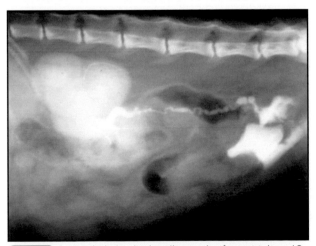

16.35 Lateral abdominal radiograph of a cat taken 10 minutes after intravenous contrast medium injection. The left ureter is slightly dilated and very tortuous, terminating in a pool of free contrast medium. The ureter was ruptured at the level of the bladder trigone.

Ultrasonography

The ureters are not seen in normal dogs and cats on ultrasonography, except for intermittent visualization of ureteral jets when ureteral urine is expressed into the bladder lumen at the trigone. However, with dilatation the ureter becomes apparent as a tubular structure distended with anechoic fluid (Figure 16.36). The dilated ureter should be followed to try to visualize a possible obstructive lesion. Ureteral calculi are a common cause and are seen as echogenic foci with distal shadowing within the fluid-filled ureter. Often the dilated portion of the ureter is tortuous, making full evaluation with ultrasonography difficult. However, it should be noted that the ureter does not always dilate significantly around the calculus, making it more difficult to visualize. Ureteral dilatation tends to begin proximally regardless of the site of ureteral obstruction and may not extend to the level of the calculus at the time of examination. Ureteral obstruction secondary to a trigone bladder mass is common and often involves both ureters. The ureters and renal pelvis should be checked carefully whenever a bladder mass is present.

Proximal ureteral dilatation may occur with pyelonephritis. A dilated, tortuous ureter may be visualized on ultrasound examination, along with adjacent free fluid, in cases of ureteral rupture. However, the most reliable diagnosis is made with excretory urography or antegrade pyelography.

Ultrasonography may be used as an alternative imaging modality for diagnosis of ectopic ureters. Although not visible in every patient, the ureterovesicular junction can often be seen as a small 'bump' projecting into the lumen of the caudodorsal bladder wall (Figure 16.37). Ureteral jets can be seen intermittently at these sites, especially with Doppler ultrasonography and intravenous administration of furosemide. The absence of a jet, and visualization of a ureter extending caudal to the bladder trigone, is consistent with ectopic ureter. Ureteral dilatation and ipsilateral hydronephrosis are often seen with concurrent ureteritis and stricture formation.

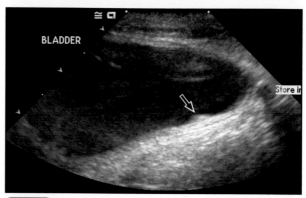

16.37 Longitudinal ultrasonogram of the urinary bladder of a healthy dog. The ureteral papilla is seen as a small echogenic protrusion into the bladder lumen (arrowed).

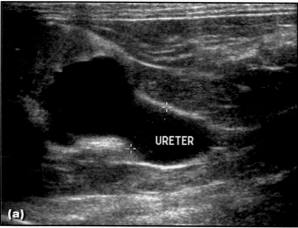

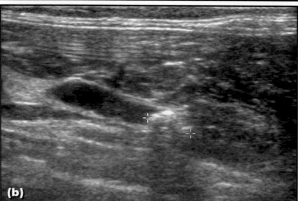

16.36 **(a)** Transverse ultrasonogram of the kidney and proximal ureter of a cat with ureteral calculi. The renal pelvis and ureter are dilated. Right is to the left and ventral is at the top of the image. **(b)** Longitudinal ultrasonogram of the distal portion of the same ureter. An echogenic calculus (between calipers) is present within the fluid-filled ureter, resulting in ureteral obstruction. Cranial is to the left and ventral is at the top of the image.

References and further reading

Ackerman N (1991) *Radiology and Ultrasound of Urogenital Diseases in Dogs and Cats.* Iowa State University Press, Ames, Iowa

Adin CA, Hergesell EF, Nyland TG, *et al.* (2003) Antegrade pyelography for suspected ureteral obstruction in cats: 11 cases (1995–2001). *Journal of the American Veterinary Medical Association* **222,** 1576–1581

Cuypers MD, Grooters AM, Williams J, *et al.* (1997) Renomegaly in dogs and cats: Part I. Differential diagnosis. *Compendium on Continuing Education for the Practicing Veterinarian* **19,** 1019–1032

Feeney DA, Barber DL, Johnston GR, *et al.* (1982) The excretory urogram: Part I. Techniques, normal radiographic appearance, and misinterpretation, *Compendium on Continuing Education for the Practicing Veterinarian* **4,** 233–240

Feeney DA, Barber DL, Johnston GR, *et al.* (1982) The excretory urogram: Part II. Interpretation of abnormal findings. *Compendium on Continuing Education for the Practicing Veterinarian* **4,** 321–329

Feeney DA, Barber DL and Osborne CA (1981) Advances in canine excretory urography. *30th Gaines Veterinary Symposium,* 8–22

Feeney DA, Barber DL and Osborne CA (1982) The functional aspects of the nephrogram in excretory urography: a review. *Veterinary Radiology and Ultrasound* **23,** 42–45

Feeney DA and Johnston GR (2007) The kidneys and ureters. In: *Textbook of Veterinary Radiology, 5th edition,* ed. D Thrall, pp 693–707. Elsevier, Philadelphia

Feeney DA, Thrall DE, Barber DL, *et al.* (1979) Normal canine excretory urogram: effects of dose, time, and individual dog variations. *American Journal of Veterinary Research* **40,** 1596–1604

Grooters AM, Cuypers MD, Partington BP, *et al.* (1997) Renomegaly in dogs and cats: Part II. Diagnostic approach. *Compendium on Continuing Education for the Practicing Veterinarian* **19,** 1213–1229

Nyland TG, Mattoon JS, Herrgesell ER, *et al.* (2002) Urinary Tract. In: *Small Animal Diagnostic Ultrasound, 2nd edn,* ed. TG Nyland and JS Mattoon, pp. 158–195. WB Saunders, Philadelphia

Rao QA and Newhouse JH (2006) Risk of nephropathy after intravenous administration of contrast material: a critical literature analysis. *Radiology* **239,** 392–397

Valdes-Martinez A, Cianciolo R and Mai W (2007) Association between renal hypoechoic subcapsular thickening and lymphosarcoma in cats. *Veterinary Radiology and Ultrasound* **48,** 357–360

17

The bladder and urethra

Alasdair Hotston Moore

Introduction

Radiographic examination remains a critical tool for diagnosis of diseases of the canine and feline lower urinary tract. Although ultrasonographic investigation is also very valuable, especially for examination of the bladder, the urethra is largely inaccessible using this modality. Radiographic examination of the urethra is a key diagnostic method, notably in male dogs and cats because of the technical difficulties of examining the urethra endoscopically in this sex.

Normal radiographic anatomy

Dog

The bladder is commonly visible on plain films because of the contrast between the soft tissue opacity of the bladder and its contents, and the fat at the pelvic canal and within the peritoneal cavity. The bladder may be entirely intra-abdominal in position (Figure 17.1a), although in around 20% of individuals the bladder neck is intrapelvic (i.e. within the bony pelvic canal) (Figure 17.1b). The bladder is a smooth oval and tapers caudally to join the urethra. Defining the normal size of the bladder is impossible because of changes with normal filling and voiding, but generally the apex is caudal to the umbilicus. It is more appropriate to relate bladder size to the history and clinical signs. For example, a small bladder is expected in a normal animal given recent opportunity to void. Conversely, a large bladder is expected in an animal subject to diuresis or fluid therapy if urination has not occurred. A full bladder in an animal with signs of urinary tenesmus is compatible with functional or anatomical urethral obstruction.

The urethra of either gender is not apparent on plain radiography because of a lack of contrast with the surrounding soft tissue. Suitable contrast studies (see below) allow visualization of the urethra from the bladder neck to the vagina or penis. In both cases, the urethral surface is smooth, although the diameter is difficult to assess accurately because the techniques do not allow control of the extent of filling.

In the bitch (Figure 17.2), the urethra joins the lower genital tract close to the vestibulovaginal junction and a ventral deviation is normal at this site. The remainder of the urethra is relatively uniform in diameter and luminal detail, although it is difficult to achieve uniform filling. In the male (Figure 17.3), three

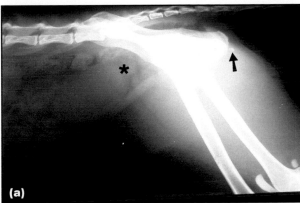

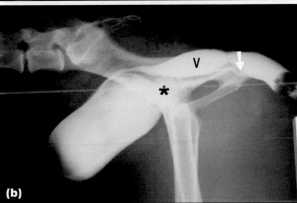

17.1 **(a)** Plain lateral radiograph of a male cat showing normal bladder size, shape and position. A urethral stone (black arrow) is also present. **(b)** Retrograde vaginourethrogram and cystogram of a bitch with an intrapelvic bladder neck (∗). The white arrow depicts the external urethral orifice. V = Vagina.

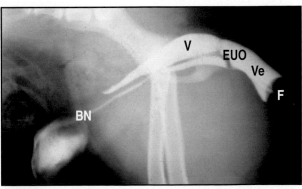

17.2 Retrograde vaginourethrogram of a normal Staffordshire Bull Terrier bitch. BN = Bladder neck; EUO = External urethral orifice; F = Bulb of the Foley catheter; V = Vagina; Ve = Vestibule.

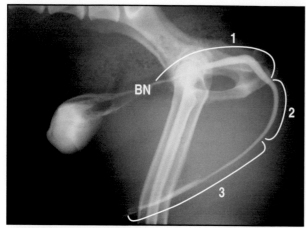

17.3 Retrograde urethrogram of a normal male dog. BN = Bladder neck; 1 = Pelvic urethra; 2 = Perineal urethra; 3 = Penile urethra.

parts of the urethra can be distinguished: the penile urethra; the perineal urethra; and the intrapelvic urethra (including the prostatic portion). Of these, the penile is the narrowest and the prostatic the widest, although this can be difficult to demonstrate radiographically.

Cat

Similar comments apply to the anatomy of the bladder and urethra in the female cat. One important difference is the consistently intra-abdominal position of the bladder neck (Figure 17.4) and the relatively long urethra compared with the dog. The male urethra is also different in anatomy because of the perineal position of the penis (Figure 17.5). The penile urethra itself is extremely narrow in the male cat.

Positional changes

The position of the bladder varies with the extent of filling; in particular, the bladder neck moves cranially as filling proceeds. This can be exacerbated by pneumocystography (see later). The urethra of the male cat may be folded when the bladder is not full, but is straightened to a variable extent during retrograde studies due to distension and tension on the prepuce during injection.

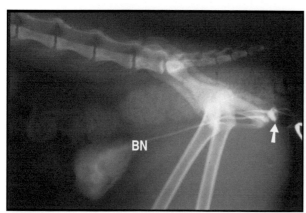

17.4 Retrograde vaginourethrogram of a normal female cat. The white arrow depicts the external urethral orifice. BN = Bladder neck.

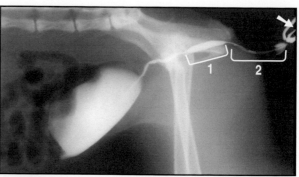

17.5 Retrograde urethrogram of a male cat. Note that this cat is a congenitally tailless Manx. Note the Allis forceps on the prepuce (arrowed). 1 = Membranous urethra; 2 = Penile urethra.

Plain radiography

Standard views are the lateral and ventrodorsal (VD) recumbent views. The lateral view (see Figure 17.1) generally provides more information than the VD view (Figure 17.6) because there is less superimposition of the surrounding skeletal structures on the lower urinary tract. However, the orthogonal views are generally a worthwhile addition. There is no expected difference in the appearance of the bladder and urethra in right or left lateral recumbency. Oblique VD views may be helpful as an adjunct to the orthogonal views to evaluate bladder and urethral lesions accurately. Horizontal beam views of the erect patient are rarely required.

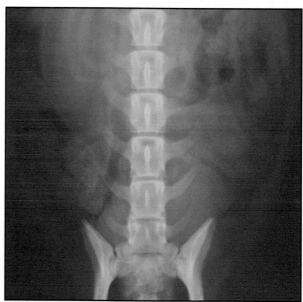

17.6 VD view of the bladder in a normal bitch. Superimposition of the pelvis and vertebrae limit the value of this view.

Normal variations

Breed variations

An intrapelvic bladder neck (see Figure 17.1b) is common in Dobermann, Old English Sheepdog and Boxer bitches. Although in most dogs and cats the bladder is spherical or oval in shape, in these breeds an oblong outline is common.

Individual variations
The bladder may not be visible in patients with little or neonatal (brown) intra-abdominal fat.

Contrast radiography

Patient preparation
Although plain radiography and ultrasonography can be undertaken with the cooperative patient conscious or sedated, most contrast examinations require the patient to be anaesthetized. General anaesthesia for these purposes allows better patient positioning, improves patient safety and avoids artefacts arising from muscle spasm during contrast medium administration or catheterization.

In addition to the normal aspects of patient preparation for anaesthesia, the descending colon and rectum should be evacuated prior to imaging. This is most appropriately achieved in dogs by administration of a phosphate enema and the opportunity for defecation before premedication. This type of enema is contraindicated in cats, and in this species low-volume lubricant or warm water enemas are preferred. It is possible to lavage the colon after induction of anaesthesia but this may result in greater contamination of the radiography suite, and additionally the presence of bubbles in the colon may produce radiological artefacts.

Plain radiographs should always be taken and inspected prior to embarking on a contrast study. This ensures that:

- Exposure factors are appropriate
- Enemas have been effective
- Contrast studies are not performed if lesions are visible on plain films.

Cystography

Pneumocystography
Pneumocystography (negative-contrast cystography) has significant limitations and is rarely used as a sole imaging examination. The procedure is straightforward:

1. Under general anaesthesia, a urethral catheter is passed in a standard clinical fashion and the urinary bladder emptied, allowing samples to be taken for culture and urinalysis at this stage.
2. The bladder is then filled with gas. The volume needed to fill the bladder is patient-specific.
3. During introduction of the gas, the bladder should be gently palpated with the finger tips through the lateral flank. The end-point is a palpably firm bladder or rebound on the syringe. Rebound is a more sensitive indicator of a full bladder with lower volume syringes (<60 ml).
4. Prior to exposure, the tip of the urethral catheter should be withdrawn into the urethra from the bladder lumen, to avoid artefact (Figure 17.7).

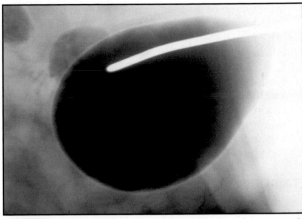

17.7 Lateral view of a pneumocystogram in a normal bitch. A metal Tiemans urethral catheter is in place but should have been withdrawn before exposure.

Although room air is commonly used for negative-contrast cystography, there is a small risk of air embolism from the technique. To reduce this hazard, some radiologists prefer to use carbon dioxide for insufflation. If carbon dioxide is utilized, administration directly from the pressurized source must be avoided.

Bladder rupture is a possible consequence of pneumocystography (Figure 17.8), but is easily avoided by attention to detail: slow insufflation, repeated gentle palpation and assessment of rebound on the dosing syringe. In addition, if a non-balloon tipped urethral catheter is used, excessive gas can escape, although this may prevent complete bladder filling.

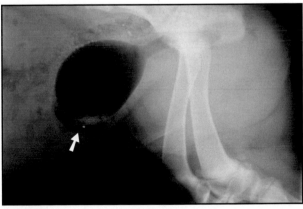

17.8 Subserosal air (arrowed) following pneumocystography in a male Newfoundland puppy. This is a consequence of over-distension of the bladder during insufflation and/or traumatic catheterization, resulting in perforation of the layers of the bladder wall.

Pneumocystography may provide the following information:

- Bladder size, but this volume is highly variable and definitive ranges of volume cannot be given
- Wall thickness, but a double-contrast cystogram is preferred
- Identification of cystic calculi, but radiolucent calculi may be occult

- Verification of an abnormal location of the bladder in cases of herniation or rupture.

However:

- Negative-contrast cystography is not a good test for the diagnosis of bladder rupture
- During pneumocystography, the bladder becomes displaced cranially into the abdomen, making it unreliable for assessment of bladder neck position.

Positive-contrast cystography

Positive-contrast cystography is carried out in a similar way to pneumocystography, except that a water-soluble iodine-based contrast agent is used. Contrast medium with a concentration of 120–400 mg I/ml is suitable. Barium should never be used. The presence of a large volume of positive contrast medium will obscure many small lesions of the bladder. The main indication for positive-contrast cystography is suspected bladder wall rupture. A second indication is to provide appropriate back pressure for a subsequent retrograde urethrogram. This back pressure will help ensure uniform urethral dilation when the catheter tip is placed in the terminal urethra.

Double-contrast cystography

This technique offers many advantages over both negative- and positive-contrast cystography. The combination of bladder distension with negative contrast medium and the presence of a small volume of positive contrast medium is the preferred technique for the diagnosis of most luminal and mural lesions.

Double-contrast cystography results in a bladder distended with negative contrast medium with positive contrast medium forming a small pool or puddle centrally (Figure 17.9). Calculi and blood clots, for example, fall into the contrast medium pool and create a filling defect. Masses of the bladder wall may result in filling defects within the contrast medium pool or be outlined by gas with positive contrast medium adhering to the surface, depending on position.

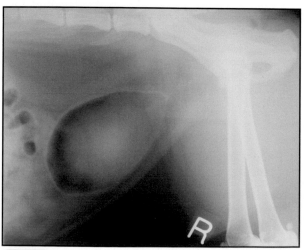

17.9 A double-contrast cystogram of a normal male cat.

Typically, the first phase of the study is a pneumocystogram (see above). Once the bladder is full, a small volume of undiluted positive contrast medium is added to create a shallow puddle to help identify small luminal lesions. In cats 1 ml of contrast medium is usually sufficient. A gradual scale of increasing volume is added to larger dogs, not exceeding 5 ml. Rotating the animal is helpful to provide coating of the bladder wall with contrast medium and to wash small lesions into the dependent contrast medium pool. However, this may result in bubble formation. To avoid this artefact an alternative is to commence with an empty bladder and introduce the positive contrast medium at this stage. This will contact the bladder surface entirely and eliminates the need to rotate the patient. The bladder is then inflated as before.

Urethrography

Urethrography is a key tool in the investigation of urethral disease, particularly when urethroscopy is not possible due to equipment or biological limitations. For all procedures, a water-soluble iodine-based contrast medium is used at a concentration of 120–400 mg I/ml.

Normograde urethrography

Normograde urethrography is occasionally indicated when retrograde studies have been unsuccessful, usually because of a failure of urethral catheterization. However, it is difficult to achieve good images because of inconsistent filling of the urethra. To obtain a normograde urethrogram, the patient must be anaesthetized. The bladder is filled with positive contrast medium and then expressed to fill the urethra during radiographic exposure. Positive contrast medium can be introduced by bladder puncture, a cystotomy tube or intravenous urography (see Chapter 16). The bladder is expressed by applying abdominal pressure with an abdominal band or paddle. Filling of the proximal urethra may be adequate for interpretation but the distal urethra, especially in the male, may be poorly filled. The technique is of limited value in most cases and does not readily allow for multiple views or repeated studies.

Conscious voiding studies are used in humans but are practically difficult in dogs and cats and the interpretation is subjective.

Retrograde urethrography

The urethra is most readily evaluated with retrograde positive-contrast studies. Retrograde urethrography in the male is a valuable technique for the investigation of dysuria and anatomical abnormalities. In either species, the principles are the same:

1. The patient is anaesthetized as the procedure is stimulating, and in addition urethral relaxation is essential to allow filling without artefactual narrowing due to muscle spasm.
2. A urethral catheter is passed to empty the bladder and the tip of the catheter is placed in the terminal penile urethra. The catheter is then pre-filled with contrast medium to avoid bubbles

in the urethra, which may mimic radiolucent stones.
3. The urethra is occluded around the catheter and the contrast medium injected.

It is important to take the radiographic exposure during injection of the contrast medium, whilst the urethra remains distended. Taking the X-ray immediately after injection results in less urethral distension and unsatisfactory studies. Appropriate radiological safety precautions are therefore essential. The operator must remain outside the primary beam and wear protective clothing. The hands of the veterinary surgeon are nearest the beam and use of appropriate catheters and lead sleeves can provide adequate protection.

In the male dog, the most suitable catheter for injection is a Foley (balloon-tipped) catheter (Figure 17.10). In almost all adult dogs, an 8 Fr (or larger) catheter can be used. The tip is placed into the penile urethra and the balloon gently inflated with saline or air sufficiently to anchor it within the distal urethra. This variation of the technique allows the hands of the veterinary surgeon to be kept well clear of the primary beam and yet produce a study with good filling of the urethra, and is preferable to holding the prepuce during injection. The hindlimbs should be pulled forward so that the femur is cranial to the tip of the penis. With the bladder filled with positive contrast medium, a single injection is all that is necessary to evaluate the entire length of the urethra. When the bladder is empty or incompletely filled, separate exposures may be necessary to evaluate the penile urethra, perineal urethra and the pelvic urethra (Figures 17.11 and 17.12). A suggested volume of contrast medium is 1 ml/kg in the dog.

In the male cat, a narrow gauge urethral catheter (3–4 Fr) is used, ideally with an end hole. A nasolacrimal cannula is particularly suitable. To secure this and maintain distension during injection, Allis tissue forceps are placed above the catheter across the prepuce (not the penis) (see Figure 17.5). A suggested volume of contrast medium for injection in a male cat is 2–4 ml in total.

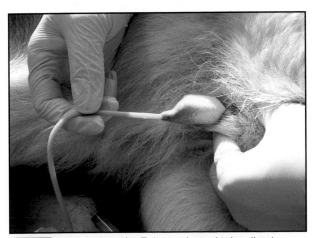

17.10 Placement of a Foley catheter in the distal penile urethra of a male dog in preparation for retrograde urethrography.

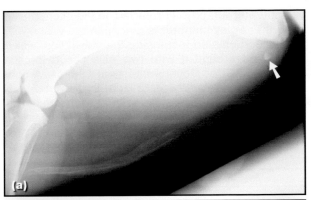
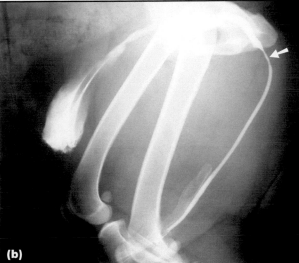

17.11 **(a)** Plain radiographic study of the penile urethra in a dog, demonstrating the 'legs forward' positioning used to remove overlying structures from the penile and perineal urethra. Note the radiopaque stone close to the tuber ischium (arrowed). **(b)** Retrograde urethrogram taken after retrograde flushing. The animal is positioned to allow evaluation of the perineal urethra in particular. There is some smooth narrowing at the ischial arch (arrowed), which may represent periurethral swelling or muscle spasm during injection.

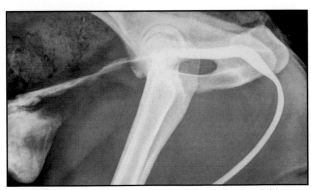

17.12 Retrograde urethrogram of a male dog with positioning, centring and exposure technique to evaluate the pelvic urethra. Note that the urethra at the level of the femoral heads is still difficult to distinguish; performing the study with a full bladder may improve contrast medium filling in this area.

Vaginourethrography
In females, direct retrograde urethrography is difficult and the presence of a catheter in the urethra obscures important detail. For this reason,

vaginourethrography is preferred. In the bitch, the tip of an 8 Fr Foley catheter is placed in the vulva, with the balloon inflated just inside the vulval lips, which are closed around it with two Allis tissue forceps (Figure 17.13) or Doyens intestinal forceps. A conventional urethral catheter is used in the cat. A sufficient volume of contrast medium (approximately 1 ml/kg) is injected to fill the vagina and then overflow into the urethra itself. As in the male, the radiographic exposure must be made during the injection.

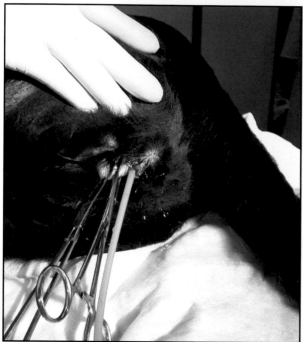

17.13 Placement of Foley catheter for retrograde vaginourethrography in a Labrador Retriever. The bulb of the catheter is inflated just inside the vulval lips, which are closed around it with two Allis tissue forceps. Ventral is to the left and the tail is to the right, with the animal in right lateral recumbency.

Ultrasonography

Bladder

Ultrasonography is particularly useful for the investigation of mural and intraluminal changes of the bladder. Ultrasonography provides useful information on:

- Bladder wall thickness and layering
- The presence of mass lesions
- The presence of calculi or sediment within the bladder lumen
- Size and shape of regional lymph nodes.

For many patients, the information provided by ultrasonography may exceed that derived from radiography. However, radiography provides additional information in relation to the surrounding bony structures and assists surgical planning by constructing a more complete picture of the anatomy; for example, the relationship of masses to the ureteral orifices. Radiography is also superior for quantifying the number of radiopaque uroliths.

Bladder wall thickness and layering

The normal bladder wall thickness on ultrasonography varies depending on the degree of distension. Whilst the wall of the distended bladder should be smooth and 1–2 mm thick, the wall of the empty bladder can be substantially thicker and folded. It is normally possible to differentiate the epithelial layer from the hypoechoic muscular layers (Figure 17.14). The epithelium is usually thin but may be thickened in the presence of inflammatory or neoplastic changes, such as polypoid cystitis or transitional cell carcinoma. Although these cannot be reliably separated ultrasonographically, polypoid cystitis is not expected to produce disruption of the layering whereas carcinomas are typically invasive. Mural haemorrhage is an uncommon cause of bladder wall thickening. This has been seen in association with systemic coagulopathies, including rodenticide intoxication, immune-mediated thrombocytopenia and disseminated intravascular coagulopathy. Mural thickening resolves quickly (1 mm/day) after reversal of the underlying cause.

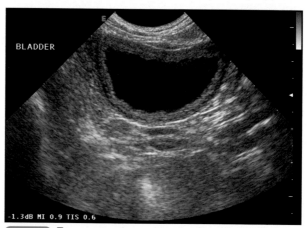

17.14 Transverse ultrasonogram of a normal canine bladder. The layering is apparent. Note the relatively hypoechoic outer muscular layer. The urine itself is anechoic due to the absence of macroscopic particles.

Bladder lumen

Ultrasonography is useful to identify calculi or smaller particles in the bladder lumen. These produce echoes which may cast acoustic shadows. Smaller particles produce a scattering pattern within the bladder lumen, sometimes likened to the appearance of a 'starry sky', or settle to produce a sediment (Figure 17.15). Whereas calculi and similar particles will move when the bladder is agitated. Less common diseases resulting in mineralization of the soft tissues of the bladder produce echogenic areas that do not displace when the bladder is manipulated. Care must be taken to avoid confusing echoes due to calculi or other particles within the lumen with those arising from side lobe or slice thickness artefacts. Artefactual echoes will usually disappear if the bladder is imaged in a different plane.

Ultrasonography is reliable for the detection of calculi within the bladder (Figure 17.16), irrespective of the mineral composition. However, it is difficult to count them reliably, so ultrasonography is therefore less useful for pre-surgical assessment than

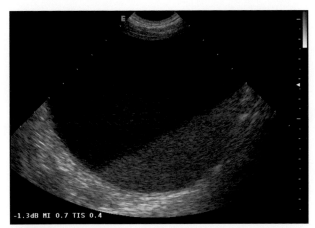

17.15 Longitudinal ultrasonogram of a canine bladder showing settled sediment, with a distinct border between the anechoic urine and the moderately echogenic debris of the small particles.

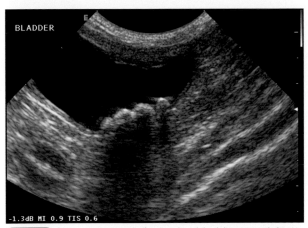

17.16 Ultrasonogram of a canine bladder containing a group of calculi. The calculi are clustered due to gravitational effects, producing bright echogenic reflections and acoustic shadowing behind.

radiography. In addition, it is not possible to ensure that no calculi are present in the urethra on ultrasound examination.

Ultrasonography is also valuable for identifying debris (Figure 17.17) within the bladder, such as blood clots or sloughed urothelium. This material is less echogenic than calculi and does not produce acoustic shadowing.

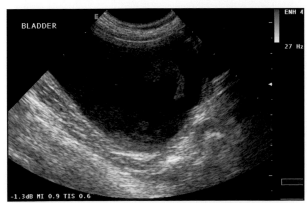

17.17 Transverse ultrasonogram of a canine bladder containing soft tissue debris floating within the lumen. Note the absence of acoustic shadowing.

Ureteric terminations

Detection of the anatomical ureteral orifice is rarely possible. However, B-mode ultrasonography, assisted by colour Doppler studies, can be used to identify the ureteral jets as they discharge into the bladder lumen (Figure 17.18). This can be used as part of the investigation of ureteral ectopia, although in many affected animals the bladder neck is intra-pelvic making the examination difficult. Examination of the ureteral orifices may also be helpful in pre-surgical planning for patients with potentially resectable bladder masses, since the requirement to consider ureteral re-implantation significantly worsens surgical outcome.

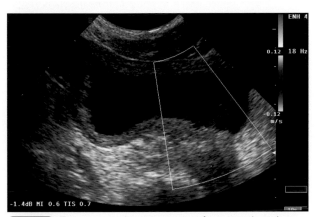

17.18 Transverse ultrasonogram of a normal canine bladder neck with superimposed colour flow Doppler highlighting a ureteral jet (red).

Urethra

Ultrasound examination of the urethra is challenging. Significant parts of this structure are inaccessible to transcutaneous ultrasonography, especially in the bitch and in cats, and endoscopic ultrasonography is not widely available. The perineal and penile urethra can be examined in male dogs, especially for detection of stones. Occasionally, the technique is valuable for identifying periurethral masses that do not produce striking changes on urethrography.

Overview of additional imaging modalities

Although magnetic resonance imaging (MRI) and computed tomography (CT) both have potential indications for imaging of the lower urinary tract, they are uncommonly applied since the combination of radiography and ultrasonography provides sufficient information for diagnosis and surgical planning in almost all cases. Both CT and MRI are used in humans for the staging of bladder neoplasms, in particular for evaluating the extension of the disease process through and beyond the bladder wall. These advanced imaging modalities are also used for evaluation of urethral and periurethral lesions. However, the cost and restricted availability of these modalities has limited their use to date in small animals.

Urinary bladder diseases

Distension

Gross distension is recognized on plain films as displacement of the apex of the intact bladder cranial to the umbilicus (Figure 17.19). A more useful judgement of bladder size is made in the light of the history of the patient. Following emptying of the bladder in the normal animal, the bladder wall contracts, maintaining an oval outline to the empty bladder. However, in patients with chronic distension or an atonic bladder, the bladder wall becomes thickened and inelastic and following emptying is folded and 'floppy' in appearance (Figure 17.20).

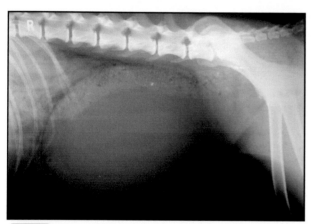

17.19 Gross distension of the bladder demonstrated on a plain lateral radiograph of a dog with a neurological cause of urinary retention.

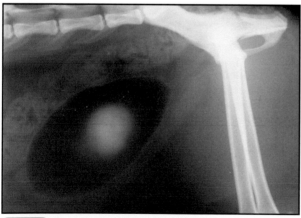

17.20 Double-contrast cystogram of an overdistended bladder in a male cat following drainage. Although the bladder has been filled to an appropriate size, the wall remains folded.

Rupture and diverticula

Most animals with bladder rupture present with collapse and clinical signs of abdominal distension. The primary finding on plain radiographs is loss of abdominal detail due to peritoneal fluid. Further imaging is required to distinguish rupture of the ureter, bladder or urethra (see below). The bladder may be ruptured and remain partially full. A visible bladder on an abdominal radiograph does not therefore preclude rupture. The preferred imaging procedure for confirmation of bladder rupture is positive-contrast cystography (see above), since this is recognized as being more sensitive than pneumocystography. As urethral rupture is an important differential diagnosis in these cases, it is often sensible to perform a retrograde urethrogram initially. The typical radiographic appearance is presence of the contrast agent in a poorly defined area outside the bladder lumen (Figure 17.21). If the contrast medium remains within a discrete structure outside the lumen, a partial thickness rupture (with intact urothelium) or diverticula should be suspected.

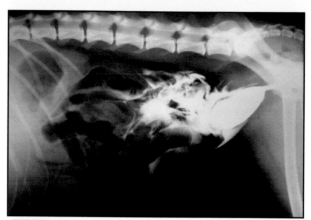

17.21 Lateral positive-contrast cystogram of a bitch following abdominal trauma. Note the positive-contrast agent outside the bladder lumen and between the serosal surfaces of other abdominal organs.

Bladder diverticula are most often seen in cats, in the position of the urachal origin at the apex of the bladder (Figure 17.22). Diverticula may be incidental findings. The diverticula seen in some cats with a history of urethral obstruction resolve following relief of the obstruction and a period of bladder decompression, suggesting that they may not be a primary cause of disease in all cases.

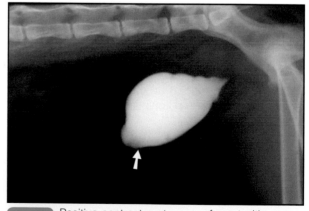

17.22 Positive-contrast cystogram of a cat with chronic urinary obstruction, illustrating a bladder diverticulum or urachal remnant (arrowed).

Mineralization

Differential diagnoses for radiopaque material in the bladder include calculi, sand, dystrophic mineralization of soft tissues or a foreign body. The terminology used for small diameter mineral debris is imprecise: 'crystals' is limited to microscopic uroliths; 'sand' refers to macroscopic uroliths that are too small to be individually identified and accurately measured;

and 'calculi' describes readily identifiable and measurable macroscopic uroliths. The radiopacity of uroliths varies with chemical composition (Figure 17.23). Sand and all calculi are echogenic on ultrasonography, irrespective of their mineral composition.

Radiopaque calculi
Struvite (magnesium ammonium phosphate) Calcium oxalate Calcium phosphate Silicate
Radiolucent calculi
Cystine Urate Xanthine

17.23 Radiopacity of calculi of differing mineral composition.

Calculi

Radiopaque calculi are typically visible on plain films. The shape of the calculi may vary according to their chemical nature, although this should not be relied upon as a guide to their composition. Struvite uroliths (Figure 17.24a) tend to be smooth, blunt-edged, faceted or pyramidal. Jackstone-shaped calculi are typically silicate, whilst oxalates (Figure 17.24b) tend to be grape-like clusters.

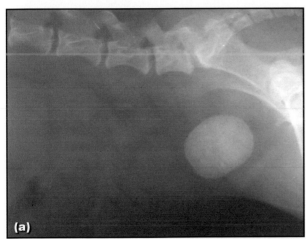

(a)

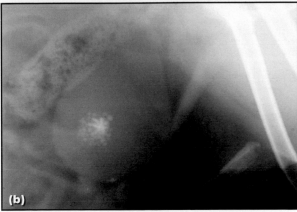

(b)

17.24 **(a)** Plain lateral radiograph of a bitch with a single large radiopaque calculus, which proved to be struvite on analysis. **(b)** Plain lateral radiograph of a bitch with a cluster of oxalate calculi.

Radiolucent calculi are by definition not visible on plain films. Pneumocystography may reveal them as soft tissue opacities within the negative contrast medium, but double-contrast cystography is often more useful. Properly performed, double-contrast cystography shows all calculi as well defined filling defects in the contrast medium pool (Figure 17.25). The presence of bubbles, which may artefactually present a similar appearance, must be considered as a differential diagnosis. Bubbles typically gather at the margin of the contrast medium pool (Figure 17.26), whereas calculi fall into the central part of the pool. In addition, bubbles often cluster and share a straight margin where they touch one another. If doubt remains, the bladder should be emptied and the study repeated or ultrasonography performed.

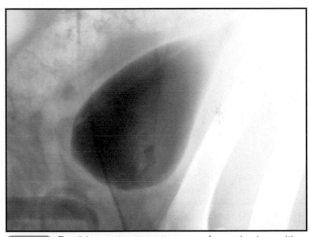

17.25 Double-contrast cystogram of a male dog with radiopaque calculi, which appear as filling defects in the small pool of contrast medium.

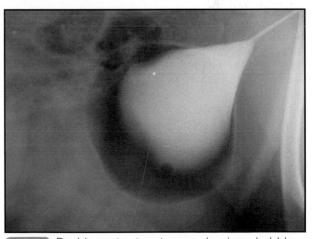

17.26 Double-contrast cystogram showing a bubble artefact. The bubble is circular and lies at the edge of the contrast medium pool.

Sand

Urine sand does not appear as discrete particles on plain radiographs but presents a somewhat diffuse and irregular increase in radiopacity within the bladder lumen (Figure 17.27a). However, on double-contrast cystography, the irregular appearance is exaggerated and a more obvious granular picture is seen (Figure 17.27b). Crystals are not visible radiographically.

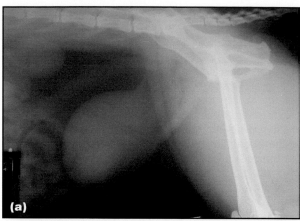

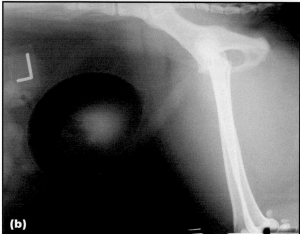

17.27 **(a)** Plain lateral radiograph of a female cat with 'bladder sand' (multiple small calculi). **(b)** A double-contrast study makes the diagnosis more apparent.

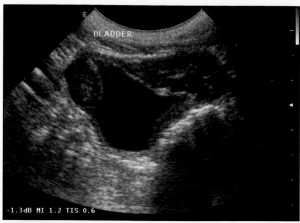

17.28 Transverse ultrasonogram of the bladder showing multiple mural masses.

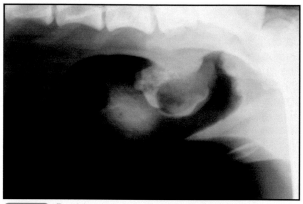

17.29 Double-contrast cystogram of a young Dobermann with an extensive rhabdomyosarcoma of the dorsal bladder wall and neck.

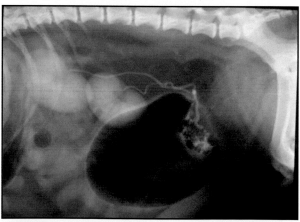

17.30 Pneumocystogram and concurrent intravenous urography of an elderly male dog with a bladder neoplasm at the trigone. Note the involvement of the trigone and the tortuosity of the left ureter; these findings are consistent with an obstruction of the ureteral orifice.

Bladder wall

Mineralization of the bladder wall is a rather non-specific finding, generally indicating dystrophic calcification. It is an uncommon change but can occur with chronic inflammation, including tuberculous cystitis, and bladder neoplasms such as transitional cell carcinoma. Cyclophosphamide-induced cystitis may also produce calcification. The presence of mural calcification should prompt a biopsy to distinguish the pathological cause. Occasionally, radiopaque urolithiasis can be confused with mural calcification. Double-contrast cystography, positional radiography and ultrasonography should allow differentiation.

Masses

Ultrasonography can be important in determining which layer or layers of the bladder wall are involved with a mass (Figure 17.28). Although most bladder masses are neoplastic, urothelial polyps may have a similar appearance. Double-contrast cystography will give the most information regarding the location and extent of such masses (Figure 17.29). Of particular importance in planning treatment is the proximity of the mass to the ureteral orifices, which limits the possibility of surgical excision. Ureteral ultrasonography or excretory urography may provide additional information (Figure 17.30).

Neoplasms

The most common neoplasm of the bladder is transitional cell carcinoma, representing over 90% of all cases. This is typically a disease of older animals. It has a predilection for development in the dorsal wall of the bladder, often at the trigone. The masses are usually solitary and focal, although satellite lesions may be present. Although urothelial in origin, the disease has often infiltrated the deeper layers at the time of diagnosis. Neoplasms are most often occult on plain radiographs, but radiographic findings on contrast studies may include:

- Distortion of the bladder outline
- Thickening of the bladder wall
- Proliferation of the epithelial surface, with increased contrast medium adherence
- Large masses may appear as filling defects in the contrast medium pool.

Much less common are soft tissue sarcomas, including leiomyosarcoma and rhadomyosarcoma. The latter is unusual in that it often affects younger animals (<1 year of age). Sarcomas arise within the muscular layers of the bladder wall and there may be no epithelial involvement. On double-contrast cystography there is a single soft tissue mass, occasionally with calcification, producing local thickening of the bladder (Figure 17.31) and there may be no contrast medium adherence if the urothelium remains intact. In animals with suspected bladder neoplasia, thoracic radiography and ultrasonography of the sublumbar lymph nodes is indicated to stage the disease.

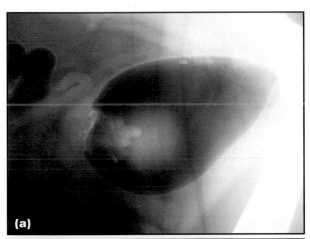

(a)

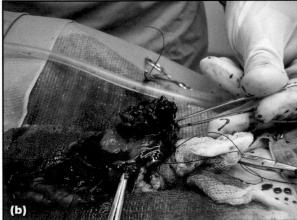

(b)

17.31 **(a)** Double-contrast cystogram of a middle-aged bitch with a mass at the bladder apex, seen as a multi-lobulated soft tissue mass with some contrast medium adherence (the urethral catheter is seen within the bladder in a dorsal location). This proved to be a rhabdomyosarcoma. **(b)** Intraoperative view during cystotomy.

Polypoid cystitis

Polypoid cystitis (Figure 17.32) is an important differential diagnosis for bladder epithelial masses. In contrast to transitional cell carcinoma, polyps are often multiple and tend to be centred on the cranioventral region of the bladder rather than the trigone. Double-contrast cystography reveals multiple soft tissue lesions arising from the urothelium, with adherence of contrast medium and forming filling defects within the contrast medium pool if sufficiently large.

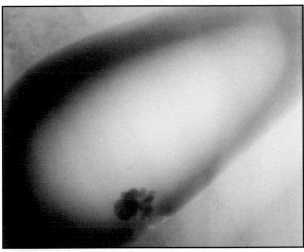

17.32 Double-contrast cystography of a dog with polypoid cystitis. A polyp is clearly visible arising from the ventral bladder wall, causing a 'cauliflower'-shaped filling defect in the contrast medium pool. More contrast medium adherence to the abnormal tissue would be apparent if less positive contrast medium was present in the bladder.

Other soft tissue masses

An important differential diagnosis for intraluminal soft tissue masses is blood clots within the bladder. These appear very similar to multiple polyps on a double-contrast study, producing irregular filling defects within the contrast medium pool (Figure 17.33). Differentiating blood clots from soft tissue masses can be difficult, although if the animal is repositioned or the bladder is drained and the study repeated, it is

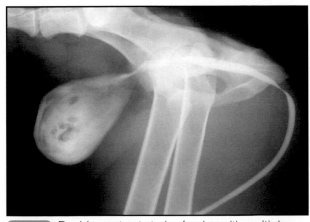

17.33 Double-contrast study of a dog with multiple blood clots in the bladder. These were due to renal haemorrhage and can be seen as multiple irregular filling defects in the contrast medium pool. A retrograde urethrogram is being carried out concurrently.

expected that blood clots will change appearance and position, whereas masses will appear similar on consecutive studies. Doppler ultrasonography may be useful for verification of a non-vascularized mass.

Less commonly, areas of bladder epithelium can separate and form soft tissue opacities within the lumen. This is seen most commonly in animals that have had a prolonged period of urethral obstruction, resulting in epithelial pressure necrosis. Double-contrast cystography demonstrates dissection of positive contrast medium into clefts under the elevated epithelium (Figure 17.34).

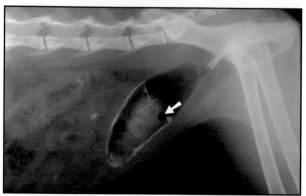

17.34 Double-contrast cystogram of a male cat with sloughing of the bladder epithelium following prolonged urethral obstruction. Contrast medium is adherent and outlines the epithelium. Note also the presence of a bubble (arrowed).

Mural air

Air within the wall of the bladder, in the absence of recent catheterization, is strongly suggestive of emphysematous cystitis. This unusual condition is due to the presence of gas-forming bacteria proliferating in the bladder, leading to deposition of gas within the bladder wall. Most commonly, emphysematous cystitis is associated with diabetes mellitus. Radiological diagnosis is straightforward, with plain films showing radiolucent pockets and streaks within the thickness of the bladder wall (Figure 17.35).

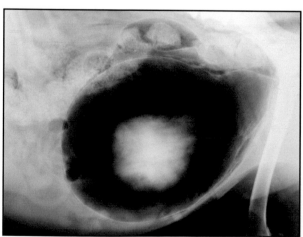

17.35 Double-contrast cystogram showing emphysematous cystitis in an English Setter bitch, associated with chronic urinary retention due to neurological disease. Note the gas streaks within the bladder wall, especially around the bladder neck.

Intramural air may also be seen following traumatic bladder catheterization, especially if the urothelium of the bladder or urethra is fragile, or if catheterization was difficult. A small amount of air may enter spontaneously, but significant amounts are only likely after attempted pneumocystography in these circumstances.

Free air within the bladder (or urethra) is almost invariably a result of catheterization or cystocentesis. Since small amounts of air can easily mimic calculi on double-contrast or positive-contrast studies (see Figure 17.26), it is important to avoid the introduction of bubbles by pre-filling the urethral catheter with contrast medium and avoiding agitation of the bladder during radiography.

Abnormal position

Pelvic bladder

In dogs of both sexes, the bladder is typically entirely intra-abdominal in position when full. Some dogs (around 20%) have an intrapelvic bladder neck. Although this may be associated with urinary incontinence (in particular urethral sphincter mechanism incompetence), it is also a common finding in normal animals and is not an invariable feature of urethral sphincter mechanism incompetence.

Hernia or rupture

The bladder can be displaced as a result of defects in the abdominal wall or perineal diaphragm. In these cases, the urethra typically becomes obstructed and the bladder forms a rounded soft tissue swelling in the affected area. The outline of the bladder itself cannot usually be distinguished from other local soft tissues. Displacement most commonly occurs into perineal ruptures, inguinal hernias and ventral abdominal wall ruptures. In suspicious cases, confirmation can be achieved by paracentesis and analysis of the contents of the swelling. Ultrasound examination can be a helpful addition to this process. The most useful radiographic approach is a retrograde urethrogram, which will highlight the position of the urethra and bladder (Figure 17.36). However, this should be undertaken with caution if the bladder is distended

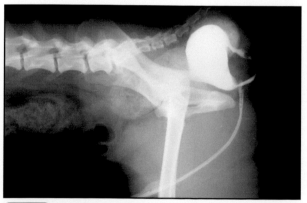

17.36 Urethrogram of perineal rupture and retroflexed bladder. The urethra is markedly kinked and partially obscured by contrast medium within the bladder. Several small air bubbles are present proximal to the tip of the urethral catheter. (Courtesy of P Holt)

and prior cystocentesis is advisable. Cystocentesis in these circumstances will also contribute to patient stabilization and may facilitate passage of a urethral catheter, which is often not possible in the presence of bladder displacement and distension.

Perineal rupture: With a perineal rupture (hernia), the apex of the bladder is retroverted into the perineum and the urethra is folded laterally or dorsally (see Figure 17.36). The prostate gland is often included in the contents of the rupture. Perineal ruptures are most commonly seen in intact male dogs.

Inguinal hernia: Bladder displacement into inguinal hernias may occur in males and females, although most commonly in entire middle-aged bitches. Inguinal herniation is rare in cats. The bladder becomes displaced into a subcutaneous position ventral to the caudal abdominal wall (Figure 17.37). The urethra is not folded but deviates ventrally to the displaced bladder neck.

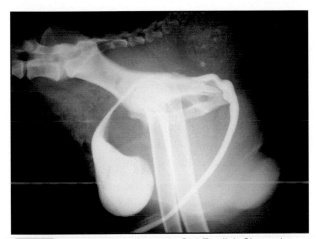

17.37 Urethrogram of a male Old English Sheepdog with an inguinal hernia and displaced bladder. (Reproduced from Holt (2008) with permission from the publisher)

Urethral diseases

Stones
The majority of urethral stones are radiopaque and will be seen on plain radiographs. Urate urethral stones, which may be found in Dalmatians and dogs with portosystemic shunts, are an exception. In the male dog, common sites of lodgement are the perineal urethra (Figure 17.38a) and the urethra immediately proximal to the os penis (Figure 17.38bc). Urethral obstruction is common in male cats. However, the region of obstruction is most often the penile urethra and the stones or plugs that cause obstruction at this site are often not sufficiently radiopaque or of sufficient size to be radiographically apparent. Urethral stones are rare in bitches and queens. Many cases of urethral obstruction by stones are managed by retrograde hydropropulsion (flushing), and radiographs are taken during and after attempts at flushing to ensure that all stones have been returned to the bladder (Figure 17.39). However, it may be difficult to count accurately the number of stones radiographically.

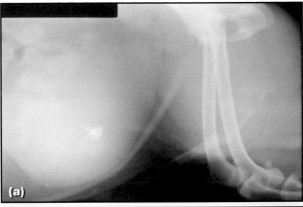

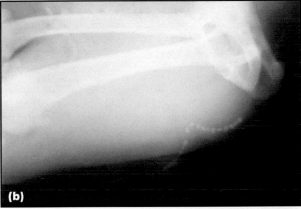

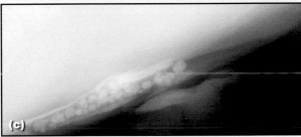

17.38 **(a)** Plain lateral radiograph of a male dog with multiple radiopaque calculi in the bladder and perineal urethra. **(b)** Plain lateral radiograph (legs forward position) showing multiple radiopaque calculi in the pre-penile urethra of a male dog. **(c)** Plain lateral radiograph of the penis of a Cavalier King Charles Spaniel with chronic urolithiasis. Multiple radiopaque calculi are visible, some of which have resulted in localized resorption of the os penis due to their longstanding nature.

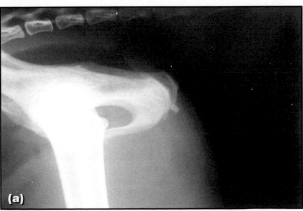

17.39 **(a)** Plain lateral pelvic view of a male cat with urethral obstruction due to a radiopaque stone in the membranous urethra. (continues) ▶

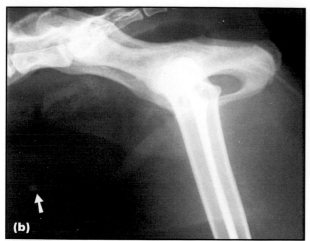

17.39 (continued) **(b)** Following successful retrograde flushing, the stone is now present in the bladder (arrowed).

Radiolucent stones are apparent on retrograde urethrography as discrete filling defects (Figure 17.40). To avoid misinterpretation, precautions should be taken to ensure that no air bubbles enter the urethra, by pre-filling the urethral catheter with contrast medium.

In male dogs, the radiologist must also take care not to mistake the fabellae, which overly the urethra on a lateral view if the hindlimbs are pulled cranially,

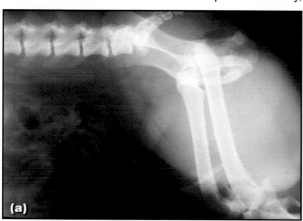

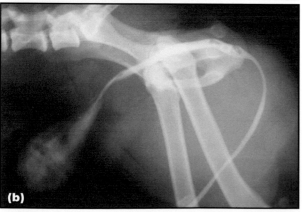

17.40 **(a)** Plain lateral radiograph of the caudal abdomen and pelvis of a male Staffordshire Bull Terrier with dysuria. No urethral stones are visible. **(b)** Positive-contrast urethrogram. Note the filling defects at the pelvic brim, which are calculi that were not visible on the plain radiograph, probably due to limited radiopacity and overlying pelvic structures.

for radiopaque calculi. In most cases, simply repeating the exposure with the hindlimbs pulled caudally will clarify the findings. A further differential diagnosis of urethral calculi on plain radiographs in male dogs is so-called 'pseudocalculi' caudal to the os penis (Figure 17.41). These are in fact separate centres of calcification of the bone and can be seen to be in line with the os penis, dorsal to the urethra.

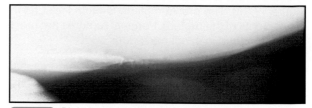

17.41 Plain lateral radiograph of the penis of a male dog, showing radiopaque 'pseudocalculi'. These are in fact separate centres of ossification caudal to the os penis.

Rupture

Urethral rupture is generally associated with a history of trauma. The trauma may be iatrogenic, following difficult catheterization in male cats. However, trauma is not always documented and clinical signs that should prompt investigation for evidence of rupture include:

- Localized bruising in the perineal, inguinal or inner thigh regions
- Localized swelling
- Localized cutaneous necrosis of the perineum and prepuce
- Ascites
- Dysuria or anuria.

Radiographic manifestations of rupture reflect the leakage of urine from the urethra into the local soft tissues. Free urine may accumulate within the peritoneal cavity if the rupture is at the bladder neck. Alternatively, more caudal lesions are associated with urine accumulation within the pelvic canal (Figure 17.42), perineum, prepuce or thigh. Distal ruptures are only apparent on plain radiographs as localized soft tissue swellings, often with disruption of tissue

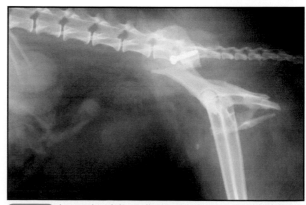

17.42 Lateral pelvic radiograph of a spaniel after a road traffic accident. In addition to multiple pelvic fractures (and prior partial orthopaedic repair) there is disruption of the soft tissue planes of the perineum, suggestive of an urethral rupture.

planes due to local inflammation and fluid accumulation. In either case, retrograde urethrography is required to establish the site of rupture. Retrograde studies may also give an indication of the extent of the urethral injury (Figure 17.43). Both of these features are important in directing decision-making during treatment. For example, perineal urethrostomy may be appropriate for ruptures of the penile urethra in male cats (Figure 17.44).

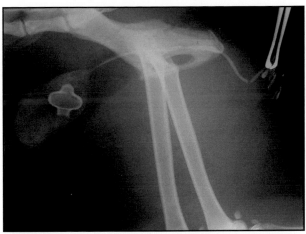

17.45 Retrograde urethrogram of a male cat 10 days after rupture of the intrapelvic urethra. The rupture has sealed but a stricture is present at the site. Additionally, a mushroom-tipped radiopaque cystotomy tube is in place.

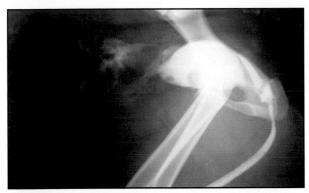

17.43 Retrograde urethrogram of a traumatized Springer Spaniel confirming the presence of two ruptures of the urethra: one at the ischial arch and one within the pelvis.

between urinations. Plain radiographs of the lower urinary tract are usually unremarkable. Sublumbar lymphadenopathy and pulmonary metastasis may be seen.

Retrograde urethrography reveals distortion of the urethral lumen. Typically there is evidence both of narrowing and erosion, classically described as presenting an 'apple core' appearance (Figure 17.46). Variable lengths of the urethra may be affected. The appearance of urethral neoplasia is similar to severe inflammatory urethral disease and unless clear evidence of metastasis is documented, biopsy samples are required to confirm the diagnosis. These may be obtained by urethroscopy or a catheter suction technique.

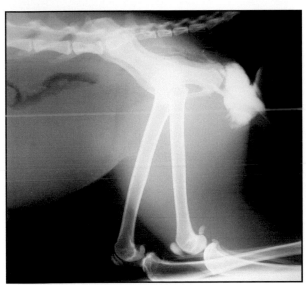

17.44 Retrograde urethrogram of a male cat with iatrogenic urethral rupture following unsuccessful attempts at catheterization. The study shows extravasation of contrast agent from the penile urethra both into the soft tissues of the perineum and into the penile vasculature. Peritoneal effusion is also present.

Radiological features of urethral rupture include leakage of contrast medium into the periurethral soft tissues. Less often, the rupture may have sealed but narrowing and irregularity of the urethral lumen may remain apparent (Figure 17.45).

Neoplasia

Neoplasia of the urethra is most commonly seen in elderly bitches. It is less common in male dogs and in cats. The clinical presentation is typically of obstructive dysuria or, less commonly, urinary frequency. Haematuria may be noted at the start of urination or

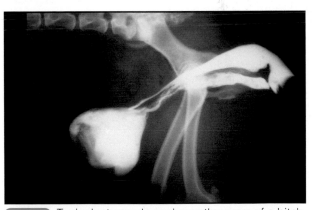

17.46 Typical retrograde vaginourethrogram of a bitch with a urethral carcinoma. Note the distortion and irregularity of the majority of the urethral length, presenting an 'apple core' appearance. Urethritis is an important differential diagnosis but carcinoma was confirmed by suction catheter biopsy in this case.

Inflammation

Inflammatory conditions include urethritis and urethral caruncle. Urethritis (Figure 17.47) is less common than urethral neoplasia but is an important differential diagnosis for animals with appropriate clinical signs. The radiographic appearance is not distinguishable from that of neoplasia and biopsy samples are indicated to confirm the diagnosis (see above).

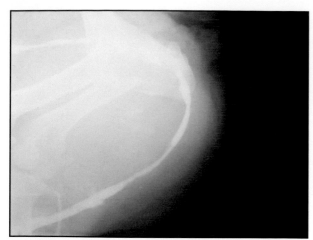

17.47 Retrograde urethrogram of a male Dachshund with diffuse urethritis. The perineal urethra is most clearly affected, with variable narrowing and urothelial irregularity.

Stricture

Urethral stricture may occur in association with neoplasia or urethritis. Radiographic features include narrowing and erosion of the urethra. There may be a history of urethral trauma, or this may be suspected if no other cause is found. In these benign cases of stricture, typically the only sign on plain radiography is bladder distension. Retrograde studies show a discrete narrowing of the urethra (see Figure 17.45), commonly with a relatively smooth urethral lumen and without evidence of erosion. The length of urethra affected is usually relatively short, although severe obstruction may prevent successful retrograde urethrography and hence determination of the extent of the stricture. Occasionally normograde urethrography can be used to assist with this, although the images are often non-diagnostic because of technical difficulties.

Developmental disease

Ureteral ectopia

In cases of ureteral ectopia, no changes are seen in the lower urinary tract on plain films but retrograde urethrography will often demonstrate retrograde filling of ectopic ureters (Figure 17.48). In most dogs, the affected ureters are intramural (see Chapter 16) and can be seen to insert in the urethra and run close to the urethral lumen (within the urethral wall) to the bladder neck. In cats, ectopic ureters (Figure 17.49) are typically extramural and can be seen as distinctly separate from the bladder neck. Although the majority of ectopic ureters are dilated in the intra-abdominal portion, this is not often apparent in the distal part associated with the urethra. The typical termination of ectopic ureters in females (dogs and cats) is the pelvic urethra (Figure 17.48), although they can pass as far distally as the urethral orifice and open alongside this at the vestibulovaginal junction (Figure 17.50). In male animals, which are less commonly affected than females, the ureters typically enter in the region of the prostatic urethra (Figure 17.51). However, it is often difficult to localize the opening site definitively, because of overlying pelvic bony structures. Less common sites of opening are the vagina and the uterus.

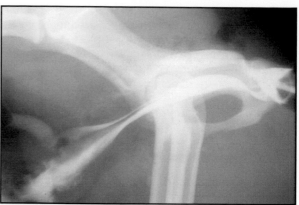

17.48 Retrograde vaginourethrogram of a young Labrador Retriever bitch with an intramural ectopic ureter. Retrograde filling of the ureter shows that it joins the urethra in the mid-pelvis. Further cranially, the ureter is seen dorsal and parallel to the urethra. The intra-abdominal ureter is seen to be less distinct (because of the lower concentration of iodine in the lumen from intravenous urography, rather than retrograde filling) and is dilated.

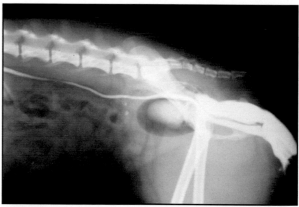

17.49 Retrograde urethrogram showing an ectopic ureter in a cat.

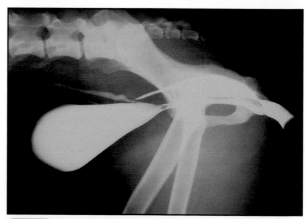

17.50 Retrograde vaginourethrogram of a Golden Retriever bitch with an ectopic ureter. In this patient the ureter joins at the urethral papilla and may be described as a vaginal ectopic ureter. At the bladder neck, a filling defect may represent a ureterocele. An intravenous urogram has already been carried out. The ectopic ureter is seen to be moderately dilated. The contralateral ureter is normal in diameter. It is not possible to distinguish which ureter is affected (left or right) and bilateral ectopia cannot be excluded.

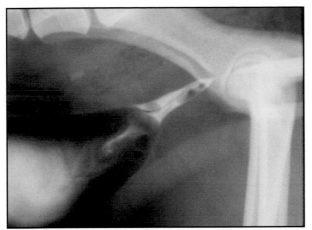

17.51 Retrograde urethrogram of a male dog with unilateral ureteral ectopia. The ureter is seen to communicate with the prostatic urethra. Regrettably, several air bubbles are present, causing artefactual filling defects.

Ureterocele

Dilatation of the intramural part of the ureter at the bladder neck is rare, and may be associated with ureteral ectopia. These may be incidental findings during investigation of urinary incontinence or occasionally are found as a cause of dysuria. In either case, plain radiography is typically unremarkable, but retrograde studies may show contrast medium within a cystic dilatation at the bladder neck (Figure 17.52). There is typically also a filling defect in the dorsal bladder lumen in this region, which represents urine within the ureterocele, separated from the bladder lumen by a thin septum of urothelium (Figure 17.53).

Diverticula

Urethral diverticula are a rare cause of urinary incontinence. They are not apparent on plain radiography, but on retrograde studies are visible as discrete out-pouchings of the urethral lumen (Figure 17.54) with a smooth urothelial surface. Most diverticula are assumed to be congenital, but they are sometimes seen in the prostatic urethra of male dogs after castration, when they may represent 'prostatic collapse'.

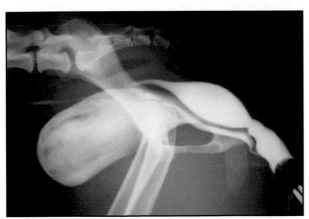

17.52 Retrograde vaginourethrogram of a Cocker Spaniel bitch with a ureterocele. Note the cystic structure at the bladder neck filled with contrast agent from the retrograde study and separated from the bladder lumen by a septum of urothelium. This is represented by a linear filling defect.

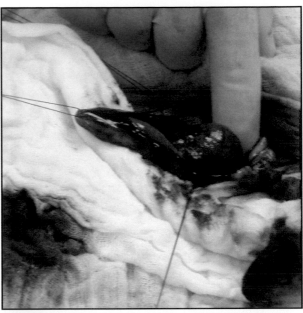

17.53 Surgical view of a ureterocele. Following a ventral midline cystotomy, the abnormal structure is seen as a distinct balloon-like fluid-filled swelling at the bladder neck.

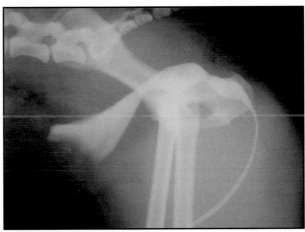

17.54 Retrograde urethrogram of a young male Cocker Spaniel with urinary incontinence. A urethral diverticulum is present in the caudal pelvic urethra.

References and further reading

Aumann M, Worth LT and Drobatz KJ (1998) Uroperitoneum in cats: 26 cases (1986–1995). *Journal of the American Animal Hospital Association* **34**, 315–324

Holt PE (1989) Positive contrast vagino-urethrography for the diagnosis of lower urinary tract disease. In: *Current Veterinary Therapy X Small Animal Practice*, ed RW Kirk, pp. 1142–1145. WB Saunders, Philadelphia

Holt PE (2008) *Urological Disorders of the Dog and Cat: Investigation, Diagnosis and Treatment*. Manson, London

Lamb CR (1997) Radiology and ultrasonography of the urinary tract. *Veterinary Quarterly* **19**, Supplement 1, s55–s56

Ragni RA and Hotston Moore A (2006) Urinary incontinence in the dog. Part 1: Diagnostic approach. *UK Vet: Companion Animal* **11**, 17–27

Scrivani PV, Chew DJ, Buffington C *et al.* (1998) Results of double-contrast cystography in cats with idiopathic cystitis: 45 cases (1993–1995). *Journal of the American Veterinary Medical Association* **212**, 1907–1909

Weichselbaum RC, Feeney DA, Jessen CR *et al.* (1998) Evaluation of the morphologic characteristics and prevalence of canine urocystoliths from a regional urolith center. *American Journal of Veterinary Research* **59**, 379–387

18

The female reproductive system

Gawain Hammond

Anatomy

The canine and feline female reproductive tract comprises internal and external genitalia:

- Internal genitalia:
  - Paired ovaries and uterine tubes (oviducts)
  - Uterus (paired horns, caudal body terminating in the cervix).
- External genitalia:
  - Vagina
  - Vestibule.

The ovaries are found close to the caudal poles of the kidneys and are generally ovoid in shape (although this is less consistent if a large follicle or corpus luteum is present). They have a cortex (containing the follicles) and a medulla. The right ovary is often found dorsal to the ascending colon, and the left ovary is located adjacent to the descending colon. The ovaries are enclosed by the ovarian bursae. The uterine tube begins as the funnel-shaped infundibulum adjacent to the ovary and continues as the ampulla then isthmus until the junction with the uterine horn. The course of the uterine tube is tortuous and lies within the wall of the ovarian bursa.

The uterus comprises two horns leading into a short body, terminating in a short thick-walled cervix. The uterine wall has three layers: an outer serosal layer (perimetrium); a muscular layer (myometrium); and an inner mucosal layer (endometrium). The uterus is generally dorsal to the small intestines, with the body lying ventral to the descending colon and dorsal to the bladder.

The vagina is long, extending through the pelvic canal. The lining of the vagina has a prominent dorsomedian fold extending from the cervix and an irregular folded appearance when non-distended. These folds end at the junction with the caudodorsally directed vestibule. The floor of the vestibule has the urethral papilla cranially and the clitoral fossa caudally. The female reproductive tract ends at the labia of the vulva.

Supporting structures

The abdominal reproductive tract is supported from the dorsal abdominal wall by the broad ligaments, which contain smooth muscle assisting in the support of the reproductive structures. The laxity in the attachments often increases with age, especially following pregnancy. The ovary is supported by proper and suspensory ligaments. The suspensory ligament is a peritoneal fold attaching the ovary to the last rib. The broad ligaments of the uterus often contain a considerable amount of fat. A peritoneal fold from the lateral aspect of the broad ligament extends through the inguinal canal, creating potential for inguinal herniation in bitches and queens.

Vascular and nervous supply

The reproductive tract gains its blood supply via two arteries. The ovarian arteries arise directly from the aorta, caudal to the renal arteries. The uterine arteries originate from the internal iliac artery. The supply from these two sources anastomose. The vestibule and vulva are supplied by the vaginal artery, also arising from the internal iliac artery. The venous drainage of the uterus and ovaries is largely via the ovarian veins, with the right draining directly into the caudal vena cava, and the left into the left renal vein. There is both a sympathetic and parasympathetic nervous supply to the reproductive tract. Sympathetic fibres generally run with the arterial supply and parasympathetic fibres arise from the pelvic nerves and pelvic plexus.

Oestrus cycle

The bitch is mono-oestrus, whilst the queen is seasonally polyoestrus. The timings of the oestrus cycles are summarized in Figure 18.1.

Stage of oestrus	Bitch		Queen	
	Average duration	Ovary	Average duration	Ovary
Pro-oestrus	9 days	Follicles	1.5–2 days	Follicles
Oestrus	9 days	Ovulation	4–10 days	Ovulation (approximately 27 h post mating)
Metoestrus	90 days	Corpus luteum	8–10 days	Corpus luteum
Anoestrus	75 days (variable)	Quiescent	3–4 months	Quiescent
Gestation period	63 days (58–68 days post mating)		63 days	

18.1 Duration of the phases of the oestrus cycle with predominant ovarian structures for the bitch and queen.

Normal radiographic appearance

Generally, the normal ovaries and uterus are not seen on plain abdominal radiographs in the non-pregnant dog or cat. If the patient is obese, then the excess abdominal fat may delineate the normal uterus as a faint linear soft tissue structure, seen between the bladder and descending colon on a lateral radiograph. The visibility of the uterus may be increased by the use of compression radiographic techniques, using a radiolucent strap or paddle to compress the area of interest. Pneumoperitoneography has also been reported to increase visibility of the abdominal viscera, but this technique has largely been replaced by diagnostic ultrasonography. If possible, withholding food for a day preceding radiography and administering enemas to clear faecal material from the descending colon will increase the visibility of organs in the caudal abdominal area. The normal non-gravid uterine diameter in the dog is around half that of the small intestine (usually about 1 cm) and is difficult to differentiate from small intestine on a plain radiograph. The normal location of the uterine body and horns in the non-gravid dog is demonstrated in Figure 18.2. The normal vagina is not seen on plain radiographs. The vulva is seen as a soft tissue shadow towards the ventral aspect of the perineum, but unless there is gross enlargement, plain radiography is unlikely to be of significant clinical utility.

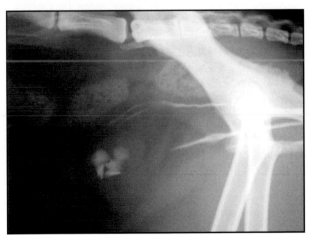

18.2 Retrograde positive-contrast study delineating the body and horns of a normal canine uterus. Radiopaque cystoliths are seen ventrally.

Contrast radiography

- Hysterosalpingography, involving the injection of positive contrast medium into the uterine lumen via a catheter passed through the cervix has been reported in the literature, but again has largely been replaced by ultrasonography.
- For the external genitalia, retrograde vaginourethrography has been widely described. The technique involves placing the inflated bulb of a Foley catheter into the vestibule to occlude the vulva. Gentle application of bowel clamps across the vulva may assist in preventing leakage. An alternative is to use a standard

urinary catheter and to gently clamp the vulval lips using a bowel clamp. Positive iodine-based contrast medium is injected via the catheter, usually 10–15 ml for a dog and approximately 5 ml for a cat, and should fill the vestibule and vagina (Figure 18.3). A degree of caution is needed, especially if using a balloon-tipped catheter, not to occlude the urethral papilla whilst completely occluding the vulva, as this risks iatrogenic damage to the vagina if excessive contrast medium is introduced (Figure 18.4).

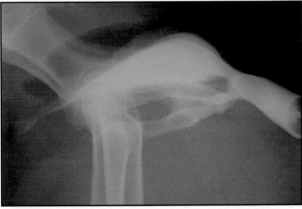

18.3 Retrograde positive-contrast vaginourethrogram of the normal lower genital tract in the bitch.

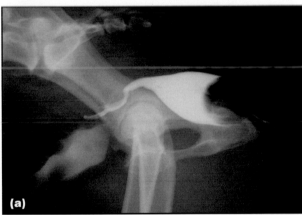

(a)

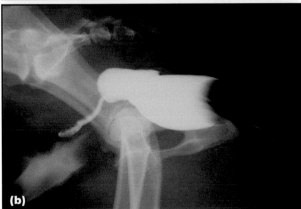

(b)

18.4 Iatrogenic rupture of the vagina during retrograde vaginourethrography due to occlusion of the urethra by the bulb of the Foley catheter. **(a)** Filling of vagina evident. **(b)** Abnormal shape of the cranial vagina, suspected to be due to dissection of the vaginal mucosa through a tear in the muscle layers. No additional filling of bladder noted. (continues) ▶

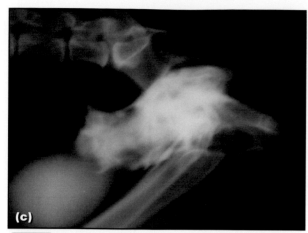

18.4 (continued) Iatrogenic rupture of the vagina during retrograde vaginourethrography due to occlusion of the urethra by the bulb of the Foley catheter. **(c)** Complete vaginal rupture, with dissection of contrast medium into the surrounding tissues. The patient was successfully managed with the placement of an indwelling urinary catheter for a few days.

- Vaginourethrography in the normal bitch demonstrates smooth margins to the vagina and vestibule. A narrowing at the junction of the vestibule and vagina, just cranial to the urethral orifice, is common. Thereafter, the vagina expands gently to a fusiform shape, then tapers cranially to the spoon-shaped paracervix. Around the time of oestrus the vagina tends to become more capacious and mucosal folds may be evident. In the normal queen, the vagina and vestibule are smooth in outline but remain narrow. Contrast medium may occasionally fill the uterine horns in the entire bitch or queen, but this is not a consistent finding.
- The use of negative contrast medium (e.g. room air, carbon dioxide) for vaginography could also be considered, and may be useful in delineating stenoses or mass lesions.

Indications

Given the generally poor visibility of the normal non-pregnant uterus and ovaries on plain radiographs, radiographic examination of the female reproductive tract is likely to be performed for one of four reasons:

1. Investigation of a palpable abdominal mass, to determine whether it involves the reproductive tract.
2. Assessment for uterine or ovarian disease where full palpation of the abdomen is not possible (i.e. due to pain, excessive size, etc.).
3. Diagnosis and/or assessment of pregnancy.
4. Investigation of vaginal or vestibular disease.

Given the mid-caudal abdominal location of the reproductive organs, and the possible distortion of the peritoneal attachments, an enlarged uterus or ovary could be palpated as a mid- or caudal abdominal mass, and may not be differentiated from other masses on palpation alone.

Ultrasonography

Ultrasonography has proven a useful diagnostic technique in the investigation of both pregnancy and disease of the female genital tract. It is in widespread use for the confirmation of pregnancy in both the bitch and queen. It can be used for examination of the internal genital organs as well as the external genitalia, but given the easy assessment of the vagina and vestibule through direct inspection and vaginography, ultrasonography of these structures is often superfluous.

The normal non-pregnant uterus and ovaries are often difficult to visualize and a high-frequency transducer (≥7.5 MHz) is ideal. The patient can be scanned in either lateral or dorsal recumbency. For the ovaries, the area caudal to the caudal pole of the kidney should be interrogated in both transverse and dorsal or sagittal planes for identification of the ovary. The position of the ovary relative to the caudal pole of the kidney is variable. They may be closely apposed or separated by up to 15–20 mm. The ovaries may not be visualized due to their small size, lack of distinction from the surrounding fat or interposed gastrointestinal structures. Canine ovaries are generally about 1.5 cm x 0.7 cm x 0.5 cm and ovoid in shape (Figure 18.5), whilst those of the queen are smaller. During pro-oestrus, follicles may be detected from days 2–7, with some reaching >1 cm in diameter as ovulation approaches. Following ovulation, the corpus luteum develops and the ovary becomes more hypoechoic and rounded, although a more irregular shape is also possible (Figure 18.6). The accuracy of ultrasonography for predicting ovulation in the bitch is still in question.

The non-gravid uterus is most easily found by searching for the uterine body between the bladder and descending colon (Figure 18.7). Visualization may be aided by using a full bladder as an acoustic window. The non-gravid uterine horns may be seen splitting cranially from the body of the uterus, but are generally difficult to identify. The horns are obscured by the small intestine and are difficult to differentiate from the surrounding fat. The different layers of the uterine wall and lumen are generally not identified, although if a small amount of fluid or mucus is present, the luminal contents may be hypoechoic/anechoic or

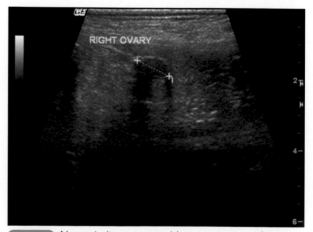

18.5 Normal ultrasonographic appearance of the canine ovary.

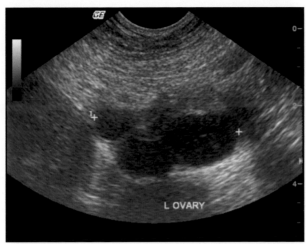

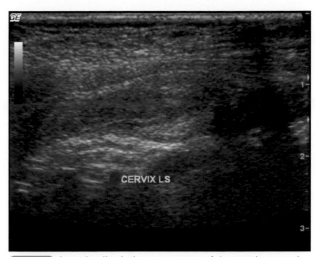

18.6 Ultrasonogram of canine ovary during metoestrus. Note the corpus luteum formation.

18.8 Longitudinal ultrasonogram of the canine cervix, which appears as a fusiform hyperechoic structure.

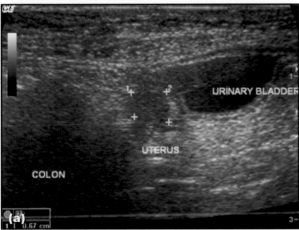

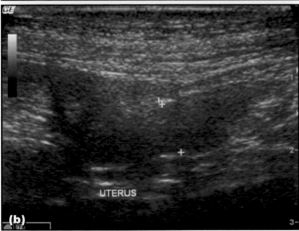

18.7 Ultrasonographic appearance of normal canine uterus. **(a)** Transverse ultrasonogram of the uterine body, demonstrating location between the bladder and descending colon. **(b)** Longitudinal ultrasonogram of the uterine body showing lack of visible layering or luminal content.

hyperechoic, respectively. The canine uterus generally measures 5–10 mm in diameter. The cervix, if seen, appears as a fusiform or linear hyperechoic structure (Figure 18.8). The uterus tends to become more hypoechoic, with occasional central hyperechoic areas, during pro-oestrus and oestrus, and this may allow slightly easier detection.

Overview of additional imaging modalities

The use of advanced imaging techniques for the female genital tract in dogs and cats is infrequently described in the literature. The use of fluoroscopy and nuclear scintigraphy has been used to measure transport through the cervix in the queen, and thermography has been used to predict ovulation in carnivores. Magnetic resonance imaging (MRI) and computed tomography (CT) should each give good anatomical imaging of the genital tract and may be considered for complicated cases, and the use of CT vaginourethrography has been reported. However, the availability and convenience of diagnostic ultrasonography renders these techniques unnecessary in the vast majority of cases.

Normal pregnancy

Both radiography and ultrasonography can be used in the assessment of normal gestation in the dog and cat, although their application will vary depending on the stage of gestation.

Radiography
The stages of radiographically visible uterine change during normal pregnancy are summarized in Figure 18.9.

Radiographic sign	Day from ovulation radiographic sign becomes visible	
	Bitch	*Queen*
Uterine enlargement	30	25–35
Shape of fetal sacs	30–40	25–35
Fetal mineralization	45	36–45

18.9 Stages of gestation and radiographic detection.

- In the bitch, uterine enlargement can generally be detected on plain radiographs on or about day 30 following ovulation.
- The individual bulges of the fetal sacs become apparent between 30 days and 40 days post ovulation.
- The uterine horns become more tubular in shape between days 38 and 45 post ovulation.
- Mineralization of the fetal skeletons is the definitive sign of pregnancy and may be seen from day 41 post ovulation, although visualization of fetal bone structures will be optimal after day 45.

Prior to the development of fetal mineralization, uterine enlargement due to pregnancy cannot be differentiated from other causes of uterine enlargement (such as pyometra) on radiographs alone. Due to the long potential life of canine sperm in the uterus (up to 7 days), the exact date of fertilization and hence exact stage of fetal development is often not known. Therefore, it is possible to have a radiograph taken at 45 days post mating that shows no evidence of fetal mineralization, yet the patient is pregnant. In these cases, diagnostic ultrasonography will often prove valuable. Once mineralization is visible, then it progresses rapidly to be clearly seen within 5 days. Therefore, a radiograph taken at 45 days post mating that shows no evidence of mineralization could be repeated 7–10 days later; if the initial radiograph is a false-negative, then the follow-up image should demonstrate clear fetal skeletons.

- In the queen, radiographically detectable uterine enlargement has been reported as early as day 19 of pregnancy, although day 25–35 is usually a more reliable guide.
- Fetal mineralization develops between day 35 and day 45.

In both species, as gestation progresses, the uterus develops a mid-ventral and caudoventral abdominal location, with resulting craniodorsal displacement of the small intestinal loops and ventral compression of the bladder. Once fetal skeletal structures are visible, radiographs generally prove a good method for assessing fetal numbers; either the number of skulls or number of vertebral columns can be counted, although care must be taken where the fetal shadows are superimposed. Fetuses normally lie in a neutral or mildly flexed position (Figure 18.10).

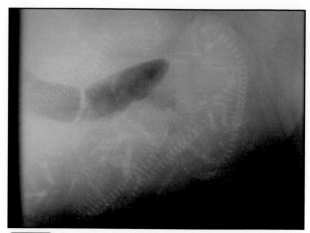

18.10 Radiographic appearance of normal canine fetal skeletons, with slight flexion of the spine and non-overlapping skull bones.

The use of ionizing radiation in diagnostic radiography does present a potential risk to the fetus. Fetal sensitivity to radiation is least in the final trimester, once organogenesis is complete. The benefits outweigh the potential risks for a radiographic study to confirm pregnancy, enumerate fetuses or to investigate other clinical problems.

Ultrasonography

Diagnostic ultrasonography allows much earlier detection of pregnancy than radiography. Although imaging of the gestational sac has been reported as early as day 10 of pregnancy in the bitch and day 11 in the queen, detection is generally easiest and most accurate between day 21 and day 35. The fetal heart beat is usually seen by day 21. Ultrasonography may be less accurate at determining fetal numbers than radiography, especially in the last trimester following fetal mineralization. Although uterine enlargement associated with pregnancy may be seen after 7 days in the bitch and 4 days in the queen, this is not a specific sign for pregnancy due to residual uterine enlargement following oestrus. Early detection of pregnancy may be further hampered by interference from gas and ingesta in the gastrointestinal tract. Optimizing the image by using the highest available probe frequency and careful patient preparation will increase the chances of early detection. The ultrasonographic detection of the stages of fetal development are summarized in Figure 18.11 and examples are shown in Figure 18.12.

Stage of fetal development	Ultrasonographic appearance	Day	
		Canine	*Feline*
Gestational sac	Anechoic cavity several millimetres across	17–20	11–14
Embryo	Echogenic structure, eccentrically located in gestational sac	23–25	15–17
Cardiac activity	Focus of fluttering echoes	23–25	16–18
Fetal movement		33–35	28–30

18.11 Ultrasonographic appearance of the stages of fetal development. (continues) ▶

Stage of fetal development	Ultrasonographic appearance	Day	
		Canine	*Feline*
Discernable head and body	Easy orientation of the fetus	28	26–28
Limb buds		35	26–28
Skeleton	Hyperechoic interfaces, developing distal acoustic shadowing as mineralization progresses	35–39	
Differentiation of internal organs	Visible heart, stomach, bladder, eyes, etc.	35–47	
Visible cardiac chambers	Identification of chambers	40	

18.11   (continued) Ultrasonographic appearance of the stages of fetal development.

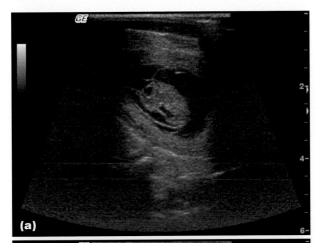

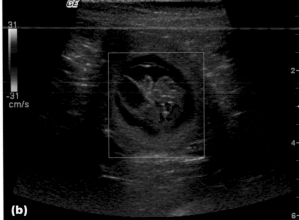

18.12   **(a)** Ultrasonogram of normal canine fetus at about 30 days of gestation. The fetus can be oriented and the eye is seen as an anechoic structure. **(b)** Colour Doppler ultrasonogram demonstrating blood flow within the fetal heart.

Assessment of fetal age

Fetal age can be approximately assessed based on the appearance of the ultrasound image (see Figure 18.11). Direct measurements can give a reasonably accurate estimate of fetal age.

- Between days 20 and 37, the most accurate method in the dog is to measure the diameter of the gestational sac (GSD), using the formula:

Gestational age (days from luteinizing hormone surge) = (6 x GSD) + 20

- After day 38, head diameter (HD) in the transverse plane is the most accurate parameter, using the formula:

Gestational age = (15 x HD) + 20

- Crown–rump length can be difficult to measure, especially in later gestation due to flexion of the fetus preventing the entire fetus being imaged in a single plane.
- The parturition date in the dog can then be calculated as:

Days before parturition = 65 – gestational age

- In the cat, after 40 days of gestation, HD is again the most useful parameter, using the formula:

Gestational age = (25 x HD) + 3

Days before parturition = 61 – gestational age

Post-partum uterus

Involution of the post-partum uterus is normally complete within 4 weeks in both the bitch and queen. The uterine wall is initially thick and irregular, and there is some luminal content of variable echogenicity (Figure 18.13). As time progresses, the walls become thinner and the amount of luminal material decreases.

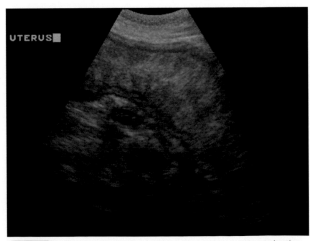

18.13   Ultrasonogram of the post-partum uterus in the early stage of involution. (Courtesy of A King)

Female reproductive system diseases

Ovary

Radiography

Ovaries of normal size and opacity are generally poorly visualized on plain radiographs. Therefore, radiography is most likely to be useful when there is either ovarian mineralization or ovarian enlargement. Although the ovaries are found close to the caudal pole of the kidneys, the ovaries have an intraperitoneal location, and enlargement or a mass of the ovary will thus appear in a mid-abdominal location on a lateral radiograph, and is likely to be lateralized on a ventrodorsal (VD) radiograph. The degree of displacement of other organs is variable and depends on the size of the mass.

- There may be ventral displacement of the small intestine. A large mass is likely to displace the ipsilateral kidney cranially, with possible rotation of the caudal pole ventrally.
- On a VD radiograph, a right ovarian mass results in medial displacement of the ascending colon and small intestine, whilst a left ovarian mass causes medial displacement of the descending colon and small intestine.

A similar radiographic appearance may occur due to masses of the head of the spleen, mesenteric lymphadenopathy, masses of the intestines or mesentery, and renal masses. Additional imaging techniques, such as ultrasonography, gastrointestinal contrast studies or intravenous urography, help to differentiate ovarian from other possible sources of a mass.

Differential diagnoses: Differential diagnoses for ovarian enlargement include:

- Neoplasia: ovarian neoplasia accounts for about 1% of canine tumours and 0.7–3.6% of feline tumours. Various forms of neoplasia have been reported in the canine ovary, including epithelial cell tumours (papillary carcinomas and adenocarcinomas, cystadenomas and undifferentiated carcinomas), germ cell tumours (dysgerminomas, teratomas and teratocarcinomas), sex-cord stromal tumours (granulosa cell tumours) and metastatic disease (rare, but reported with mammary, intestinal and pancreatic carcinomas and lymphosarcomas). Feline ovarian neoplasms are most commonly dysgerminomas, but granulosa cell tumours, teratomas and epithelial tumours have also been reported. Neoplasms may be bilateral and have variable metastatic rates. Thoracic radiographs should be obtained to evaluate the patient for pulmonary metastases. Some ovarian diseases result in peritoneal effusion, in which case ultrasonography will be more useful than radiography. Some ovarian tumours may also result in pleural effusion
- Ovarian cysts (follicular and luteal)
- Haematoma
- Hydrovarium.

Most causes of ovarian enlargement will result in a soft tissue opacity mass (Figure 18.14). However, mineralization may be seen with teratomas and teratocarcinomas, which may include bony tissue (including formed teeth and skeletal structures) (Figure 18.15). Dystrophic mineralization has also been reported in other ovarian neoplasms.

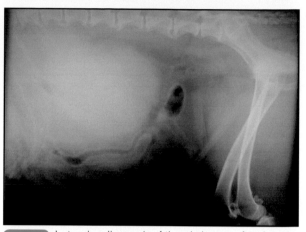

18.14 Lateral radiograph of the abdomen of an intact bitch, demonstrating a large rounded soft tissue mass in the dorsal mid-abdomen with ventral displacement of intestinal structures. The left renal shadow can be seen superimposed on the mass. An ovarian neoplasm was found at exploratory surgery.

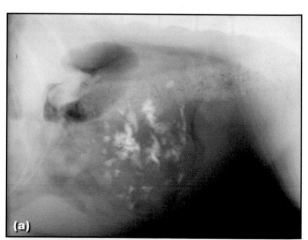

(a)

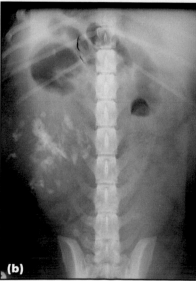

(b)

18.15

(a) Right lateral and **(b)** VD radiographs of the abdomen of an intact bitch, demonstrating a large soft tissue mass with irregular mineralization in the right mid-abdomen. The mass is causing displacement of the intestines and compression of the cranial pole of the bladder. (continues) ▶

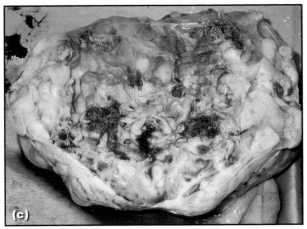

18.15 (continued) **(c)** A teratoma was confirmed on histopathology, and contained hair clumps and sheets of cartilage and foci of bone.

Ultrasonography

Ultrasonography can be used to assess ovarian masses in conjunction with radiography, but also allows assessment of ovarian disease where there has not been significant enlargement of the ovary. For a mass detected on plain radiography, ultrasonography may allow identification of the ovarian origin of the mass, based on the location relative to the kidney and uterine horn. Assessment of the structure of the mass is also possible, with cystic changes (Figure 18.16) being differentiated from more solid tissue.

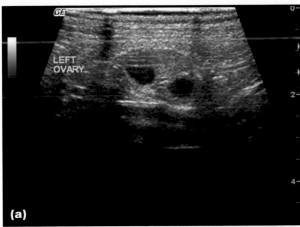

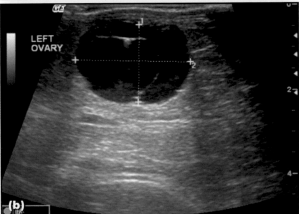

18.16 Ultrasonograms of cystic changes in the ovary. **(a)** Two small cystic areas in the ovary. **(b)** Cyst occupying the entire ovary.

Ultrasonography is also useful in examining the remainder of the abdomen for evidence of metastatic spread in the case of neoplasia.

Ultrasonography is the imaging modality of choice for suspected disease where the overall size of the ovary has not increased, and is therefore unlikely to produce recognizable changes on abdominal radiography. This may allow detection of cystic or cavitary lesions, such as benign ovarian cysts or haematomas. Early detection of ovarian neoplasia may also be possible with ultrasonography, revealing a solid mass, or a mass with cavitary areas (granulosa cell tumour, teratoma, adenocarcinoma) or areas of mineralization (teratoma) (Figures 18.17).

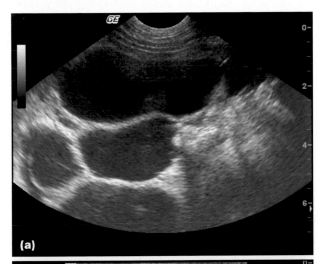

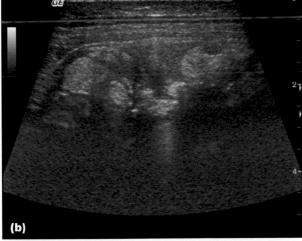

18.17 Ultrasonograms of the bitch in Figure 18.15, demonstrating the heterogenous nature of an ovarian teratoma. **(a)** Cystic areas. **(b)** Solid tissue with acoustic shadowing.

Uterus

Herniation

The extension of the broad ligament of the uterus through the inguinal canal does lead to the possibility of uterine herniation (see above). Herniation may be congenital or acquired (e.g. during gestation). The extra-abdominal mass is usually easily detected on clinical examination, but radiography and ultrasonography are useful in determining the nature of the herniated organs.

Endometrial disease

Canine endometrial hyperplasia–pyometra complex is a common disease, resulting from an abnormal response to progesterone with subsequent infection leading to pyometra. In older patients (>6 years) cystic endometrial hyperplasia usually precedes pyometra, whilst in younger bitches it is possible to develop pyometra without underlying endometrial disease.

Ultrasonography: This is the optimal imaging technique for diagnosing both cystic endometrial hyperplasia and pyometra. Cystic endometrial hyperplasia alone may not result in radiographically visible enlargement of the uterus, and pyometra is generally conveniently diagnosed using ultrasonography, minimizing the use of ionizing radiation.

- Cystic endometrial hyperplasia is generally seen on ultrasonographic examination as a diffuse thickening of the uterine wall, with multiple anechoic areas contained within the wall (Figure 18.18). This finding is diagnostic for cystic endometrial hyperplasia.

- As pyometra develops, fluid collects in the lumen of the uterus. The uterine horns are usually symmetrically affected, but this is variable and only one horn may be affected. Hence, it is important to check for uterine distension on both sides of the abdomen.
- The fluid is usually hypo- to anechoic, but may contain echogenic material that has a swirling pattern in real time.
- If mildly dilated, the uterine horns can be of a similar size to loops of small intestine (Figure 18.19a). However, the layered appearance of the intestinal wall should be visible (uterine wall layers are generally not visible on ultrasonography) and the intestinal loops will usually show some peristaltic activity. Another method for differentiating the uterus from the intestine is to trace the uterine horns caudally to the bifurcation.
- The uterus may be massively distended, in which case the uterine wall is likely to be very thin (Figure 18.19b).

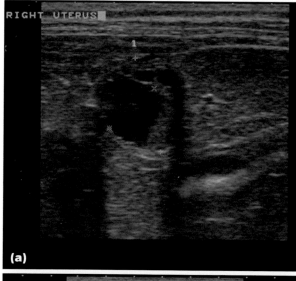

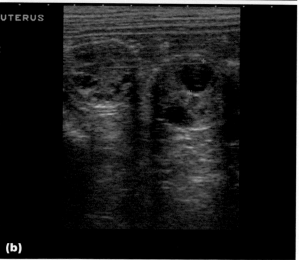

18.18   Ultrasonograms of cystic endometrial hyperplasia, demonstrating **(a)** large cystic areas within the uterine wall and **(b)** the diffuse nature of disease (both uterine horns are affected).

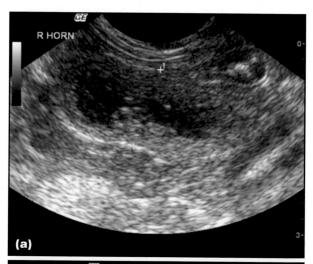

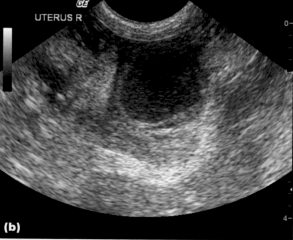

18.19   Ultrasonograms demonstrating the appearance of pyometra. **(a)** Mild dilatation of the uterine horn with echogenic fluid. A transverse view of a loop of jejunum is seen at the right of the image, demonstrating the differing appearance of the walls of the uterus and small intestine. **(b)** A more dilated uterine horn containing echogenic fluid.

Differential diagnoses: Differential diagnoses for a fluid-filled uterus (with no visible fetal structures) include hydrometra (usually anechoic fluid), haemometra and mucometra (both likely to be echogenic fluid), but these are much less common than pyometra. Aspiration of the dilated uterus is not recommended due to the risk of peritoneal contamination.

If the uterus is distended sufficiently, it may be seen on plain abdominal radiographs.

- Mild distension will lead to the uterine body becoming visible between the descending colon and bladder neck. However, the uterine horns may be lost amongst the loops of small intestine (Figure 18.20a).
- Greater distension will lead to the uterine horns becoming visible, usually as a convoluted soft tissue mass caudal to the small intestines and cranial to the bladder. The small intestines may be displaced cranially (Figure 18.20b).

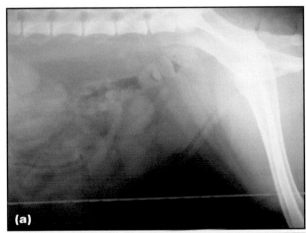

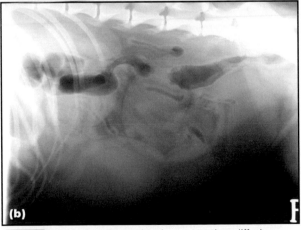

18.20 Lateral radiographs demonstrating differing degrees of pyometra. **(a)** Moderate distension of the uterus, with separation of the bladder and descending colon and occupation of the caudoventral abdomen by coiled soft tissue loops. **(b)** Severely distended loops of uterus occupying the ventral and caudal abdomen, with dorsal displacement of the intestines.

Differential diagnoses for general uterine enlargement with soft tissue opacity on radiography include: pregnancy prior to fetal mineralization; post-partum uterine enlargement (may be seen for 1–2 weeks following parturition); hydrometra; mucometra; and haemometra.

Rarely, an emphysematous pyometra develops and is seen on radiographs as tubular structures containing gas or mixed gas and soft tissue/fluid (and must be differentiated from intestinal gas) (Figure 18.21). This has been associated with *Clostridium perfringens* and *Pseudomonas aeruginosa* infection, and may be linked with metritis or fetal death.

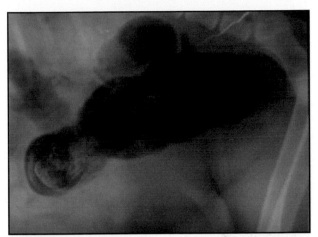

18.21 Lateral radiograph showing marked gaseous distension of the uterus with faintly visible fetal skeletal structures within the lumen. (Courtesy of the University of Bristol)

Stump pyometra

Stump granuloma or stump pyometra can be difficult to diagnose without the use of ultrasonography. Typically, ultrasonography shows a heterogenous mass lesion between the bladder and descending colon, immediately cranial to the pelvic inlet, but small lesions may be difficult to identify (Figure 18.22a). Radiographs may show a soft tissue mass effect between the bladder and descending colon, often with a focal loss of serosal detail (Figure 18.22b). Contrast medium within the bladder and/or descending colon may be helpful to highlight the lesion (Figure 18.22c). This is an area where advanced imaging (CT and MRI) may be of use.

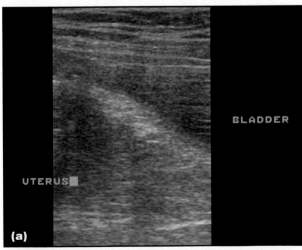

18.22 Stump pyometra. **(a)** Ultrasonogram showing a hypoechoic moderately defined mass dorsal to the bladder neck. (continues)

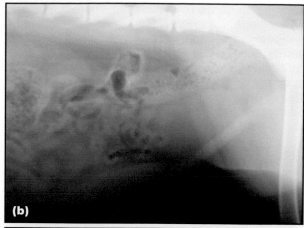

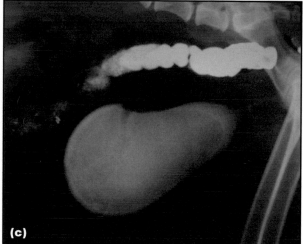

18.22 (contined) Stump pyometra. **(b)** Lateral radiograph of the caudal abdomen showing an ill defined soft tissue mass between the bladder neck and descending colon. (Courtesy of M Sullivan) **(c)** Lateral radiograph of the caudal abdomen showing a soft tissue mass between the contrast medium-filled bladder and contrast medium-filled rectum. (Courtesy of the University of Bristol)

Focal uterine enlargement

Focal uterine enlargement may be seen on either ultrasonography or plain radiography. Differential diagnoses include early pregnancy with a small litter size, focal pyometra and uterine neoplasia. Ultrasonography is most useful in confirming the involvement of the uterus and diagnosing the cause of enlargement. Displacement of other organs depends on the location and size of the lesion. Focal wall thickening on ultrasonography may result from neoplasia or uterine granuloma or abscess. Differential diagnoses for generalized and focal uterine enlargement are presented in Figure 18.23.

Uterine neoplasms are fairly uncommon in both the bitch and queen (0.3–0.4% of all neoplasms in the bitch, 0.2–1.5% in the queen). Most canine uterine neoplasms are mesenchymal (leiomyomas, 85–90%; leiomyosarcomas, 10%), but adenomas/adenocarcinomas, fibromas/fibrosarcomas and lipomas also occur. Most feline uterine neoplasms are adenocarcinomas, but leiomyomas/leiomyosarcomas, fibromas/fibrosarcomas, lipomas and lymphosarcomas have also been reported.

Generalized uterine enlargement
Pregnancy prior to fetal mineralization
Post-partum uterus prior to complete involution
Pyometra
Mucometra
Haemometra
Hydrometra

Focal uterine enlargement
Pregnancy with a small number of fetuses, prior to fetal mineralization
Localized pyometra
Stump pyometra or granuloma of uterine body (seen between the bladder and descending colon)
Uterine neoplasia

18.23 Differential diagnoses for generalized and focal uterine enlargement without evidence of fetal structures.

Abnormal findings during pregnancy

Both radiography and ultrasonography are useful in the investigation of abnormalities during gestation. These may include fetal distress and death, fetal mummification and dystocia.

Fetal distress: This is most easily assessed by measuring the fetal heart rate using ultrasonography. Normal fetal heart rate is roughly twice that of the bitch or queen, but this may be reduced by fetal hypoxia (e.g. as a result of dystocia). M-mode ultrasonography is a useful method for assessing heart rate.

Fetal death: Fetal death may be determined using ultrasonography or radiography. Ultrasonographic assessment of fetal viability is based on verifying cardiac activity. Other signs include fetal movement and appropriate development of the fetus relative to the expected stage of gestation. Ultrasonography is generally more reliable than radiography for detecting recent fetal death.

Radiographic evidence of fetal death is only generally apparent after skeletal mineralization has occurred. Signs may include:

- Intrafetal or perifetal gas
- Fetal disintegration (lack of normal arrangement of bones)
- Demineralization of fetal bones
- Overlapping of the cranial bones (the Spalding sign)
- Abnormal fetal position (e.g. hyperextension).

Care must be taken as some of these changes may be mimicked by overlying intestinal gas or superimposition of multiple fetuses, and distortion of the skull bones may occur if the skull is passing into the pelvic canal, as in dystocia.

Fetal mummification: When the fetus dies, mummification may ensue. This is demonstrated by compaction of the skeletal structures and increased radiopacity (Figure 18.24). This may be seen with ectopic pregnancies, as the fetus appears in an abnormal location. In these cases, there is often a peritoneal effusion obscuring the fine detail, and it is

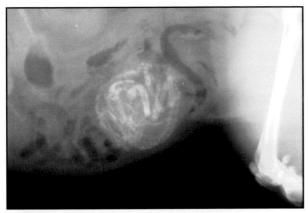

18.24 Radiographic appearance of fetal mummification. Note the increased radiopacity of the fetus and the abnormally flexed appearance. (Courtesy of M Sullivan)

difficult to differentiate fetal mummification from acute uterine rupture.

Fetal death before 25 days probably results in resorption of the fetus, whilst after 35 days abortion is more likely. An aborted fetus quickly loses the normal ultrasonographic appearance and is usually expelled within a few days.

Dystocia: This condition may most usefully be assessed using radiography. Causes that may be identified on radiographs include fetal malpresentation and fetal oversize, pelvic canal obstruction (e.g. previous pelvic fracture) and uterine inertia (failure of fetuses to approach the pelvic inlet). Radiography should also be performed if there is a query about retained fetuses. Ultrasonography can be used to assess fetal distress (see above) and may also allow detection of uterine inertia.

Cervix

The cervix is generally poorly identified with diagnostic imaging and is likely to present an obviously abnormal appearance only when a large mass is present. In these cases, the definition of the cervical end of the vagina will be lost on retrograde vaginography (Figure 18.25), and there may be a mass effect separating the bladder and descending colon.

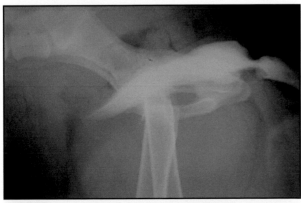

18.25 Lateral positive-contrast retrograde vaginourethrogram showing an ill defined margin to the cranial end of contrast medium column at the interface with the cervix. A cervical neoplasm was found at exploratory surgery.

Vagina and vestibule

The vagina and vestibule are often adequately examined by direct inspection or vaginoscopy, and hence diagnostic imaging is not needed in every case of vaginal disease. The limited access for standard ultrasound probes also reduces the use of ultrasonography for examining vaginal lesions, and plain radiography is similarly of little benefit. However, contrast radiography can still play an important role in assessing the external genitalia, especially when lesions are located in the more cranial region of the vagina. Vaginography or vaginourethrography may assist in the diagnosis of stenosis or strictures, hypoplasia or aplasia, fistulas and masses.

Vestibulovaginal stenosis

A septum or annular narrowing is present at the vestibulovaginal junction, which may result from incomplete perforation of the hymen or hypoplasia of the genital canal. The clinical importance of vestibulovaginal stenosis (Figure 18.26) is unclear, and mild to moderate narrowing is commonly seen as an incidental finding. However, severe stenosis has been implicated in recurrent lower urinary or genital tract infections due to the retention of pooled urine in the vagina proximal to the stenosis. There may also be difficulties encountered during parturition.

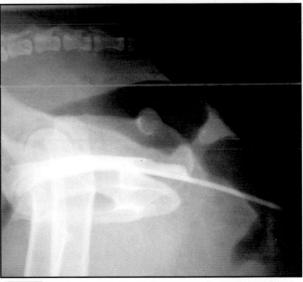

18.26 Lateral radiograph following positive-contrast urethrography and pneumovaginography showing vestibulovaginal stenosis. A soft tissue narrowing between the vagina and vestibule is clearly demonstrated by the negative contrast medium.

Vaginal aplasia

Vaginal aplasia results in failure of development of the vagina and can be seen as a lack of vaginal filling on vaginography (Figure 18.27).

Vaginitis

Vaginitis can occur in intact or neutered bitches, and less commonly in queens, and may result from bacterial or viral infections and chemical or mechanical irritation, generally presenting with a vulval discharge. Vaginitis is likely to be diagnosed by cytology and vaginoscopy. However, on positive-contrast vagino-

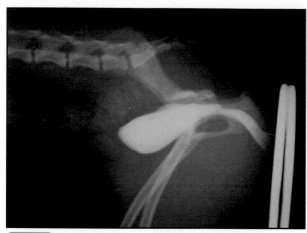

18.27 Lateral positive-contrast retrograde study demonstrating vaginal aplasia. Note the lack of contrast medium filling the lower genital tract.

graphy, vaginitis results in an irregular margin to the interface between the luminal contrast medium and the mucosa of the vagina (Figure 18.28).

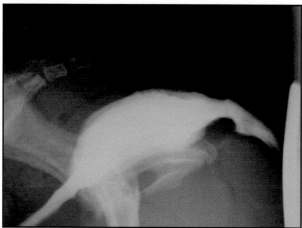

18.28 Lateral retrograde vaginourethrogram demonstrating irregular margins to the mucosa of the vagina (especially dorsally). This appearance is consistent with vaginitis.

Vaginal fistulas

Vaginal fistulas may develop between the vagina and rectum, leading to recurrent vaginal or urinary infections. Fistulas may be congenital or traumatic in nature. They may be demonstrated using vaginography, when defined extravasation of contrast medium occurs into the rectum.

Ureteral ectopia

Rarely, ectopic ureters may insert into the lower genital tract, and vaginography is likely to show retrograde filling of the ureter from the point of insertion to the external genitalia.

Vaginal and vulval masses

Possible causes of masses in this region include:

- Vaginal hypertrophy: most commonly occurs in younger bitches, with brachycephalic breeds predisposed to this condition. It results in a thickening of the lining of the vagina, which is

seen as a corrugated appearance on vaginography (Figure 18.29). The vagina may also be enlarged
- Vaginal oedema
- Vaginal or uterine prolapse: usually results from a congenital weakness of the supporting tissues, although hyperoestrogenism due to cystic ovaries has also been implicated. Uterine prolapse may also be associated with parturition
- Vaginal or vestibular polyp
- Vaginal or vestibular neoplasm: neoplastic lesions of the vagina or vestibule include leiomyomas, fibromas, polyps and leiomyosarcomas. Most (>80%) are reported as benign. Whilst caudal masses are likely to be easily accessible to visual inspection, contrast radiography may be considered to delineate more cranial masses. Vaginal masses usually appear as filling defects in the contrast medium pool and are frequently smoothly marginated (Figure 18.30)
- Clitoral hypertrophy
- Cyst
- Abscess
- Haematoma.

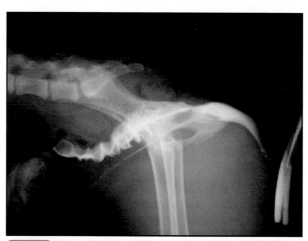

18.29 Lateral retrograde vaginourethrogram showing corrugated irregular filling of the vagina, which is overlong. This appearance is consistent with vaginal hyperplasia.

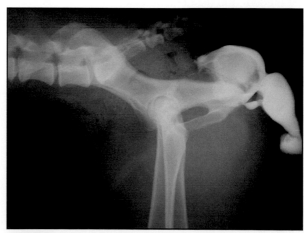

18.30 Lateral retrograde vaginourethrogram showing a large ventral rounded filling defect in the caudal vagina. A vaginal mass was confirmed on vaginoscopy.

There is little published work studying the use of ultrasonography in vaginal disease, and direct inspection and radiography are likely to offer more information. However, both ultrasonography and radiography are vital if there is concern for systemic or metastatic disease associated with vaginal lesions.

Miscellaneous conditions

Uncommon conditions of the female reproductive system are often congenital and include intersexuality. These patients may present due to clitoral hypertrophy and radiography of the perineal area may show an os clitoris. Duplication of the reproductive tract is rare.

Mammary glands

The canine and feline mammary glands are located ventrally. There are generally five pairs of glands in the bitch and four pairs in the queen, although some variation is possible. The cranial glands are supplied by branches from the axillary and internal thoracic arteries, and the caudal glands by branches from the deep circumflex iliac and caudal superficial epigastric arteries. Both arteries and veins show multiple anastomoses. Lymphatic drainage of the cranial glands is to the axillary and sternal nodes, and the caudal glands drain to the inguinal nodes. The normal mammary gland cannot be distinguished from the surrounding fascial planes and skin on radiographs, although this area may seem more swollen close to parturition and during lactation. The use of ultrasonography to assess mammary glands has been reported. The normal mammary gland has a homogenous appearance on ultrasonography around the time of parturition.

Mammary gland diseases

Mammary neoplasia
Mammary neoplasia is extremely common in the bitch. The incidence of neoplasia is significantly reduced by ovariohysterectomy, and can be increased by the use of injectable progestins for oestrus suppression. The risk of malignant neoplasms is 0.05% if the animal is spayed prior to the first oestrus, 8% if spayed after the first season, and 26% if spayed later than the second season. Spaying at any age seems to reduce the risk of benign neoplasms. Neoplasms are approximately 50% malignant histologically, although the tumour behaviour may not match this. The majority of canine mammary neoplasms are epithelial tumours or carcinomas of various types, although sarcomas (e.g. fibrosarcomas, osteosarcomas) do occur less frequently. Benign neoplasms are most often fibroadenomas, with simple adenomas and benign mixed tumours also occurring.

Mammary neoplasia in the queen is much more likely (>85%) to be malignant, but occurs at less than half the frequency of the bitch. Siamese cats seem to show an increased risk of mammary neoplasia. There is an effect of early neutering, with a sevenfold reduction in incidence reported when ovariohysterectomy is performed at 6 months of age. The

majority of feline mammary neoplasms are adenocarcinomas.

Diagnostic imaging: This does not have a huge role to play in the assessment of primary mammary neoplasia; palpation and histopathology are likely to be more important. However, radiography is indicated if there is a risk of metastatic disease. Mammary neoplasia can spread to the lungs or to the draining lymph nodes. Thoracic radiographs should be evaluated for pulmonary metastases and for sternal lymphadenopathy. In the queen, metastatic spread to the pleura has also been reported. If the neoplasm involves the caudal mammary glands, then the sublumbar lymph nodes should be evaluated using radiography and/or ultrasonography.

Mineralization of mammary lesions has been reported, and is more often associated with benign lesions than with malignant disease. Mineralization may be seen on survey radiographs along the ventral abdomen (Figure 18.31) and as distal acoustic shadowing on ultrasonography. If it is necessary to demonstrate mineralization within a mammary mass using radiography, then oblique views skylining the mammary mass could be used, but these are rarely indicated.

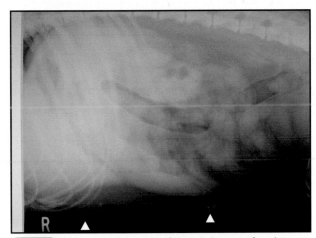

18.31 Lateral radiograph of the abdomen of an intact bitch, showing dilated loops of uterus occupying the caudoventral abdomen (pyometra was confirmed at exploratory surgery) and multiple mineralized opacities ventral to the abdominal wall. These were confirmed as multiple mineralized mammary gland tumours (arrowheads).

The use of ultrasonography to assess primary mammary neoplasms gives a good representation of the tissue composition of the neoplasm. In addition, the use of Doppler ultrasonography demonstrates the vascularity of the mass. However, the extent of local invasion is not accurately portrayed using ultrasonography. Ultrasonographic assessment of sternal adenopathy is more sensitive and specific than radiography.

Mastitis
On ultrasonography, an inflamed mammary gland will generally appear enlarged, heterogenous and irregular. With severe cases, bubbles of gas may be seen, and abscessation has been reported.

References and further reading

Bartels JE (1978) Radiology of the genital tract. In: *Radiographic Diagnosis of Abdominal Disorders of the Dog and Cat*, ed. T R O'Brien, pp. 615–659. WB Saunders, Philadelphia

Boyd JS (1971) Radiographic identification of the various stages of pregnancy in the domestic cat. *Journal of Small Animal Practice* **12**, 501–506

Chatdarong K, Kampa N, Axner E, *et al.* (2002) Investigation of cervical patency and uterine appearance in domestic cats by fluoroscopy and scintigraphy. *Reproduction in Domestic Animals* **37**, 275–281

Crawford JT and Adams WM (2002) Influence of vestibulovaginal stenosis, pelvic bladder and recessed vulva on response to treatment for clinical signs of lower urinary tract disease in dogs: 38 cases. *Journal of the American Veterinary Medical Association* **221**, 995–999

Davidson AP, Nyland TG and Tsutsui T (1986) Pregnancy diagnosis with ultrasound in the domestic cat. *Veterinary Radiology* **27**, 109–114

Dennis R, Kirberger RM, Wrigley RH and Barr F (2001) *Handbook of Small Animal Radiological Differential Diagnosis*, pp 193. WB Saunders, Philadelphia

Diez-Bru N, Garcia-Real I, Martinez EM, *et al.* (1998) Ultrasonographic appearance of ovarian tumours in 10 dogs. *Veterinary Radiology and Ultrasound* **39**, 226–233

Durant BS, Ravida N, Spady T, *et al.* (2006) New technologies for the study of carnivore reproduction. *Theriogenology* **66**, 1729–1736

Dyce KM, Sack WO and Wensing CJG (2002) The pelvis and reproductive organs of the carnivores. In: *Textbook of Veterinary Anatomy, 3rd edn*, ed. KM Dyce *et al.*, pp. 435–453. WB Saunders, Philadelphia

England GCW (1999) Diseases of the reproductive system. In: *Textbook of Small Animal Medicine*, ed. JW Dunn, pp. 574–611. WB Saunders, Philadelphia

Feeney DA and Johnston GR (2002) The uterus, ovaries and testes. In: *Textbook of Veterinary Diagnostic Imaging, 4th edn*, ed. DE Thrall, pp 603–614. WB Saunders, Philadelphia

Ferretti LM, Newell SM, Graham JP, *et al.* (2000) Radiographic and ultrasonographic appearance of the normal feline postpartum uterus. *Veterinary Radiology and Ultrasound* **41**, 287–291

Hernandez JL, Besso JG, Rault DN, *et al.* (2003) Emphysematous pyometra in a dog. *Veterinary Radiology and Ultrasound* **44**, 196–198

Johnson CA (1991) Diagnosis and treatment of chronic vaginitis in the bitch. *Veterinary Clinics of North America: Small Animal Practice* **21**, 523–531

Johnston SD, Root Kustritz MV and Olson PNS (2001) Disorders of the feline vagina, vestibule and vulva. In: *Canine and Feline Theriogenology*, ed. SD Johnston *et al.*, 472–473. WB Saunders, Philadelphia

Klein MK (2001) Tumours of the Female Reproductive System. In: *Small Animal Clinical Oncology, 3rd edn*, ed. SJ Withrow and EG MacEwen, pp. 445–454. WB Saunders, Philadelphia

Kyles AE, Vaden S, Hardie EM, *et al.* (1996) Vestibulovaginal stenosis in dogs: 18 cases. *Journal of the American Veterinary Medical Association* **209**, 1889–1893

Lyle SK (2007) Disorders of Sexual Development in the Dog and Cat. *Theriogenology* **68**, 338–343

Manothaiudom K and Johnston SD (1991) Clinical approach to vaginal/vestibular masses in the bitch. *Veterinary Clinics of North America: Small Animal Practice* **21**, 509–521

Mattoon JS and Nyland TG (2002) Ovaries and uterus. In: *Small Animal Diagnostic Ultrasound, 2nd edn*, ed. TG Nyland and JS Mattoon, pp. 231–249. WB Saunders, Philadelphia

Nagashima Y, Hoshi K, Tanaka R, *et al.* (2000) Ovarian and retroperitoneal teratomas in a dog. *Journal of Veterinary Medical Science* **62**, 793–795

Nyman HT, Nielsen OL, McEvoy FJ, *et al.* (2006) Comparison of B-mode and Doppler ultrasonographic findings with histologic features of benign and malignant mammary tumors in dogs. *American Journal of Veterinary Research* **67**, 985–991

Ragni RA (2006) What is your diagnosis? Vaginal oedema/hyperplasia or vaginal prolapse. *Journal of Small Animal Practice* **47**, 625–627

Rivers W and Johnston GR (1991) Diagnostic imaging of the reproductive organs of the bitch: methods and limitations. *Veterinary Clinics of North America: Small Animal Practice* **21**, 437–466

Rutteman GR, Withrow SJ and MacEwen EG (2001) Tumors of the mammary gland. In: *Small Animal Clinical Oncology, 3rd edn*, ed. SJ Withrow and EG MacEwen, pp. 455– 477. WB Saunders, Philadelphia

Sforna M, Brachalente C, Lepri E, *et al.* (2003) Canine ovarian tumours: a retrospective study of 49 cases. *Veterinary Research Communication* **27 Suppl 1**, 359–361

Thilagar S, Vinita WP, Heng HG, *et al.* (2006) What is your diagnosis? Small intestinal and colon obstruction; emphysematous pyometra. *Journal of Small Animal Practice* **47**, 687–688

Wang KY, Samii VF, Chew DJ, *et al.* (2006) Vestibular, vaginal and urethral relations in spayed dogs with and without lower urinary tract signs. *Journal of Veterinary Internal Medicine* **20**, 1065–1073

19

The male reproductive system

Margaret Costello

Prostate gland

Anatomy

The normal prostate gland in the dog is centred at the bladder neck and proximal urethra, and completely encircles the urethra. In the cat, there is a long portion of preprostatic urethra between the bladder neck and the prostate gland, and the gland is very small and does not completely encircle the urethra ventrally. The normal prostate gland is a bilobed structure with a dorsal groove and internal septum dividing the gland into right and left lobes, which are further subdivided into lobules by septae. The prostate gland is rounded ventrally and more flattened dorsally.

Normal variations

Breed variations: Scottish Terriers are reported to have a prostate gland up to four times the size of other similarly sized and aged dogs.

Individual variations: Overall size of the prostate gland varies between individuals and is highly dependent on hormonal status. The normal prostate gland enlarges from birth to puberty and maturity. Hyperplasia of the prostate gland begins in early middle age (4–5 years) and in old age fibrosis and atrophy may occur.

Normal radiographic anatomy

Dog

Plain radiography: In order to visualize the prostate gland optimally, a separate radiograph of the caudal abdomen is required centred 1–2 cm cranial to the hip joint. A low kV technique will maximize soft tissue contrast. In medium and large dogs a grid should be utilized. A lateral radiograph is usually the most helpful with a ventrodorsal (VD) view offering limited additional information.

The normal prostate gland is recognized by its relationship to the surrounding organs, in particular the urinary bladder. Clear visualization also relies on a moderate amount of abdominal fat to distinguish the prostate gland from other soft tissue opacities. A triangle of fat is usually seen ventrally between the urinary bladder cranially and the prostate gland caudally. Often the caudal margin of the prostate gland is not seen. The dorsal margin of the prostate gland may not be clearly seen due to border effacement, although its approximate size is usually determined by location of the colonic contents. If the animal is immature, has been neutered, given oestrogen therapy or if there is some localized fluid in the region of the bladder neck, the prostate gland may not be visualized.

The exact position of the prostate gland varies depending on the state of distension of the bladder. It will be cranial to the pubic brim (i.e. intra-abdominal) if the bladder is quite full. If the bladder is minimally distended, then the prostate gland may be intrapelvic and caudal to the pelvic brim, and therefore difficult to visualize on the lateral view. On a VD radiograph, the prostate gland is adjacent to the pubic brim either in the midline or to one side, being a small ovoid structure of soft tissue radiopacity. Visualization of the prostate gland in either view will be further affected by the degree of faecal distension of the colon. The prostate gland is likely to be completely obscured by a full rectum in the VD view.

Cat

The normal prostate gland in the cat is not visualized radiographically. Prostatic disease is extremely uncommon in the cat and is not discussed further.

Contrast radiography

Positive-contrast retrograde urethrography

Technique: The prostatic urethra and many diseases of the parenchymal prostate gland can be evaluated with positive-contrast retrograde urethrography. For details on the technique, see Chapter 17.

Normal findings: The normal prostatic urethra should be reasonably uniformly distended and smooth in outline with no major filling defects. A normal tiny filling defect is sometimes visible in the dorsal wall of the urethra at the centre of the prostate gland, representing the colliculus seminalis, which is where the vas deferens and the prostatic ducts enter the urethra. The urethra may appear slightly wider in the centre of the prostate gland and may taper a little at the cranial and caudal margins of the prostate gland. The extent of central dilatation may vary depending on the pressure applied during the contrast medium injection, and a degree of normal variation from animal to animal is to be expected. Changes in the degree of distension must be interpreted with caution. The adjacent bladder neck should be carefully assessed and should be smoothly tapering.

Occasionally, intraprostatic reflux of contrast medium can occur in a normal dog. The reflux should only outline normal prostatic ducts. Abnormal reflux is a non-specific finding and may occur with prostatitis, abscesses, cysts or neoplasia.

Contrast urethrography is helpful when trying to decide whether the prostate gland is asymmetrically enlarged. It also helps to distinguish the location of the urinary bladder and its position relative to the prostate gland, as this is not always possible to determine from plain radiographs, especially where there is extensive prostatomegaly. Equally, ultrasonography may be confusing when more than one bladder-like structure is apparent.

Ultrasonography

Equipment

A 7.5–10 MHz microconvex curvilinear or sector probe is ideal for transabdominal imaging of the prostate gland. Transrectal ultrasonography would enable much better image clarity of the prostate gland, but the technique has disadvantages including the necessity for sedation or general anaesthesia and the need for specialized equipment.

Technique

The animal can be examined in lateral or dorsal recumbency. A full bladder aids evaluation as it pulls the prostate gland cranially. Occasionally, a standing position may aid visualization of the intrapelvic prostate gland as the bladder, if moderately distended, will 'drag' the prostate gland into the abdomen. Another technique is to perform a rectal examination and cranially displace the prostate gland by digital manipulation if it is proving difficult to examine transabdominally.

- The transducer is placed on the caudal abdominal wall, to one side of the prepuce and cranial to the pubis.
- The normal canine prostate gland is examined by locating the bladder neck. This may involve angling the probe caudally if the prostate gland is partly or wholly intrapelvic, in which case a dorsal plane scan is obtained. Otherwise, the prostate gland is examined in both transverse and longitudinal planes.

Indications

The indications for ultrasonographic examination of the prostate gland include:

- Haematuria
- Recurrent urinary tract infection
- Prostatomegaly
- Caudal abdominal pain
- Dyschezia or dysuria
- Caudal abdominal mass
- Haemospermia
- Orchitis
- Pyrexia of unknown origin.

Normal ultrasonographic appearance

The normal prostate gland surrounds the trigone of the bladder and proximal urethra. In transverse section it is semi-ovoid with a flattened dorsal surface adjacent to the rectum, and more rounded ventrally. The ultrasonographic appearance varies with age, hormonal status and equipment settings. The prostate gland normally has a homogenous parenchymal pattern with a fine texture and medium echogenicity, although this is variable (Figure 19.1a).

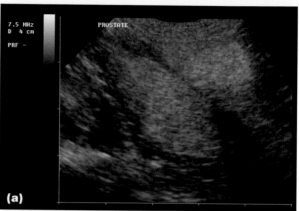

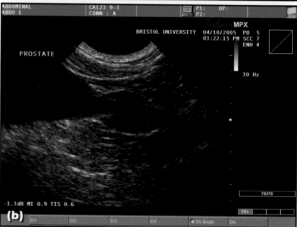

19.1 Sagittal ultrasonograms of **(a)** a normal prostate gland and **(b)** a prostate gland in a neutered dog.

The prostate gland has a bilobed appearance divided by the urethra, which runs in the centre or slightly dorsally. The bilobed appearance is apparent in transverse section. The dorsal and ventral capsules may also be appreciated in this view. In addition, edge shadowing is seen at the margins of the prostate gland in transverse section. The prostate gland appears more round to ovoid in sagittal section. The individual lobules are not discerned. On sagittal section the urethra runs obliquely through the prostate gland. The urethra appears as a hypoechoic structure. A normal urethra is not usually dilated as it passes through the prostate gland, although some dilatation may be evident in dogs under general anaesthesia.

Very rarely, the ductus deferens may be observed as hypoechoic linear echoes coursing obliquely through the dorsal part of the prostate gland. Small cystic lesions (<1 cm diameter) are usually considered to be normal, representing accumulations of prostatic secretions.

In neutered animals the prostate gland is small and more hypoechoic (Figure 19.1b). Exactly how small the prostate gland becomes after neutering depends on the age at which the animal was neutered. Prostate glands are smallest in animals neutered before puberty.

Dorsal to the prostate gland, the descending colon will be appreciated as a highly echogenic linear region in sagittal section or as a semilunar-shaped region in transverse section. The pubic bone is ventral to the prostate gland and creates a hyperechoic line with a strong acoustic shadow. Prostatic size is quite variable. Measuring the size of the prostate gland is of most value when following the course of a disease, be it progression or resolution.

Overview of additional imaging modalities

Computed tomography (CT) and magnetic resonance imaging (MRI) are likely to be useful modalities for imaging any extension of prostatic diseases (e.g. localized lymphadenopathy, local and distant spread of neoplasms). Currently, availability and cost preclude the day-to-day use of these techniques for imaging the prostate gland.

Determination of prostate gland size

Radiography
The prostate gland normally lies within the pelvis but with moderate distension of the bladder it may be intra-abdominal. The prostate gland should not exceed 70% of the distance between the sacral promontory and the pubis on a lateral radiograph, or one half of the width of the pelvic inlet on a VD view. Compression of adjacent structures, such as the descending colon and rectum, may be appreciated radiographically and provide an indication of prostatic enlargement.

Ultrasonography
Transabdominal ultrasonography is a simple and quick technique for the estimation of prostatic size. Studies have shown a relationship between prostatic size and both age and bodyweight. The prostate gland was 2.2 cm in length by 2.2 cm in depth as measured by ultrasonography in 8 dogs (age range 2–4 years) weighing between 7 kg and 30 kg. Due to the great variation in possible size of the normal prostate gland, *serial* examinations may provide the most reliable information when monitoring a disease process.

Prostatic diseases

Change in size

Increase in size: Generalized enlargement of the prostate gland (Figure 19.2) produces cranial and ventral displacement of the urinary bladder along the floor of the abdominal cavity. The colon may be displaced dorsally on the lateral view and laterally (right or leftward displacement) on the VD view. The colon lumen may taper if the prostatomegaly is extreme, and proximally it may be over-distended with faecal material causing obstipation (Figure 19.3).

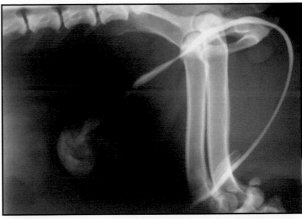

19.2 Lateral radiograph showing generalized prostatomegaly.

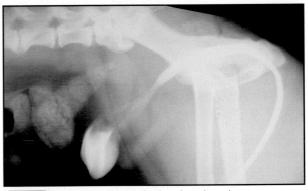

19.3 Lateral radiograph showing dorsal prostatomegaly. There is evidence of obstipation with the colon being dorsally displaced. The lumen of the colon is narrowed. The contrast medium highlights the ventral position of the urethra within the prostate gland.

Extreme prostatomegaly may cause dramatic cranial displacement of the abdominal contents. The prostate gland usually lies on the floor of the abdomen as it enlarges, resulting in cranial and dorsal displacement of the abdominal organs. Prostatomegaly may also be largely contained within the pelvis (Figure 19.4) and therefore difficult to assess, except for its effect on the rectum.

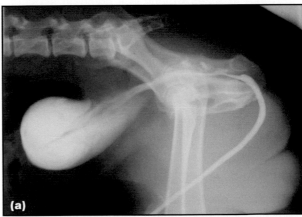

(a)

19.4 **(a)** Lateral view of a retrograde contrast study showing reflux of contrast medium into a largely intrapelvic prostate gland and irregularity of the urethral lumen. Pallisading new bone is present on the vertebral bodies of L5, L6 and L7. The histological diagnosis was a prostatic adenocarcinoma. (continues) ▶

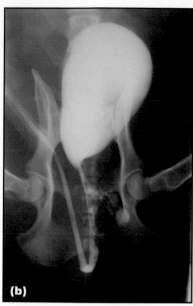

(continued)
(b) VD view of a retrograde contrast study showing reflux of contrast medium into a largely intrapelvic prostate gland and irregularity of the urethral lumen. Pallisading new bone is present on the vertebral bodies of L5, L6 and L7. The histological diagnosis was a prostatic adenocarcinoma.

(b)

Asymmetrical enlargement of the prostate gland (e.g. cysts, neoplasia) may cause variations in the displacement pattern of the bladder. A cyst or abscess extending dorsally, may compress the bladder ventrally against the floor of the abdomen so that it loses contact with the colon. A lesion causing ventral prostatomegaly may elevate the bladder dorsally away from contact with the abdominal wall. The bladder may also be cranially displaced.

Conditions such as acute prostatitis and neoplasia do not usually cause massive prostatomegaly. Severe prostatomegaly is much more likely to be due to prostatic hyperplasia, cysts or abscesses.

Even when the prostatomegaly is extreme, the margins of the prostate gland usually remain sharp. If the margins are indistinct in the presence of a moderate amount of abdominal fat, this is suggestive of a more aggressive process such as prostatitis or neoplasia. Abscesses generally have sharp margins, but some will result in a localized peritonitis and therefore have indistinct margins.

Decrease in size: Atrophy is a common sequel to neutering. The rate of prostate gland size change after neutering and the final size are not consistent. A neutered male is likely to have a very small prostate gland, and may be difficult to identify if the animal was neutered at a very young age. Atrophy may also occur secondary to Sertoli cell neoplasia or secondary to oestrogen therapy. Atrophy is also seen as a degenerative change associated with old age. On radiographs the prostate gland will be small or indiscernible.

Change in opacity

Increased opacity: The normal prostate gland has a soft tissue opacity, as does a mildly enlarged prostate gland. As enlargement becomes more severe, the radiopacity of the prostate gland may become heterogenous. Mineralization within the prostate gland is an unusual finding and warrants further investigation through ultrasonography and biopsy. It is more

commonly associated with neoplasia than with chronic diseases such as prostatitis.

Mineralization of a paraprostatic cyst (Figure 19.5) is another differential diagnosis for a mineralized mass in the caudal abdomen. Frequently, the mineralization has a pattern creating an 'eggshell'-type appearance.

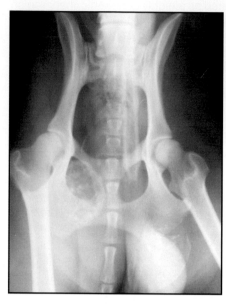

VD radiograph showing two mineralized paraprostatic cysts within bilateral perineal hernias.

Decreased opacity: Gas opacities within the prostate gland are suggestive of severe infection from gas-producing bacteria. Reflux from a negative- or double-contrast cystogram is possible if such a study has been performed. In this situation, the reflux is not necessarily an indication of serious disease and usually indicates dilated prostatic ducts.

Abnormalities of contrast studies

Assessment of the path of the urethra within the prostate gland necessitates a contrast study (see Figure 19.3). If the urethra is asymmetrically positioned within an enlarged prostate gland, this indicates the presence of a mass lesion. If the urethra has a stricture or mucosal irregularity, then this suggests aggressive disease. Extravasation of contrast medium occurs where there is cavitary disease within the prostate gland, which is communicating with the urethra. Absence of extravasation does not rule out cavitary disease. Severe extravasation of contrast medium into cavitary lesions is suggestive of neoplasia (see Figure 19.4).

Metastases

The commonest malignant neoplasms of the prostate gland are adenocarcinoma and transitional cell carcinoma. The most common metastatic sites are the regional lymph nodes and adjacent bony structures. Often only the bones or lymph nodes are affected. Carcinomas of the prostate gland spread readily to the local regional lymph nodes; usually the medial iliac and hypogastric lymph nodes. This causes ventral displacement of the terminal descending colon or rectum.

The most common appearance of metastatic lesions to the bone is purely proliferative, seen most often on the ventral surfaces of the caudal lumbar vertebral bodies. The appearance may be of smooth or pallisading new bone on the mid-ventral vertebral body (see Figure 19.4) and is quite different from spondylosis, which is smooth and projects from the vertebral endplates. Bony reaction is also sometimes seen on the sacrum, the wings of the ilium and the shafts of the femur. Histologically there may be lytic lesions, although this is rarely appreciated radiographically. Metastatic spread to the thorax often occurs in the later stages of the disease. Metastatic spread to the long bones is also common. Prostatic carcinoma has been reported in conjunction with hypertrophic osteopathy (Marie's disease).

Benign prostatic hyperplasia

Benign prostatic hyperplasia is the most common canine prostatic disorder. It is a presumptive diagnosis in all middle-aged to older intact male dogs. Histologically, it has been shown to be present in 100% of entire dogs >7 years old. However, many dogs will never show clinical signs.

Prostatomegaly commonly results secondary to glandular hyperplasia. The enlargement is usually symmetrical with smooth margins. If diffuse enlargement is present, the normal bilobed appearance of the prostate gland may be lost. The ultrasonographic changes may include varying degrees of subtle heterogeneity to the parenchyma. Heterogeneity may be present with or without obvious enlargement. The texture may be smooth or coarse. Scattered hyperechoic foci may be present, thought to be secondary to fibrosis or vascular changes. Mineralization is not usually seen, unless concurrent disease is present. Parenchymal cysts of varying size and number may also be present (cystic hyperplasia) (Figure 19.6).

The overall parenchymal appearance may become quite heterogenous, making a diagnosis of benign prostatic hyperplasia difficult. The capsule of the prostate gland should be intact and there should be no evidence of lymphadenopathy. However, it is not possible to differentiate benign hyperplasia from neoplasia or prostatitis on the basis of the ultrasound examination alone. Concurrent disease conditions are common in older dogs. Frequently hyperplasia, neoplasia and prostatitis co-exist in the same prostate gland. Biopsy is required for definitive diagnosis and complete staging. Biopsy samples should be taken from multiple areas within the prostate gland to ensure a complete assessment of all co-existing diseases. If there is lymphadenopathy, usually the lymph node biopsy accurately reflects the most serious disease in the prostate gland.

Cysts

Parenchymal cysts: Parenchymal cysts may occur in benign prostatic hyperplasia. These cysts may occur secondary to dilated acini and ducts and can be acquired or congenital. They may also be seen with prostatitis (Figure 19.7) and neoplasia. True cysts have smooth walls and anechoic contents with distal acoustic enhancement. Multiple small cysts may create the appearance of a hyperechoic parenchyma because of the acoustic enhancement. If the walls are

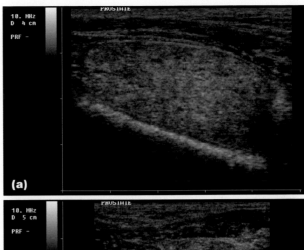
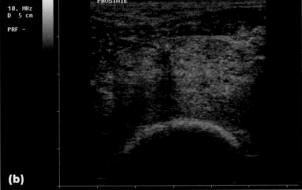

19.6 **(a)** Sagittal and **(b)** transverse ultrasonograms showing the typical appearance of benign prostatic hyperplasia. Note the multiple small cysts throughout the prostatic parenchyma. The hyperechoic interface deep to the prostate gland is the descending colon.

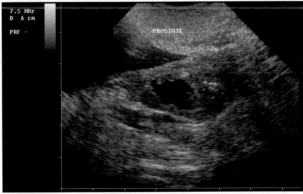

19.7 Ultrasonogram of prostatitis. An irregular cyst is present dorsocranially and hyperechoic specks (likely to represent mineralization) are seen just caudal to the cyst. The prostate gland is hypoechoic with poorly defined margins.

irregular and the contents echogenic, abscess or haemorrhage must be considered. True cysts may become infected. Aspiration with cytology and culture are required for definitive diagnosis.

Paraprostatic cysts: Paraprostatic cyst is a term used to describe a cyst located outside the prostatic parenchyma. They are derived from remnants of the uterus masculinus, vestigial Mullerian ducts or subsequent to prostatic haematoma. There is usually a stalk connecting them to the prostate gland. These cysts vary in size, shape and location, but may appear as a second bladder-like structure in the caudal abdomen either cranial to, alongside or caudal to the urinary bladder. It can be difficult to determine which structure is the urinary bladder if the cyst is very large. Careful evaluation of the bladder neck and prostate gland position can help in differentiating the bladder from a cyst, but a cystogram or retrograde urethrogram may be necessary in order to positively identify which structure is the urinary bladder. Sometimes the walls of paraprostatic cysts are calcified, creating an 'eggshell' appearance on radiographs.

Typically, on ultrasound examination a paraprostatic cyst will appear as a fluid-filled anechoic to mildly echogenic structure with variable wall thickness. Where the walls are mineralized they appear highly echogenic. Septations may also be present. The cysts are variable in size but can be very large occupying much of the caudal abdomen, and may extend into the pelvic cavity and into perineal hernias. Paraprostatic cysts may become infected, resulting in the contents appearing very echogenic. Occasionally, paraprostatic cysts may be largely solid, but have a mixed echogenicity. When paraprostatic cysts are diagnosed, the prostate gland and testes must be carefully evaluated for concurrent disease.

Prostatitis

Bacterial prostatitis in intact male dogs is quite common and may be acute or chronic. Concurrent urinary tract infection predisposes an animal to prostatitis or it can be an extension of testicular or epididymal disease. Fungal prostatitis is extremely rare.

Prostatomegaly is generally present with the enlargement being symmetrical or asymmetrical. Determining the various contributions of the concurrent benign prostatic hyperplasia and prostatitis may be difficult. The parenchyma usually has a heterogenous appearance. There may be focal or multifocal poorly defined hypoechoic areas, and a variable number of cysts or cyst-like structures may be present. Some cysts may have quite echogenic contents. One or more large cyst-like structures with irregular thickened walls and echogenic contents may indicate an abscess. Small foci of mineralization may be present with chronic prostatitis (see Figure 19.7) but this finding is seen more commonly with neoplasia.

Focal fluid accumulation may be present in the caudal abdomen. Regional lymphadenopathy may also be present, although this is unusual and generally only mild. Serial ultrasound examination during treatment may show resolution of the changes in the prostate gland, including shrinkage in the size of the prostate gland if neutering is chosen as part of the treatment regime. The testes should also be examined as infection may spread there or they may be the primary cause of the infection. Occasionally, prostatitis may resemble benign prostatic hyperplasia and have a fairly homogenous appearance. Definitive diagnosis often requires fine-needle aspiration and culture.

Abscesses

Abscesses may form as a sequel to acute or chronic prostatitis (see above). Infection of benign cysts is common. It is even possible for the entire prostate gland to become abscessated.

Neoplasia

Neoplasia of the prostate gland is relatively uncommon in the dog and extremely rare in the cat. Prostatic carcinoma is seen in middle- to old-aged, medium- to large-breed, intact and neutered dogs. Prostatomegaly in a neutered animal, especially with evidence of mineralization, is very suggestive of neoplasia. Adenocarcinomas and transitional call carcinomas are the commonest tumour types. These tumour types may be difficult to differentiate histologically and are not distinguishable ultrasonographically. Lymphoma is very uncommon.

Ultrasonographically, the prostate gland is typically asymmetrically enlarged and irregular with a heterogenous parenchyma (Figure 19.8). There may be multiple hyperechoic foci, some of which may be

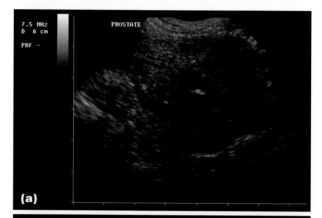

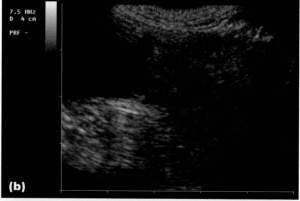

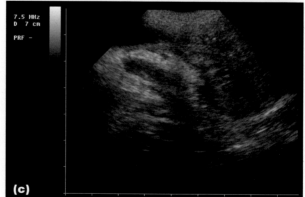

19.8   Ultrasonograms of a prostatic mass. **(a)** An enlarged hypoechoic prostate gland with an unclear capsular margin, **(b)** irregularity at the trigone of the bladder and **(c)** haziness dorsocranially, highly suggestive of neoplasia. The histological diagnosis was a prostatic adenocarcinoma.

associated with distal acoustic shadowing, indicating mineralization. The presence of mineralization is highly suggestive of neoplasia. Cavitary lesions may be present, giving an appearance not dissimilar to prostatitis. Particular care should be given to assessing the prostatic capsule as neoplastic disease commonly causes capsular disruption.

Metastatic neoplasia causes regional lymphadenopathy, involving the hypogastric, medial iliac and lumbar aortic lymph nodes. The enlargement may be quite severe. Metastasis to the lumbar vertebrae can cause smooth or irregular proliferative lesions of the ventral surfaces of the vertebral bodies. Radiography is useful to confirm these findings. Biopsy of the prostate gland or lymph nodes is required to confirm the diagnosis. Neoplastic seeding has been reported using either fine-needle aspirate or tissue core biopsy techniques, particularly with transitional cell carcinoma.

Atrophy

The prostatic parenchyma usually appears uniformly hypoechoic.

Testes and scrotum

Radiography

Radiographic examination of the testes and scrotum adds little to a thorough clinical examination. Ultrasonography allows more detailed assessment of this area, in particular the testes. Radiography is of value where a retained testicle has undergone neoplastic transformation, causing an abdominal or inguinal mass. Where the retained testes are of normal size they will not be identified radiographically.

Ultrasonography

Technique

A 10–15 MHz linear probe is the most useful for evaluation of the testes. The probe should be placed directly on each testicle in turn. If using a sector type probe, a gel block may be used as a standoff in order to examine the testes. Alternatively, each testicle can be used in turn as a standoff to examine the other (i.e. whilst holding the testes, the probe is placed on the upper testicle to examine the lower testicle). If using a high-frequency linear probe a standoff is not required. The testes should be scanned in transverse, longitudinal and dorsal planes.

Indications

The indications for ultrasonographic examination of the testes and scrotum include:

- Prostatic disease
- Feminization syndrome
- Infertility
- Palpable mass
- Testicular asymmetry
- Atrophy
- Pyrexia of unknown origin
- Scrotal swelling
- Localized retained testicles.

Normal ultrasonographic appearance

The paired testes are contained within the scrotum separated by the median septum. They are covered by connective tissue, which radiates septa centrally to join the mediastinum testis. These septa divide the testes into lobules. The epididymis comprises a head, body and tail. The head lies at the cranial pole of the testis, the body is located along the lateral and dorsal aspect of the testis, and the tail is positioned caudally to the testis.

The normal testis is moderately echogenic with a fine even echotexture (Figure 19.9). A thin peripheral hyperechoic line may be visible, which represents the visceral and parietal tunics. The mediastinum testis is a central hyperechoic linear structure in the mid-sagittal plane and a focal hyperechoic structure in the transverse plane. The head and body of the epididymis are nearly isoechoic with the testicle, whilst the tail is hypoechoic (sometimes appearing almost anechoic) and has a coarser echotexture. The head is in a cranial position, and the body can be followed caudally from it in both sagittal and transverse planes. The tail is found in a caudal location.

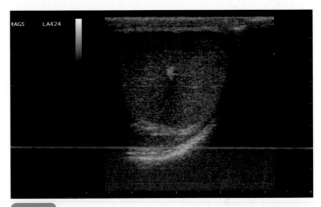

19.9 Transverse ultrasonogram of a normal testicle.

Testicular diseases

Neoplasia

Neoplasia of the testes is the second most common tumour in male dogs, although rare in cats. Most neoplasms are benign and of these interstitial (Leydig) cell tumours are the most common. Other neoplasms include seminomas and Sertoli cell tumours. Cryptorchid animals are reported to be at 13 times greater risk of developing a Sertoli cell tumour or seminoma, and may develop these neoplasms at a relatively young age. Multiple concurrent neoplasms may also occur. Many Sertoli cell tumours are functional and often metastasize to the regional lymph nodes, liver and lungs.

The ultrasonographic appearance of the various testicular neoplasms is variable. Large lesions will cause testicular enlargement and obliterate the mediastinum testis and the epididymis.

- Interstitial cell tumours (Figure 19.10) are the most common. Generally, they are composed of small hypoechoic nodules that can be singular or may become confluent. Bilateral interstitial cell tumours commonly occur.

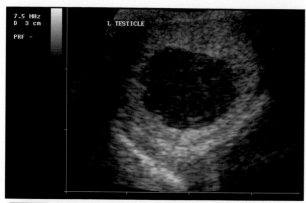

19.10 Ultrasonogram of a focal hypoechoic testicular mass. The histological diagnosis was an interstitial cell tumour.

- Sertoli cell tumours may cause testicular enlargement with atrophy of the contralateral testicle if the tumour is producing oestrogen. They tend to have a mixed echogenicity.
- Seminomas (Figure 19.11) are often large and solitary, causing testicular enlargement. Generally, the appearance of a seminoma is hypoechoic relative to normal testicular echogenicity, but this is not always the case. Seminomas tend to be unilateral.
- Neoplasms of cryptorchid animals are typically Sertoli cell tumours. The masses tend to be quite large and irregular and have a mixed or complex echogenicity. Seminomas also occur in cryptorchid animals.

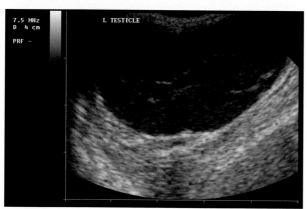

19.11 Ultrasonogram of a testicular tumour. Note the large mass occupying most of the testicle. The histological diagnosis was a seminoma.

Orchitis

Orchitis is often seen concurrently with epididymitis. Infection is likely to occur retrograde along the ductus deferens. Penetrating wounds may also cause orchitis, but this is much less common. Secondary abscess formation is common. The testicular walls may be thick or thin, and the contents vary in echogenicity. The testicular parenchyma may become diffusely patchy. The testicle and epididymis are usually enlarged. Fluid may be seen around the testicle. Chronic infection may result in a small testicle of mixed echogenicity. Orchitis may appear very similar to a neoplasm, but localized fluid accumulation is much less common in neoplasia.

Testicular torsion

Testicular torsion is more common in enlarged, intra-abdominal, neoplastic testes. The characteristic appearance is of a diffuse increase in echogenicity with capsular thickening, epididymal and spermatic cord enlargement, and scrotal thickening. It may be difficult to differentiate testicular torsion from orchitis.

Atrophy

The testicle is smaller than normal. The parenchyma may be normal or hypoechoic. Atrophy may be an ageing change, it may occur in one testicle secondary to a Sertoli cell tumour in the other testicle, or it may occur with a retained testicle. Non-neoplastic retained testicles tend to be very small and difficult to identify; they may be located anywhere from just caudal to the kidneys to the inguinal canal.

Scrotal diseases

Hernia

Herniation of the small bowel may be confirmed by seeing the loops of intestine in the scrotal sac. Radiographically, the presence of tubular gas lucencies within the scrotum is diagnostic of intestinal herniation. Ultrasonographically, the intestines may be identified by the distinctive layered appearance and peristalsis. Peritoneal fat also may herniate into the scrotum. Fat is usually hyperechoic compared with the normal testicle. Any herniated organ may become strangulated or necrotic, leading to local inflammation or fluid formation.

Penis

Radiography

The only part of the penis identifiable on plain radiographs is the os penis. It is seen on the ventral aspect of the abdomen on the lateral view. On a properly positioned VD view, the prepuce overlies the vertebrae and is difficult to identify. Oblique views demonstrate the structure more clearly. Radiography of the penis is of little value compared with a thorough clinical examination, except for evaluation of penile urethral calculi (see Chapter 17). Fractures and osteomyelitis of the os penis have also been described.

References and further reading

Atalan G, Barr FJ and Holt PE (1999) Comparison of ultrasonographic and radiographic measurements of canine prostatic dimensions. *Veterinary Radiology* **40**, 408–412

Atalan G, Holt PE and Barr FJ (1999) Ultrasonographic estimation of prostate size in normal dogs and relationship to bodyweight and age. *Journal of Small Animal Practice* **40**, 119–122

Bell FW, Klausner JS, Hayden DW, *et al.* (1991) Clinical and pathologic features of prostatic adenocarcinoma in sexually intact and castrated dogs: 31 cases (1970–1987) *Journal of the American Veterinary Medical Association* **199**, 1623–1630

Cartee RE and Rowles T (1983) Transabdominal sonographic evaluation of the canine prostate *Veterinary Radiology* **24**, 156–164

Feeney DA, Johnston G, Klausner JS, *et al.* (1987) Reports of reproductive studies: canine prostatic disease-comparison of radiographic appearance with morphologic and microbiologic findings: 30 cases (1981–1985) *Journal of the American Veterinary Medical Association*

190, 1018–1026

Krawiec DR and Heflin D (1992) Study of prostatic disease in dogs: 177 cases (1981–1986). *Journal of the American Veterinary Medical Association* **200**, 1119–1122

Lattimer JC (1998) The prostate gland In: *Textbook of Veterinary Diagnostic Radiology, 3rd edn*, ed. DE Thrall, pp. 499–511. WB Saunders, Philadelphia

LeRoy BE and Lech ME (2004) Prostatic carcinoma causing urethral obstruction and obstipation in a cat. *Journal of Feline Medicine and Surgery* **6**, 397–400

Parry NMA (2007) The canine prostate gland: Part 1 Non-inflammatory diseases. *UK Vet* **12**, 1–4

Parry NMA (2007) The canine prostate gland: Part 2 Inflammatory diseases. *UK Vet*, **12**, 37–41

Index

Index

Index

Index